T0190132

"My excitement for this book cannot be overstated. As our society more fully grapples with the complexities of health communication laid bare during the COVID-19 pandemic, and students from all disciplines want to become more knowledgeable about issues of health communication, this text will provide a solid, informed, and sensitive look at our field. This book, which nicely incorporates both the breadth and depth of our field, will serve as a useful resource for faculty teaching upper level health communication classes to students from all backgrounds. It is one that not only mentions but also deeply and actively grapples with issues of diversity, discrimination, medical ethics, and access issues across its fifteen chapters. Nowhere is this more clear than in the inclusion of the Montgomery family story, a companion narrative to accompany the textbook chapters that will be a phenomenal pedagogical feature for engaging with undergraduates. I look forward to adopting this book the next time I teach health communication."

— **Katharine J. Head**, *Indiana University-Purdue University Indianapolis, USA*

"I have been using the first edition of this book since it was published, and I am eager to adopt the second edition, *Health Communication: Research and Practice for a Diverse and Changing World*. Health communication is a diverse, dynamic, and rapidly developing field of study. To capture the many facets of our field and translate them within a context of higher education is no small feat. Having thoroughly reviewed this second edition, I believe that Drs. Nancy Harrington and Rachael Record have developed a textbook that will accomplish that feat. One of the ways the authors address the conundrum of competing against material that becomes rapidly outdated is to center chapters within more overarching theoretical approaches, which are then supported by individual research studies. For example, I may be biased as a scholar of technology and media adoption, but nothing seems to lose its shelf life quite so quickly as 'new' communication technology research, *unless* the research is well supported theoretically. Thus, although media consumption, technology use, broadband access, etc. are deeply interwoven with health and communication, chapters *about* these topics (e.g., 'new technologies in health communication,' 'internet and eHealth') quickly become outdated. The authors have addressed this issue in multiple ways, for example, focusing on health information seeking (online and offline), which will ensure usability for many years to come. Finally, *Health Communication: Research and Practice for a Diverse and Changing World* follows the lead of the subtitle change. In the second edition authors both add and reorder information to prime readers to think about how others may experience health and engaged a strategy that I hope will help those of us who adopt this textbook to inspire discussion and action that will achieve each decade of the U.S. government's Healthy People goals - 'improve the health and well-being of people.' All people."

— **Kate Magsamen-Conrad**, *The University of Iowa, USA*

"*Health Communication: Research and Practice for a Diverse and Changing World*, piloted in my 300-level Introduction to Health Communication course, was very well received by a large and diverse group of students ranging from communication to kinesiology majors. The students particularly appreciated the relevant and timely content, health justice-based case studies, and the narrative flow of the text. I am confident and excited about utilizing this textbook as a resource for my future classes."

— **Rati Kumar**, *San Diego State University, USA*

Health Communication

This thoroughly revised second edition covers the major areas of research, theory, and practical application in health communication.

This textbook takes an in-depth approach to health communication by analyzing and critically evaluating research conducted across multiple paradigmatic perspectives and focusing on translational application of research findings. Using the story of the Montgomery family, a biracial, multigenerational family, and their health experiences as a case study, chapters explore topics including patient–provider communication, health communication in the media, ethical issues, and public health crises. New chapters cover the potential for communication to address discrimination in healthcare settings, health information seeking, social support and caregiving, and the relationship between health and environmental communication. Chapters offer pedagogical features that will prove useful to students and instructors of health communication, such as summary boxes, theory tables, suggestions for in-class activities, discussion questions, and lists of additional resources.

Developed for use in advanced undergraduate and master's level health communication and public health courses, this text represents the breadth and depth of health communication theory and research as it exists today.

Online resources for instructors including additional theory tables, PowerPoint slides, test questions and assignments, sample syllabi, and lists of additional resources are available at https://www.routledge.com/9781032100470.

Nancy Grant Harrington is a Professor of Communication in the College of Communication and Information at the University of Kentucky, USA.

Rachael A. Record is an Associate Professor of Communication at San Diego State University, USA.

Health Communication

Research and Practice for a Diverse and
Changing World

**Nancy Grant Harrington and
Rachael A. Record**

2nd Edition

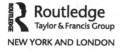
Routledge
Taylor & Francis Group

NEW YORK AND LONDON

Designed cover image: Ash Garrison

Second edition published 2024
by Routledge
605 Third Avenue, New York, NY 10158

and by Routledge
4 Park Square, Milton Park, Abingdon, Oxon, OX14 4RN

Routledge is an imprint of the Taylor & Francis Group, an informa business

First edition published by Routledge 2014

Library of Congress Cataloging-in-Publication Data
Names: Harrington, Nancy Grant, author. | Record, Rachael A., 1986– author.
Title: Health communication : research and practice for a diverse and changing world /
Nancy Grant Harrington, Rachael A. Record.
Description: 2nd edition. | New York, NY : Routledge, [2024] | Preceded by
Health communication / edited by Nancy Grant Harrington. 2015. |
Includes bibliographical references and index.
Identifiers: LCCN 2023006539 (print) | LCCN 2023006540 (ebook) |
ISBN 9781032102603 (hardback) | ISBN 9781032100470 (paperback) |
ISBN 9781003214458 (ebook)
Subjects: MESH: Health Communication | Professional-Patient Relations—ethics |
Social Factors | Communications Media
Classification: LCC R118 (print) | LCC R118 (ebook) | NLM WA 590 | DDC
613—dc23/eng/20230505
LC record available at https://lccn.loc.gov/2023006539
LC ebook record available at https://lccn.loc.gov/2023006540

ISBN: 9781032102603 (hbk)
ISBN: 9781032100470 (pbk)
ISBN: 9781003214458 (ebk)

DOI: 10.4324/9781003214458

Typeset in Bembo Std
by codeMantra

Access the Support Material: https://www.routledge.com/9781032100470

To Dan O'Hair, our dear friend, colleague, and mentor, who thoughtfully wrote the foreword to the first edition of this book. May your selflessness and dedication to mentoring students, faculty, and staff stand as an example to all who follow you.

You are gone too soon.

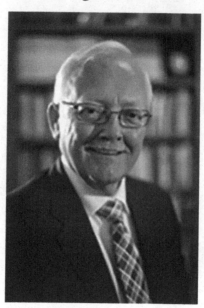

Contents

Preface

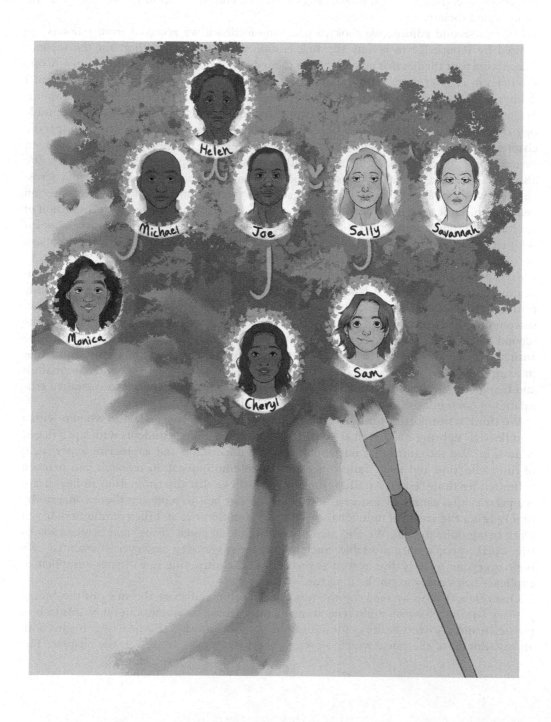

Welcome to the second edition of *Health Communication: Theory, Method, and Application*, which is now titled *Health Communication: Research and Practice for a Diverse and Changing World*. The first edition of this text, published in 2015, was written to provide a theory, method, and metatheory-driven review of health communication scholarship for upper-division and master's level students in communication and related disciplines. It was designed to fill a gap between textbooks written for lower-division courses and *The Routledge Handbook of Health Communication*, which is more suited for graduate studies. This second edition represents our effort not only to update the material, certainly necessary after nearly a decade, but also to better meet the needs of the post-pandemic undergraduate audience and more directly confront the challenges of health communication in our complex and complicated society.

For this second edition, we took to heart the feedback we received from scholars recruited by Routledge to review the first edition and provide direction for the second. There were four themes that emerged from the reviews. First, reviewers noted some inconsistencies in chapter voice and style due to the nature of the edited textbook. After much deliberation, we decided that the second edition would be an authored text to allow for greater control and consistency across chapters. Second, reviewers noted that the technology chapters were out of date and limited. Our solution was to no longer include specific chapters on technology but to mention in every chapter how technology comes into play in various contexts and how it influences health communication processes and outcomes. We also took a similar approach with social media, including research on social media across chapters when applicable instead of having a specific section on the topic in the chapter on health communication in the media. Third, reviewers called for a more direct discussion of practical and translational applications of textbook content. This recommendation, coupled with feedback we had received from instructors over the years indicating that the emphasis on metatheory was perhaps beyond what was needed for an undergraduate text, led us to address paradigmatic perspectives only in Chapter 1 as part of providing a foundation for health communication scholarship and put our emphasis in remaining chapters on study findings and their implications. Finally, reviewers called for greater attention to challenges surrounding discrimination in healthcare. This became a central part of our vision for the second edition. We have added a new chapter on discrimination and what it means to be antiracist in health communication, and we have infused findings related to discrimination in its multiple forms in every chapter. In addition, as a way of rejecting white nationalism and being allies to our students and colleagues of color, we have chosen to capitalize ethnicities of color but use lower case for the white racial identity.

We think it's important for us to acknowledge that we are two cis white women with a middle-class upbringing, as well as being first-generation college students with a privileged education. We recognize that our ability to fully understand and appreciate experiences of discrimination and their significance for health communication research and practice is limited by those lenses. As allies, though, we believe that discrimination in healthcare is a priority that cannot be ignored, and so we did our best to represent those concerns by highlighting the voices of individuals from these communities and the community-driven work being done therein. We also recognize that talking about "isms" and bias can sometimes make people uncomfortable. Such talk in today's society, however, is essential. We hope everyone realizes this, as well as realizing that confronting one's biases—implicit or explicit—helps everyone in the long run.

One other change we made to the text is to develop and share the story of the Montgomery family, a biracial, multigenerational family whose daughter, Cheryl, wants to be a physician and discovers health communication along her journey. Each chapter begins with an installment of the story, which serves to highlight topics covered in the chapter. The main characters, most of whom are included in the family tree pictured at the start of this preface, were illustrated by a graduate of the University of Kentucky College of Fine Arts. Because health and illness are embodied and experienced through narrative, we hope the Montgomery family's story will provide an opportunity for readers to delve deeper into the concepts covered in the chapters.

Organization and Features of the Book

This textbook has 15 chapters organized into six sections. The first section, *Understanding Health Communication Foundations*, includes an introductory chapter on health, healthcare, and the discipline of health communication and a chapter on discrimination and health communication. The second section, *Being a Patient*, contains chapters on patient–provider communication; patient experiences of uncertainty, decision making, coping, and health literacy; and health information seeking. The third section, *Caring for Patients*, includes chapters on healthcare provider roles and perspectives, social support and informal caregiving, and end-of-life communication. The fourth section, *Health Communication Challenges*, addresses mental health and mental illness, intercultural health communication, and ethical issues in health communication. The fifth section, *Societal-Level Health Communication Concerns*, covers health communication in the media, environmental health communication, and public health crises. The last section, *Looking Forward*, offers a chapter focused on practical information for students wishing to continue their studies in health communication, find a career in health communication, or become allies in efforts to end discrimination and promote patient empowerment.

This book has several pedagogical features that facilitate its use as a textbook. Each chapter has summary boxes to highlight main points of the chapter. **Key terms** are in boldface throughout the text. The theories guiding the research studies presented in each chapter are summarized in theory tables that list the name of the theory (or model or framework), provide a summary of the theory's principles, and offer a reference for further reading. Each chapter also has suggestions for in-class activities and discussion questions.

Changes to the Second Edition

We've touched on several of the changes to the second edition already, but we present them here in bulleted form for ease of reference.

- The book is authored instead of edited.
- The book's title has been updated to reflect changes in content and emphasis.
- The literature has been updated.
- Although many of the concepts covered in the book could apply to multiple chapters, chapters have been organized to avoid overlap.
- Chapters no longer emphasize the metatheoretical or paradigmatic perspectives of the research reviewed but instead emphasize study findings and their implications.
- There is a stand-alone chapter devoted to discrimination and health communication, and issues of discrimination are addressed in each chapter.
- There is not a stand-alone chapter on technology; instead, technology is addressed in each chapter as applicable. Likewise, there is not a specific section on social media in the chapter on health communication in the media; instead, research on social media is included across chapters when applicable.
- Each chapter includes a theory table for ease of reference.

- There are expanded online resources, including a comprehensive theory table to provide opportunities for instructors to highlight additional theories they might like to include during lectures or possible student assignments.
- Each chapter begins with an installment of the Montgomery family narrative as a way to bring some of the topics addressed in each chapter to life.

Student Evaluations

We were fortunate to be able to pilot test most of the chapters of the book with undergraduate students. We collected evaluations on the chapters, asking students what they liked most and least about each one, what they found confusing, what parts they thought should be longer or shorter, and whether there was anything they would change. We also asked students to rate the chapters along several dimensions (e.g., interest, relevance, writing style). Overall, 89% of students found the chapters to be somewhat or extremely interesting, 90% found them to be somewhat or extremely easy to follow, 94% reported learning some or a lot, and 92% felt the chapters would help them some or a great deal in real life as a patient, caregiver, or employee in the healthcare industry.

Online Resources

Online resources are available for students and instructors. Students will be able to download files from the textbook's page on the Routledge website. Materials include a list of additional resources for each chapter, such as movies and documentaries, podcasts and TED talks, and other relevant resources (e.g., websites, YouTube videos). There is also a table consolidating all the theories that were included in the chapter theory tables and adding other relevant theories that did not get addressed in the chapters. The student section also includes the full Montgomery family narrative with color images, as well as the notes for each installment. Instructors will be able to access chapter quizzes, reflection assignments, PowerPoint® slide decks, and sample syllabi through Routledge's Instructor Hub, whose link is also available on the book's page on the Routledge website.

Audiences for the Book

As with the first edition, this textbook is targeted toward upper-division undergraduate and master's level students in health communication and other social and behavioral sciences, as well as students in the health professions. We anticipate that programs in communication will be most likely to adopt the book; however, other social and behavioral science disciplines such as health education and public health may also find the book to be of interest. Avid health communication scholars of any background also may be interested in the book.

As you adopt *Health Communication: Research and Practice for a Diverse and Changing World* for your courses, we hope you find it engaging and easy to use. We hope your students like it, as well. We've done our best to be undergraduate friendly. If you have any feedback you'd like to share, we'd love to hear from you. Best wishes for a successful class!

Special Thanks

We have several people to thank. First, thank you to all the chapter authors from the first edition of this book. Your work was outstanding, and we are grateful for your contributions. Special thanks also go to our amazing artist, Ash Garrison, whose talent brought the Montgomery family characters to life. Thanks, as well, to Rachel Crick, Brittany White, Courtney White, and Dr. Brittany Lash for providing invaluable feedback on the Montgomery family narrative. Thank you to Max Groznick for providing helpful assistance with chapter evaluations during pilot testing. And special thanks to Dr. Rati Kumar for allowing us to pilot our chapters in her health communication course. Finally, we want to thank Alexandra de Brauw, publisher, and Sean Daly, senior editorial assistant. We are grateful to them and to Routledge/Taylor & Francis Books for making this second edition possible.

Nancy Grant Harrington
Rachael A. Record

Unit I

Understanding Health Communication Foundations

Meet Dr. Cheryl Montgomery

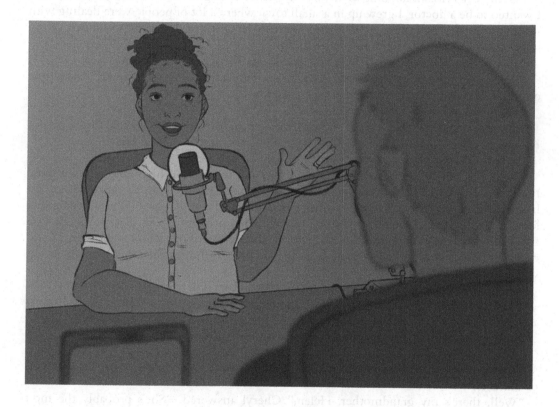

Cheryl sat nervously in her chair, wishing her palms would stop sweating. Over the past few years, she'd already done a number of successful interviews. But this would be her first time discussing the more personal aspects of her life. Despite the butterflies in her stomach, she was really looking forward to this interview. And following a nod from the host, she saw the light in the studio turn red, indicating they were recording.

"Welcome, folks, to episode 323 of *The People Who Made Me*. I'm Bryce Thomas Patrick, your host. If you're new to the show, each week we listen to the personal journey of someone who is changing the world. But we don't just ask them about what they've done. We want to know about all the people who helped them along the way. And today, we have with us Dr. Cheryl Montgomery, the 40-year-old visionary who's changing the world through community health. Welcome, Dr. Montgomery!"

"Thanks, Bryce. I'm very excited to be here," Cheryl replied.

"Not as excited as we are to have you here," Bryce responded. "Now, Dr. Montgomery, I'm sure you know the drill. We ask our guests to talk us through their stories and tell us

DOI: 10.4324/9781003214458-2

how they found themselves on such unique and impressive career paths. And with you, we've started off really strong. You're a double doctor? An MD *and* a PhD?" Bryce said with eyebrows raised and hands out. "Wow!"

"Well, yes," Cheryl said, blushing a bit. "I started out wanting to be a doctor, but then I discovered health communication. So after I earned my MD, I went back to school to earn my PhD. Given what I wanted to do, it made sense."

"That sounds like a lot of school, but pretty awesome," Bryce laughed. "Now, not to spoil the end of the story, but you're a renowned expert in environmental breast cancer research, and you're the founder and director of the *Helen Montgomery Community Clinic for Breast Cancer Awareness and Prevention*. Where did this journey start for you?"

"Well," Cheryl said, nodding as she decided where to begin. "I knew at a young age that I wanted to be a doctor. I grew up in a small town where a lot of people were dealing with so much disease and illness and so many health complications. I wanted to be part of the solution, to help the people in my community."

"That's a big dream for a kid. Were people generally supportive?" Bryce asked.

"My family was," Cheryl replied. "But some of the adult figures in my life at the time didn't think I had what it took to become a doctor."

"You're joking, right?" Bryce asked.

"I'm not, actually," Cheryl said. "When I was a junior in high school, I told my counselor I wanted to be a doctor. Believe it or not, she said it wouldn't be a good fit for me."

"What? Clearly, she was wrong," Bryce replied.

"Well, yes, but I didn't know that at the time. As a teenager in high school, it felt more likely that I was wrong. But when I told my dad about what she said, he literally said, 'To hell with that!' and 'You can be anything you damn well want to be!'" Cheryl recounted, lowering her voice to sound more like her dad. "He's protective like that. He made sure that I didn't let the counselor make assumptions about me—about who I was or what I was capable of. Because of his encouragement, I ended up enrolling at the top university in our state—with a scholarship."

"Well, that's a great start to a dream path," Bryce observed.

"It sure was," Cheryl smiled. "So like a lot of eighteen year olds, I went off to college as a wide-eyed first year student, ready to take on the world and feeling invincible."

"Ready to take on the world, with a little push from your dad," Bryce noted.

"That's right," Cheryl said, smiling. "My dad, Joe."

"And who else? Who else played a role in your journey? Or should I say, who's your cast of characters?"

"Well, there's my grandmother, Helen," Cheryl answered. "She's probably the most important person in my story, especially as far as my research into breast cancer goes."

"And how would you describe Helen?" Bryce asked.

"Vibrant. Warm. Feisty. She was the whole package," Cheryl answered, feeling her eyes get a little teary as she thought about her favorite person.

"And there's my stepmom, Sally," Cheryl continued. "She adopted me shortly after she and my dad got married. I would describe her as creative and dedicated to her family. She's definitely the heart of the Montgomery family."

"Any brothers or sisters?" Bryce asked.

"One. My sibling, Sam, who's actually my stepmom's child. And my dad adopted him as well."

Bryce nodded. "Younger or older?" he asked

"Younger," Cheryl laughed. "By seven years. And despite not being genetically related, I'd say we had a very typical sibling relationship. Sam drove me crazy, and I'm sure I did the same. But we're really close."

"So, he was pretty young when you left for college?" Bryce asked.

"Eleven," Cheryl said, nodding. "It was hard to leave them at home and go off to college. But I knew that's what I needed to do, for me."

"Of course," Bryce acknowledged. "So, anyone else we should know about?"

"Well," Cheryl said, thinking for a moment. "My Uncle Michael and cousin Monica. They're both in healthcare, too. I call Uncle Michael my Jiminy Cricket, and Monica, well, she's my rock. She's the strongest person I know. And my Aunt Savannah. She was Sally's sister, but she really loved being around our family, so we took her in…despite her rougher edges." Cheryl cleared her throat a bit. "And then there are my two best friends, Nathian and Liz. We met during our first year of college and bonded for life. Funny enough, Liz was pre-med with me, and Nathian was majoring in health communication, so it all kind of fit. And those are my people."

"Okay, perfect," Bryce replied. "So, we have your people, and we know that if you hadn't ignored that high school counselor, you might not be sitting here right now. So, what else, Dr. Montgomery? Tell us your story."

"Well," Cheryl began. "I guess it begins about twenty years ago as I went off to college…"

1   Introduction to Health, Healthcare, and Health Communication

Welcome to health communication! We want to start off this learning adventure with two healthcare jokes.

- A man calls the doctor's office and says frantically, "My wife is pregnant, and her contractions are only two minutes apart!" "Is this her first child?" the doctor asks. "No, you idiot!" the man shouts. "This is her husband!"
- A patient goes to the doctor for a follow-up visit. The doctor says, "You look much worse than you did last week! I said you should smoke a maximum of five cigarettes a day!" The patient replies, "That's exactly what I did! And it wasn't easy—because up until now, I didn't smoke at all!"

We hope these jokes gave you a bit of a chuckle. But they're meant to do more than tickle your funny bone. We shared them to highlight how easy it is to think you're asking simple questions or making clear requests when there's actually still plenty of room for misinterpretation. The cases above are arguably harmless, but there are multiple examples of when miscommunication has led to much more serious outcomes. That's something everyone wants to avoid, and it's where the discipline of health communication comes into play (although it's much broader than that). We're glad you're here to learn how.

 We, your authors, have several goals for this book. We want it to offer you a cutting edge, comprehensive presentation of health communication research focusing on a range of essential topics, including patient–provider communication, health information seeking, social support, ethical issues, public health crises, and more. We want it to reveal the challenges and complexities inherent in health and healthcare, including discrimination in its multiple forms, and the kinds of contributions health communication research can make to improve and advance society. And we want it to help you appreciate that although certain principles of health communication apply broadly, the experience of health and illness also is highly personal, affecting each person and their lived lives in unique ways.

 When you realize that most of the illness, injury, and premature death in the world can be prevented—and that competent communication is essential to that process—you know that the discipline has a crucial role to play. We're going to use this introductory chapter to lay the groundwork for the chapters to come by reviewing foundational topics in health and health communication. First, we'll provide an overview of perspectives on health. This section will include a critical look at the American healthcare system and a review of the United Nation's sustainable development goals and the U.S. government's *Healthy People* initiative. It will give you an idea of the nature of the healthcare landscape that must be navigated and the health goals that everyone should be working toward to the extent that they are able. Next, we'll provide an orientation to the discipline of health communication,

DOI: 10.4324/9781003214458-3

which will include a brief history of how the field began. This section also will include a discussion of theory, methods, metatheoretical paradigms, and multidisciplinary, interdisciplinary, and translational research. Finally, we'll talk some about the organization of the book and its pedagogical features. Let's begin, shall we?

Perspectives on Health

Although people may think that being healthy just means not getting sick, health is actually much more than that. The World Health Organization (WHO; 1948) defines **health** as "a state of complete physical, mental and social well-being and not merely the absence of disease or infirmity" (para. 2). From this perspective, you can think of health holistically and consider what is called **whole person health**. The National Center for Complementary and Integrative Health (NCCIH; 2021, para. 1) explains:

> Whole person health involves looking at the whole person—not just separate organs or body systems—and considering multiple factors that promote either health or disease. It means helping and empowering individuals, families, communities, and populations to improve their health in multiple interconnected biological, behavioral, social, and environmental areas. Instead of treating a specific disease, whole person health focuses on restoring health, promoting resilience, and preventing diseases across a lifespan.

Whole person health recognizes that for people to be healthy, healthcare providers, stakeholders, and policymakers must work to promote positive health in all aspects of society, including promoting "healthy behaviors, environments, and policies to maintain health and prevent, treat, and reverse chronic diseases" (NCCIH, 2021, para. 6). The NCCIH lists five exemplar health programs prioritizing a whole health perspective. One of them is the Whole Health Institute (n.d.), which was founded in 2019 to address "physical, mental, emotional, and social well-being by working with health systems, partners, employers, and communities" (para. 1, "About" section). This institute approaches healthcare through a *whole healthcare delivery model*, which they describe as follows (n.p., "Home" section):

- The patient's journey from the time they seek health care to treatment and everything in between
- Reinforced by touchpoints of care that are rooted in evidence-based, whole health approaches
- Delivered by a cross-functional team that assesses individual's needs across a range of physical, mental, behavioral, and social dimensions
- Activated by the individual, who is empowered by self-care tools and resources
- Made financially sustainable through value-based payment models

The perspective of whole person health is a reminder that every human is part of a larger system where everyone's health and health behaviors influence and, for better or worse, are influenced by everyone else's health and health behaviors. These are called **individual-level factors**. For example, if you get a vaccine, it reduces your risk of getting sick, which means you are less likely to get other people sick. At the same time, if you smoke cigarettes, it doesn't just increase your risk of lung cancer—it can increase the risk of lung cancer for anyone who smells the smoke. But it's not just individual-level behaviors that affect health. It's systems-level factors, too.

Systems-level factors are external influences on an individual's health and health behaviors. They are largely outside of an individual's control. They include social, cultural, mass media, organizational, governmental, and environmental factors, many of which operate without people even realizing their impact. We'll be addressing many of these factors in forthcoming chapters, including social determinants of health in Chapter 2. The two we focus on in this chapter are the healthcare systems within which people seek and receive care and efforts to address systemic factors in order to promote health both nationally and globally. We turn to those topics now.

Healthcare in the United States

Healthcare is provided to individuals within healthcare systems, and these systems vary dramatically based on where you live in the world. In a fascinating account of healthcare systems around the globe, T. R. Reid (2010) compares several nations' approaches to medical treatment and payment for services. There are core variations across the systems based on whether (a) healthcare providers and payers (e.g., insurers, Medicare, Medicaid) are private or run by the government, (b) costs are financed through employers/employees, taxes/premiums, or out-of-pocket expenditures, (c) the systems are non-profit or for-profit, and (d) every citizen is covered or not. Considering these factors in the United States, there is a mix of private and government-run providers and payers; costs are financed every which way, with large amounts coming out-of-pocket from patients; there is a mix of for-profit and non-profit entities; and not every citizen is covered (even with the **Affordable Care Act**, also known as Obamacare). Henry Aaron, a leading healthcare economist at the Brookings Institution, said,

> I look at the U.S. health care program and see an administrative monstrosity, a truly bizarre mélange of thousands of payers with payment systems that differ for no socially beneficial reason, as well as staggeringly complex public systems with mind-boggling administered prices and other rules expressing distinctions that can only be regarded as weird.
>
> (Reid, 2010, pp. 43–44)

This quote might be from over a decade ago, but it still is true today.

If Americans were getting exceptional healthcare from this "weird" system, then it might be worth it, but they're not. Did you know that the United States is the only developed nation that doesn't provide some form of universal healthcare to all its citizens? And that medical bankruptcy is unheard of in other developed nations? In the United States, though, even with Obamacare in place, a study by David Himmelstein and colleagues (2019) found that from 2013 to 2016, approximately 530,000 Americans each year declared bankruptcy due to medical bills. Outlandish medical bills are such a problem in the United States that National Public Radio (NPR) and Kaiser Health News (2018–present) co-produce a podcast series called *Bill of the Month* that highlights a personal or family experience with outrageous medical bills "in order to shed light on U.S. health care prices and to help patients learn how to be more active in managing costs" (para. 1).

When comparing large healthcare systems to each other, Reid (2010) explains that healthcare systems can be evaluated along dimensions of cost, quality, and choice. He cites several sources of data to make the claims that "Among the world's developed nations, the United States stands at or near the bottom in most important rankings of access to and quality of medical care" and "The one area where the United States unquestionably leads the world is in spending" (p. 9). In other words, Americans are spending more money for poorer quality and less access. The U.S. healthcare system has more similarities to developing nations' systems than it does to developed nations' systems.

Harvard economist William Hsiao observed that "the creation of a national health care system involves political, economic, and medical decisions, but the primary decision to be made is a moral one" (Reid, 2010, p. 215). Unlike every other developed nation on the planet, the United States has taken a moral stance that not all of its citizens deserve healthcare. Because of that choice, people suffer and die needlessly. Reid wrote his book in the hopes that the United States could learn from other countries that spend less money on healthcare yet have better health outcomes and universal access, but he fears that his argument will fall on deaf ears because of American exceptionalism, or the belief that "our strong, wealthy and enormously productive country…doesn't need to borrow any ideas from the rest of the world" (pp. 12–13). We think that's dreadfully shortsighted. We recommend that you consider reading Reid's (2010) book and see if you want to become a part of working toward the change the U.S. system desperately needs. Part of that change involves national and global efforts to promote health. Let's start with the global level.

United Nations Sustainable Development Goals

The **United Nations (UN) Sustainable Development Goals (SDGs)** call on "Governments and all stakeholders to take transformative actions, individually and collectively, for people, planet and prosperity, while strengthening universal peace in larger freedom" (UN, 2022, p. 7). The goals were developed over two years of extensive consultation with stakeholders around the world and adopted at the September 25–27, 2015 meeting at the UN headquarters in New York. The 17 goals include global economic, social, and environmental dimensions (see Table 1.1). Now that there are more than eight billion people on the planet, these goals are more important than ever.

Table 1.1 United Nations Sustainable Development Goals

Goal 1. End poverty in all its forms everywhere

Goal 2. End hunger, achieve food security and improved nutrition and promote sustainable agriculture

Goal 3. Ensure healthy lives and promote well-being for all at all ages

Goal 4. Ensure inclusive and equitable quality education and promote lifelong learning opportunities for all

Goal 5. Achieve gender equality and empower all women and girls

Goal 6. Ensure availability and sustainable management of water and sanitation for all

Goal 7. Ensure access to affordable, reliable, sustainable and modern energy for all

Goal 8. Promote sustained, inclusive and sustainable economic growth, full and productive employment and decent work for all

Goal 9. Build resilient infrastructure, promote inclusive and sustainable industrialization and foster innovation

Goal 10. Reduce inequality within and among countries

Goal 11. Make cities and human settlements inclusive, safe, resilient and sustainable

Goal 12. Ensure sustainable consumption and production patterns

Goal 13. Take urgent action to combat climate change and its impacts

Goal 14. Conserve and sustainably use the oceans, seas and marine resources for sustainable development

Goal 15. Protect, restore and promote sustainable use of terrestrial ecosystems, sustainably manage forests, combat desertification, and halt and reverse land degradation and halt biodiversity loss

Goal 16. Promote peaceful and inclusive societies for sustainable development, provide access to justice for all and build effective, accountable and inclusive institutions at all levels

Goal 17. Strengthen the means of implementation and revitalize the global partnership for sustainable development

---

Note. From United Nations (n.d.a).

Acknowledged as "a supremely ambitious and transformational vision" with "unprecedented scope and significance" (UN, n.d.b, n.p.), the SDGs officially came into effect on January 1, 2016, with the goal of being accomplished by 2030. Meeting these goals would mean improved health and well-being for people in every corner of the world. The essential role of communication in establishing, maintaining, and promoting the partnerships and infrastructures necessary to accomplish these goals is clear. To show how, we'll highlight just a few of the success stories as reported in the latest *SDG Good Practices* report (UN, 2022).

- The RecyclesPay Educational Project in Nigeria, run by the African Clean-up Initiative, involves the national, regional, and local governments, the private sector, recycling institutions, local schools, and low-income communities in addressing SDGs 1, 3, 4, 6, 10, 11, 13, 14, 15, and 17. Its main objective is to raise enough money from recycling to pay the school fees of more than 10,000 vulnerable students. One of the enabling factors helping this program is "access to the internet and tech tools for easy communication with beneficiaries and stakeholders" (UN, 2022, p. 29).
- The Deqing County Rural Digital Governance System in the Zhejiang Province of China, run by the Deqing Big Data Development Administration, involves the regional and local governments along with rural communities, including farmers, in addressing SDGs 1, 2, 3, 6, 8, and 9. Its main objective is to improve rural spaces through the use of industry, government, and the rural information structure. Efforts include improving farmers' digital literacy through, in part, creating "a new carrier for online social communication for villagers" (UN, 2022, p. 32).
- The SINERGI Project in Indonesia, run by the Rajawali Foundation, involves the U.S. Agency for International Development, the Center for Public Policy Transformation, the Central Java Provincial Government, private sector and non-governmental organizations, and youth coalitions in addressing SDGs 4, 5, 8, 10, and 17. Its main objective is to promote coordination among stakeholders to help vulnerable young people living in poverty enter the labor market. When COVID-19 threatened to cripple the project because of reduced availability of low-skilled labor positions, the project team worked with youth to establish "an infrastructure of communication to gather real-time updates on the levels of employment at the grassroots level" (UN, 2022, p. 36).
- The Transforming Exploitation and Saving Through Association (TESTA) program in India, run by the Vilpa Foundation, involves the national, regional, and local governments, police departments, prosecutors, the judiciary, legal services, legal volunteers, social workers, and nongovernmental organizations in addressing SDGs 5, 8, 16, and 17. Its main objectives are to increase the conviction rate for sex trafficking cases in India and to prevent women and girls from being forced into sex trafficking. This project requires immense coordination and communication among numerous operatives involved in stopping sex trafficking, something they achieved by applying a collective impact model to secure a commitment from all involved.

Hundreds of similar projects are being conducted across the globe under the UN's SGD agenda, and all of them benefit from strategic, coordinated communication among the individuals and organizations involved. The same is true of the communication supporting and promoting the U.S. Healthy People initiative, which has an agenda focused on the health of U.S. citizens.

The U.S. Healthy People Initiative

The **Healthy People initiative** in the United States began in 1979 when U.S. Surgeon General Julius Richmond published *Healthy People: The Surgeon General's Report on Health*

Promotion and Disease Prevention. In the first chapter of his report, Dr. Richmond noted that improvements to American health would not come from more medical care and spending but "through a renewed national commitment to efforts designed to prevent disease and promote health" (U.S. Public Health Service, 1979, p. 1). An analysis of the factors contributing to the 10 leading causes of death in the United States had revealed that "as much as half of U.S. mortality in 1976 was due to unhealthy behavior or lifestyle; 20% to environmental factors; 20% to human biological factors; and only 10% to inadequacies in health care" (p. 9). Recognizing that prevention reduces healthcare costs, improves the quality of people's lives, and literally saves lives, Dr. Richmond issued a call "to enhance both individual and national perspective on prevention through identification of priorities and specification of measurable goals" (p. 13). In response, in 1980 the Office of Disease Prevention and Health Promotion (ODPHP) published *Healthy People 1990*, which included "the first set of ambitious, measurable 10-year objectives for improving health and well-being nationwide" (ODPHP, 2021, para. 2). These reports have been updated each decade, making *Healthy People 2030* the fifth iteration of the report.

The goals and objectives of the Healthy People reports have evolved considerably over the years. Whereas the 1990 report focused on decreasing overall death and increasing older adults' independence, the 2000 report specified three goals: increasing the healthy life span (not just reducing death), reducing health disparities, and increasing access to preventive services. *Healthy People 2010* increased emphasis on improved quality of life and aimed to eliminate health disparities, not simply reduce them. *Healthy People 2020* specified four ambitious goals (ODPHP, 2021, para 5):

- Attain high-quality, longer lives free of preventable disease, disability, injury, and premature death
- Achieve health equity, eliminate disparities, and improve the health of all groups
- Create social and physical environments that promote good health for all
- Promote quality of life, healthy development, and healthy behaviors across all life stages

And now *Healthy People 2030* is in place. This latest report "builds on knowledge gained over the last 4 decades and has an increased focus on health equity, social determinants of health, and health literacy—with a new focus on well-being" (ODPHP, 2021, para. 6).

In total, *Healthy People 2030* has 358 core objectives across numerous categories: health conditions (e.g., heart disease and stroke, foodborne illness), health behaviors (e.g., family planning, sleep), populations (e.g., adolescents, people with disabilities), settings and systems (e.g., environmental health, housing and homes), and social determinants of health (e.g., economic stability, neighborhood and the built environment). There are also objectives designated as developmental or research, but it's the core objectives that are backed by data collected from reliable and valid measures at the national level. This makes it possible to track whether the objectives are being met and where efforts might be falling short. The status of each core objective is reported as (a) having baseline data only, (b) meeting or exceeding the target, (c) improving, (d) having little or no detectable change, or (e) getting worse. We encourage you to visit the Healthy People website to learn the status of the objectives. If you do, you'll see that progress is being made on many fronts, the result of more than four decades of concentrated effort, but there is a lot more progress that needs to be made.

For progress to happen, there needs to be work on several fronts. We need individuals to modify their health behavior to reduce risk and promote well-being. We need healthcare providers to promote health and prevent, not just treat, diseases and conditions that lead to premature death and chronic illness and disability. We need legislation, regulation, and social sanctions to make the physical and social environment healthier. And we need to address systemic issues that perpetuate discrimination and lead to health disparities in historically marginalized groups. Furthermore, we need everyone—patients, family members, healthcare providers, allied health professionals, advocates, policymakers, and stakeholders—to understand and appreciate the principles of competent communication and put those principles into practice. And while we're at it, we need to better educate the public on the benefits of implementing a single-payer, non-profit healthcare system that provides access to care for all Americans—just like every other developed nation.

At the center of all of this is health communication. So, if this book can raise your awareness of health communication research and practice, increase your understanding of how health communication operates in people's daily lives, and help you take an active role in the promotion of health and prevention of disease, then we, as your textbook authors, will be happy. We also will be happy if you gain an understanding of the discipline of health communication, itself, so let's turn to that topic now.

Perspectives on Health

A comprehensive perspective on health recognizes that health involves the whole person in their physical and social environments and that multiple factors at both the individual level and systems level influence health and illness.

Healthcare systems of developed nations vary along four core dimensions:

- Whether healthcare providers and payers are private or government-run
- Whether costs are financed through employers/employees, taxes/premiums, or out-of-pocket expenditures
- Whether the systems are non-profit or for-profit
- Whether every citizen is covered or not

The U.S. Healthy People initiative and the United Nations Sustainable Development Goals are national and global efforts to promote health.

An Orientation to Health Communication

In the early 1970s, a small group of communication scholars began meeting at the annual convention of the **International Communication Association (ICA)** to discuss shared research interests in health communication. In 1972, they requested that ICA recognize them as a special interest group called "Therapeutic Communication." At the 1978 convention, wanting to reflect a broader scope of interest in health beyond therapeutic communication, they voted to change the group's name to "Health Communication," and given growth in membership, they were granted division status. Thus, the field was born (Kreps et al., 2022). Today, health communication is one of the most vibrant, complex, and significant areas of research and practice in contemporary society. As many scholars have noted, and as we have already pointed out, health communication affects all persons throughout their lives, whether through interpersonal conversations about health, exposure to health images and information through the workplace or the media, or involvement in the healthcare system. As health issues become more pressing in society, the interest in health communication and the roles for health communication scholars and practitioners will only increase.

Before we get ahead of ourselves, let's tell you what exactly we mean by "health communication." If you scan the literature, you will find several definitions from various sources. We're going to cut to the chase and share the definition we presented in the first edition of this textbook: **Health communication** is the study of messages that create meaning in relation to physical, mental, and social well-being. We derived this definition from two sources. First, the **National Communication Association (NCA)** provides a definition of communication, stating that it is the study of "how people use messages to generate meaning within and across various contexts" (NCA, n.d., para. 1). Central to this definition is the idea that people use messages to create meaning, not simply exchange information. Messages and meanings constitute the heart of communication. Second, our definition is consistent with the WHO (1948) definition of health provided above, which emphasizes physical, mental, and social well-being.

Definition of Health Communication

Health communication is the study of messages that create meaning in relation to physical, mental, and social well-being.

With the definition of health communication in hand, we, as students and researchers, can branch out in all directions. We can consider health communication processes, such as information dissemination, persuasion, and instruction. We can consider the people involved in health communication, such as patients and providers. We can consider goals such as disease prevention and health promotion. And, of course, we can consider communication channels, such as interpersonal communication, mass communication, online information, and social media. We're going to consider all of that and more in this book. We'll be looking at health messages across a variety of contexts, channels, and purposes, and we'll cover the physical, mental, and social aspects of health. In doing so, we're going to be presenting a wide range of theory-driven research from multiple disciplines, including psychology, nursing, medicine, public health, and, of course, communication. As you read about the various studies presented in each chapter, it will be helpful for you to have an understanding of communication as a social science, so let's lay some quick, but solid, groundwork in theory, methods, metatheory, and research.

Some Groundwork in Theory

We'll begin with theory. We've noticed that people in general don't seem to care too much for theory. This could be because they consider being theoretical the opposite of being practical. But Kurt Lewin, a noted psychologist who was one of the "forefathers" of the communication discipline (Schramm, 1997), is known for having said that there's nothing as practical as a good theory. Why is a good theory practical? Because it helps to guide research. Although you could just decide to study some communication phenomenon with no theoretical guidance whatsoever, how would you know where to begin? How would you know what questions to ask? How would you know what's important to look for? How would you make sense of the data you gather? How would you even know what kind of data to gather? You wouldn't. Although atheoretical research can be valuable in a descriptive sense, to be able to make useful contributions to the discipline's knowledge base, it's wise to make use of **theory**, or "an organized set of concepts and explanations about a phenomenon" (Littlejohn, 2001, p. 19).

Table 1.2 Theoretical Frameworks in Health Communication

Theory/Model	Brief Summary	Citation
Communication Infrastructure Theory	An ecological model that describes how communication infrastructures within neighborhoods, called storytelling networks (STNs), influence individual and community-level health outcomes. STNs are composed of community organizations, geo-ethnic media, and neighborhood residents that are situated within a communication action context.	Kim and Ball-Rokeach (2006)
Digital Divide	A gap exists between individuals advantaged by the internet and individuals relatively disadvantaged by the internet because of differences in access and utilization.	Rogers (2001)
Health Belief Model	People's health behavior is influenced by five beliefs (perceived susceptibility to disease, perceived severity of disease, perceived benefits of engaging in the behavior, perceived barriers to engaging in the behavior, and self-efficacy) and motivated by internal and external cues to action.	Rosenstock (1974) and Rosenstock et al. (1988)
Integrated Model of Behavioral Prediction	Attitude toward a behavior, subjective norms about what other people do, and perceived behavioral control predict behavioral intention, which predicts behavior. Skills and environmental constraints moderate the ability of intention to predict behavior.	Fishbein and Ajzen (2010)
Multiple Goals Theory	Conversations involve task, identity, and relational goals, and these goals sometimes conflict. Messages that resolve conflicting goals are more competent than those that prioritize one goal at the expense of others.	Caughlin (2010)

Note. See *Supplemental Online Theory Table* for additional theories/models.

Health communication research is guided by many different theories, which you'll see reflected in the studies we present in upcoming chapters. For now, we want to introduce you to some exemplar theories or models that have informed a great deal of work in the area (see Table 1.2). We'll begin with one of the earliest and most influential: the health belief model. **The health belief model (HBM)** was developed by several social psychologists in the 1950s while they were working for the U.S. Public Health Service (Rosenstock, 1974). They were trying to figure out why people were not engaging in common sense preventive health behaviors, such as screenings and immunizations, even though these services were available at low or no cost. The researchers determined that people's health beliefs played a substantial role in their behavior. In short, the HBM states that people's health behavior will be influenced by four beliefs: *perceived susceptibility* to disease, *perceived severity* of disease, *perceived benefits* of engaging in the behavior, and *perceived barriers* to engaging in the behavior. In addition, internal or external *cues to action*, such as developing a cough or seeing a public service announcement, can motivate behavior. Irwin Rosenstock and colleagues (1988) later added a fifth belief to the model, *self-efficacy*, or a person's belief that they can successfully execute the behavior. According to the model, for people to be motivated to engage in a health behavior, their perceived susceptibility, severity, benefits, and self-efficacy need to be high, and their perceived barriers need to be low. There also should be helpful cues to action to prompt the behavior. Let's consider a hypothetical example to make this a little clearer.

Let's say that Tim and Barry are college roommates. They keep hearing about how everyone needs to keep up to date with COVID-19 vaccines (an external cue to action). Tim thinks he's impervious to disease (low susceptibility) and that if he did catch the virus, it wouldn't be that bad (low severity). Plus, he thinks the vaccine won't work (no benefits) and it may actually hurt him because the whole pandemic is a government conspiracy anyway (a barrier). Plus, he's not so sure he could track down a vaccination clinic (self-efficacy). Thus, Tim does not get vaccinated. Barry believes the exact opposite of Tim and gets vaccinated and boosted as recommended. Later, Tim starts to notice he can't smell the delicious pizza that Barry brought home for dinner (an internal cue to action). He starts feeling bad and getting sicker by the day (more internal cues to action). Barry finally convinces him to go see a doctor, who diagnoses him with COVID-19. Tim asks for the vaccine at that point, and the doctor says, "That's not the way vaccines work." Whereas Barry's beliefs allowed him to engage in preventive behaviors, Tim's beliefs did not.

The next model we'll discuss is another highly influential one. The **integrated model of behavioral prediction (IMBP)** was developed over many years by Martin Fishbein and Icek Ajzen (2010), and it reflects what is called the **reasoned action approach (RAA)**. The core principles of the RAA are that (a) people's intention to behave precedes their actual behavior and (b) several factors influence intention. Importantly, "reasoned" action in this approach does not mean objectively rational action; instead, people decide for themselves what they think is reasonable on an individual basis. The first version of what ultimately became the IMBP was called the **theory of reasoned action (TRA)**. The TRA said that *attitude toward the behavior* and *subjective norms* about what other people do would predict *behavioral intention*, which then would predict *behavior*. The second version of the RAA was called the **theory of planned behavior (TPB)**. The TPB added *perceived behavioral control*, or the extent to which people believe they have control over the behavior and can accomplish it (basically, self-efficacy), as a predictor of intention. Finally, after years of research using the TRA and TPB, the IMBP was presented as a comprehensive model of behavioral prediction. It added two factors—*skills* and *environmental constraints*—as potential moderators of the intention–behavior relationship (a moderator is a variable that either strengthens or weakens the relationship between two other variables). We'll demonstrate how the IMBP works with a quick hypothetical example.

Jill has decided it's time to start eating healthier. She likes the idea of eating nutritious foods (attitude), most of her friends and relatives eat nutritious foods (subjective norms), and she believes that she'll be able to shop for and cook nutritious foods (perceived behavioral control). So, her behavioral intention is very high. Unfortunately, when she visits her grocery store with an eye toward fresh fruits and vegetables, whole grains, and lean meat and fish, she discovers that the selection is quite limited and the foods are expensive (environmental constraints). She buys what she can afford and brings it home. Her attempt at cooking Brussels sprouts and salmon, though, is a dismal failure (skills). Despite her high behavioral intention, Jill decides she's stuck with processed foods and does not change her behavior.

Next, we're going to move away from models that focus on individual behavior to those that have a more macro-level focus. We'll start with **communication infrastructure theory (CIT)**. CIT is an ecological model that describes how communication infrastructures within neighborhoods, called **storytelling networks (STNs)**, influence individual and community-level health outcomes (Kim & Ball-Rokeach, 2006). STNs are composed of community organizations, geo-ethnic media, and neighborhood residents. They are situated within what is called a *communication action context*, which describes neighborhood characteristics that promote or impede communication within STNs (e.g., resources for families and children, public spaces such as libraries and parks, neighborhood appearance and safety, ethnic and cultural diversity). CIT was originally developed to examine ecological influences on civic engagement, but it evolved to recognize the impact of such engagement on individual and community health. In short, "When a communication action context facilitates a strong neighborhood STN, positive health outcomes are experienced at both the individual and community level" (Wilkin et al., 2010, p. 611).

Knowing this, researchers have used CIT to guide intervention work to improve the health of individuals and communities across the nation. Holley Wilkin and colleagues (2010) describe several such projects. For example, researchers have developed multiethnic communication maps of neighborhoods in Los Angeles, California to provide information on communication resources to communities. They've identified STNs in Atlanta, Georgia to help healthcare providers locate and enroll qualified residents into a healthcare assistance program. And they've studied how STNs have helped individuals in Alabama overcome low health literacy by accessing community-level communication resources and protecting themselves during a hurricane by using STNs as a resource for preparedness activities.

The last theory we'll share is not so much a full-fledged theory (yet) as a concept: the digital divide. The term **digital divide** was coined in the mid-1990s to refer to the fact that there was a gap between people who had access to **information and communication technology (ICT)** and those who did not (Rogers, 2001). This divide raised serious concerns about equity because information and communication underwrite knowledge, and knowledge is power. As digital divide research progressed, the idea of unequal access to technology expanded to include concerns about attitudes toward and motivation to use technology, knowledge and skills to use technology, how frequently and for what purpose technology was being used, and the ability to maintain and update the technology as needed. Several communication theories speak to digital divide concepts, but one that is especially suited is Jan van Dijk's (2013) **resources and appropriations theory**, which considers the diffusion, acceptance, and adoption of ICTs. The theory's premises are as follows (van Dijk, 2013, p. 33):

1. Categorical inequalities in society produce an unequal distribution of resources.
2. An unequal distribution of resources causes unequal access to digital technologies.
3. Unequal access to digital technologies also depends on the characteristics of these technologies.
4. Unequal access to digital technologies brings about unequal participation in society.
5. Unequal participation in society reinforces categorical inequalities and unequal distributions of resources.

By *categorical inequalities*, van Dijk (2013) means *personal characteristics* such as age, race, and health (with older, minority, and unhealthy individuals being disadvantaged) and *positional characteristics* such as employment and education (with unemployed or low wage/low skill workers and those with less education being disadvantaged). In short, van Dijk's theory explains how the digital divide deepens itself through a feedback loop wherein categorical inequalities and unequal distribution of technological resources lead to unequal participation in society, which in turn reinforces categorical inequalities and unequal distribution of technological resources. But how does this impact health? Let's consider an example of living in poverty during the COVID-19 pandemic.

People living in poverty have fewer resources than others, which means they often have inconsistent access to the internet and other mediated information services, if they have access at all. Throughout the COVID-19 pandemic, national and international guidelines for avoiding infection changed as scientists learned more and updated their knowledge about the virus. These science-based updates were disseminated on credible digital and internet-based platforms. People with access to these platforms would receive this information, but people without access would not. Not having current information could increase the risk of getting COVID-19. If people caught the virus, they might end up hospitalized and unable to work, possibly even losing their job. With increased medical bills and fewer paychecks, it would be even harder for them to access digital and internet-based platforms to gain information to help keep them healthy and safe. Thus, the cycle perpetuates itself.

Some Groundwork in Methods

Now that your head is sufficiently spinning from theory, it's time for some methods to bring you back down to earth. **Methods** are simply the strategies researchers use to study phenomena of interest. Methods are often grouped broadly into quantitative and qualitative approaches. **Quantitative methods** require data in numerical form so that the data can be analyzed through statistical techniques. The goal of quantitative research usually is to make generalizations about groups of people or phenomena along a set of relevant variables. The variables need to have clear conceptual and operational definitions. A **conceptual definition** describes the meaning of a variable, pretty much like a dictionary definition. An **operational definition** describes how you will measure your variable. For example, if you used the WHO's (1948) conceptual definition of health for a study, you would need to measure physical, mental, and social well-being. **Qualitative methods** require data that allows for in-depth analysis of the socially constructed meanings of language and behavior. The goal of qualitative research usually is to develop a rich understanding of human experiences. Although some scholars will debate the relative merits of quantitative versus qualitative research, a lot of researchers use both methods to provide a more holistic understanding of their topic of study. This approach is called **mixed-methods research**.

Some Groundwork in Metatheoretical Paradigms

In addition to theory and method, researchers also ground their work in metatheoretical paradigms. A **paradigm** is a way of looking at the nature of the social world. We're not going to get into the weeds with this, but we will state that there are three common paradigmatic approaches in health communication research: scientific, interpretive, and critical-cultural. All have merit, and all make important contributions to the body of health communication knowledge. To give you an idea of how, we're going to take a moment to briefly describe each paradigm and present an exemplar study from within the paradigm.

The **scientific paradigm** states that there is one objective reality that exists independent of human beings and that researchers can work without bias to reveal this reality. It doesn't matter that human behavior is complex and each person is a unique individual; there are regularities underlying who people are and what they do, and research conducted from the scientific perspective is out to identify those regularities. As you might expect, scientific researchers embrace quantitative methods such as experimental and survey research and content analysis to gather numerical data that can be analyzed through statistical techniques.

A great example of research that represents the scientific paradigm is a social media study by Nicole Kashian and Susan Jacobson (2020). The researchers were interested in exploring the relationship between engagement in a Facebook support group for Stage IV breast cancer patients, factors related to social media engagement, and health expectations of the members. They used the optimal matching model of stress and social support and the strength of weak ties theory, as well as the construct of perceived homophily, to explore user engagement (as measured by Facebook analytics) and participants' expectations about their health outcomes (e.g., believing they will live longer as a result of participating in the support group). Kashian and Jacobson hypothesized positive relationships between engagement and optimal social support, tie strength, and homophily, as well as between engagement and health expectations, and they posed a research question asking what factors best predicted engagement. Using content analysis of Facebook posts and anonymous survey data from 74 women who belonged to the private Facebook group, they found support for all hypotheses except the relationship between homophily and engagement, and they found that optimal social support was the factor that best predicted engagement. This study fits the scientific paradigm because of its focus on isolating and assessing how variables are related to one another in predictable and generalizable ways.

The **interpretive paradigm** states that there are multiple subjective "truths" that are socially constructed by humans in everyday interaction and that the researcher plays an active role in constructing these truths. Interpretivist research strives to uncover and understand these subjective, situated meanings of human behavior. Interpretive researchers employ qualitative methods such as interviewing and participant-observation, gathering detailed, descriptive data that they can mine for meaning.

A terrific example of research from the interpretive perspective is a study by Shou Zhou and colleagues (2022) that identified perceived challenges related to COVID-19 prevention and vaccination among ethnic minorities during the pandemic. Guided by the PEN-3 theoretical model, the researchers gathered formative data that could be used to develop a public health campaign to promote COVID-19 prevention behaviors and increase vaccination uptake. They interviewed 18 participants who self-identified as Latino American or Hispanic (LA), African American or Black (AA), and American Indian or Alaska Native (AI/AN), and they identified themes surrounding pandemic-related challenges, perceptions of COVID-19 vaccines, and campaign messaging preferences. They found that participants from all three ethnic groups faced similar challenges related to their social lives and finances as a result of the pandemic, but they also found important differences among ethnicities, such as being particularly concerned about work-related stress (AA) or mental health issues (LA). In terms of perceptions of the vaccines, the researchers found shared beliefs that vaccines could prevent the spread of the virus and stop the pandemic, as well as shared concerns over side effects and how quickly the vaccines were developed, but again, they also found differences among ethnicities, such as concerns about lack of vaccine knowledge (LA), wanting to see public officials and government leaders get vaccinated first (AA), and ensuring equitable access to vaccination (AI/AN). Finally, there were consistent shared beliefs among the different groups about message features that could increase vaccination acceptance and uptake, such as designing positive, prosocial messages that included cultural practices and emphasized protecting family members. Identifying multiple perspectives like these is a primary goal of the interpretive paradigm.

Finally, the **critical-cultural paradigm** is similar to the interpretive paradigm, but it distinguishes itself by its focus on **power**, or the social, political, economic, and cultural means of oppression by the haves of the have-nots. Its methods strive to give voice to people who have been marginalized and to empower them to create social change. In the health communication context, the critical-cultural paradigm forces researchers to question the assumptions they make about what it means to be healthy or sick and who has the authority to say what counts as health promotion or disease prevention behavior (Dutta & Zoller, 2008). Further, it encourages researchers to find ways to change the system to promote greater fairness and equality. #PowerToThePeople!

An excellent example of health communication research from the critical-cultural perspective is work by Comfort Tosin Adebayo and colleagues (2022). These researchers noted that Black women in the United States experience pregnancy-related complications at a significantly higher rate than women of other races and that Black women are three to four times more likely to die from pregnancy-related complications than non-Hispanic white women. Guided by critical race theory, the researchers examined structural barriers within the U.S. healthcare system that limit Black women's access to quality care during prenatal and postnatal doctor's visits. For almost a year, the researchers interviewed Black women seeking maternal care in Milwaukee, Wisconsin, which "ranks as the most racially segregated metropolitan city in the U.S." and where "maternal mortality rates were five times higher among African American women compared to non-Hispanic White women in the city" (Adebayo et al., 2022, p. 1138). Following an extensive analysis of their data, the researchers used narratives to highlight problematic experiences of Black women stemming from the white-centric nature of the biomedical model of healthcare, unfair treatment based on health insurance, provider dismissiveness of pain, and the perception of Black women as a charity case. Adebayo et al. note that "Centrally woven throughout the narratives of women in this study is the experience of a racially insensitive healthcare system" (p. 1140). Examining social structures to identify discriminatory systems is a primary goal of the critical-cultural perspective.

The Nature of Health Communication Research

Health communication scholars rely on numerous theories to guide the design of their research studies. They use quantitative and qualitative methods to conduct their research. Research can be conducted from scientific, interpretive, or critical-cultural paradigmatic perspectives. Health communication research can be multidisciplinary or interdisciplinary, and research results can be translated to have a positive impact on the health and well-being of society.

In addition to understanding how theory, methods, and metatheoretical paradigms help to guide health communication research, it's important to appreciate how different academic disciplines contribute to the body of knowledge in health communication and the extent to which they work independently or collaboratively. Health communication is a very broad field, and many researchers from many disciplines have contributions to make. Depending on how they work together (or not) leads to taking a multidisciplinary or interdisciplinary perspective on the research (Parrott & Kreuter, 2011). **Multidisciplinary research** involves scholars from two or more disciplines *independently* investigating the communication dimension of a health problem. For example, researchers from medicine, pharmacy, and communication may each independently study cost-of-care conversations between patients and physicians. In doing so, they'll bring their unique disciplinary knowledge to bear on the research question. Disciplinary knowledge is important, of course, and can certainly offer important and diverse perspectives on a research problem. A completely independent approach, however, especially for complex questions regarding human communication and health behavior, can substantially limit scientific understanding.

This was the conclusion reached by Nancy Harrington and colleagues (2020) in their systematic review of 54 cost-of-care conversation studies. They reviewed this literature to determine (a) how cost-of-care conversations are conceptually and operationally defined in the literature, (b) the extent to which theory was used to guide cost conversation research, (c) the major methodological characteristics of cost conversation studies, and (d) whether findings from the literature could be used to inform the development of communication strategies to guide cost-of-care conversations between patients and providers. After completing their review, they were left with the impression that the literature did not offer an evidence base for developing communication strategies for having effective cost conversations. Instead, the research was heavily descriptive (e.g., results described the length of cost conversations or whether the patient or physician initiated them) and overwhelmingly atheoretical (only three of the 54 studies were guided by theory).

Harrington et al. (2020) suspected that the reason for this might be that few communication scholars had been involved in conducting the studies. To find out whether their suspicion was correct, they had one of their research assistants track down the educational degrees of the study authors (thanks, Tianen!). He was able to identify the educational degrees of 220 of the 252 authors. How many do you think had PhDs in communication? Four. That's not even two percent. Harrington et al. argued that health communication scholars need to be involved in cost-of-care conversation research teams because their training equips them "to understand the complexities and nuances of message production and exchange in the creation of shared meaning between communicators" (pp. 8–9) and because the communication discipline offers "a wealth of theoretical frameworks that can be brought to bear to help describe, explain, and eventually guide cost conversations" (p. 8). In other words, when studying a communicative behavior, it's advisable to include someone on the research team who is credentialed in the communication discipline. This conclusion highlights the essential role of interdisciplinary research.

Interdisciplinary research involves researchers from two or more disciplines working *collaboratively* to investigate a health problem or the communication aspect of a health problem. The important difference here is that the researchers are working in teams whose members bring different types of expertise to the problem and who can learn from one another to better inform the research. An outstanding example of interdisciplinary health communication research comes from Lauren J. Van Scoy, a medical doctor, and Allison M. Scott, a communication scholar, who began working together to study end-of-life decision making among family members in intensive care units. Van Scoy, a practicing pulmonary and critical care physician, had substantial experience talking to families about end-of-life decisions and had witnessed the exceptional challenges families faced in having these discussions and reaching sound decisions about end-of-life care. She knew that having conversations about a patient's wishes and recording those wishes in a legal document called an advance directive helped patients avoid unwanted care that could prolong unnecessary suffering (see Chapter 8). She sensed that the quality of conversations played a role in making good decisions, yet no matter how much she searched the medical literature, she could find no measure of communication quality, only measures of communication quantity (e.g., number of conversations, length of conversations). Finally, she took a chance and Googled "communication quality measure"—and she found Scott's research on end-of-life conversations.

Scott knew that the research on end-of-life decision making consistently showed that *quantity* of conversations was not related to completing advance directives. She argued that it was conversational *quality*, not quantity, that mattered. Her work was guided by **multiple goals theory**, a theory that explains how people who craft their messages to address task, identity, and relational goals have higher quality communication than those who ignore these goals (Caughlin, 2010). Through extensive observational research with parent/adult child dyads having conversations about end-of-life decision making, Scott was able to demonstrate that the conversations that addressed the task goal of discussing end-of-life decisions, the identity goal of liking and respecting the other person, and the relational goal of affirming the relationship were positively related to satisfaction with the conversation and feelings of hope but negatively related to hurt feelings and relational distancing (Scott & Caughlin, 2014). Subsequent longitudinal analysis showed that such high-quality conversations led participants to have a greater mutual understanding of end-of-life preferences, greater relationship satisfaction and closeness, and a greater likelihood of having completed an advance directive one year after the initial conversation (Scott, 2022).

Van Scoy read all of Scott's research in one night and called her the next day. They've since established a research partnership that has been remarkably successful. They have received major grants from the National Institutes of Health (e.g., "Association between Communication Quality during ICU Family Meetings and Patient Health Outcomes," "Engaging Underserved Communities in End-of-Life Conversations: A Cluster, Randomized Controlled Trial," "Communication Quality Analysis of End-of-Life Discussions by Clinicians") and have published multiple articles in top-tier journals (e.g., Van Scoy et al., 2016, 2017). In addition, they've developed a sophisticated assessment tool that's now being used by other researchers to code for conversation quality (Van Scoy et al., 2022), and they've directly shared their message about the value of using a multiple goals framework to guide clinical conversations with a group of nearly 20,000 practicing clinicians (Scott & Van Scoy, 2020). Furthermore, they're working on an intervention to promote quality advance care planning conversations that can be used in clinical practice so that their research will have a positive impact on patients' and families' lives. This success is the result of embracing an interdisciplinary approach that included perspectives from both medicine and communication.

Having a positive impact on people's lives is the ultimate goal of health communication research. It's a process called **research translation**: taking study results and translating them from research contexts to actual community and practice settings. For too long, academic researchers have been gaining knowledge only to have that knowledge end up in a journal on a dusty bookshelf. Sharing new knowledge with other researchers through journals is absolutely fine and part of what establishes disciplines and advances science. However, publication should not be an ending point, it should be a starting point. Indeed, translating knowledge to practice is what allows health communication research to make contributions to the promotion of health and well-being, and these days researchers are more aware of that than ever. There are multiple examples of health communication research that has been translated for large-scale impact. Because we could spend the rest of this chapter talking about these translational programs of research and the outstanding scholars doing this work, we instead provide a concise summary in tabular form (see Table 1.3). If you want to know more about any of these researchers and their work, feel free to send us an email, and we'll put you in touch.

Table 1.3 Communication Scholars and Their Translational Research

Communication Scholar	Translational Accomplishment
Wayne Beach, PhD in Interaction Analysis from the University of Utah	Dr. Beach led the production of two videos depicting the experience of breast cancer, *When Cancer Calls…* and *A Journey Through Breast Cancer*. The first presents the phone conversations from a family's journey through a mother's cancer diagnosis, care, and death. The second is a documentary centered on the fears, uncertainties, and hopes of a woman navigating cancer treatments. Both films have been disseminated through several outlets, including PBS, and seen by millions of viewers.
Erin Donovan, PhD in Communication from the University of Illinois at Urbana-Champaign	Dr. Donovan studies ways to improve the quality of informed consent documents by reducing sources of uncertainty and making information more comprehensible. The template for informed consent that she developed was officially added to the Texas Administrative Code as part of the state's regulatory revision of consent procedures, going into effect statewide in 2020.
Mohan Dutta, PhD in Mass Communication from the University of Minnesota	Dr. Dutta uses a culture-centered approach to develop interventions to improve the lives of historically marginalized and disenfranchised people by fostering culturally-based participatory strategies to address unequal health policies. He has completed projects on food insecurity, poverty and health, health among migrant workers in low-skilled sectors, health of transgender sex workers, and cardiovascular health among African Americans.

(Continued)

Table 1.3 Continued

Communication Scholar	Translational Accomplishment
Lynn Harter, PhD in Communication Studies from the University of Nebraska	Dr. Harter co-hosts *Defining Moments*, a podcast featuring research-based illness narratives published in the discipline's flagship journal, *Health Communication*. To date, there have been 35 episodes, with reviews describing the podcast as phenomenal and innovative, as well as a necessity to hear. The podcast is available through WOUB Public Media on NPR One.
Michael Hecht, PhD in Communication from the University of Illinois Michelle Miller-Day, PhD in Human Communication from the Arizona State University	Drs. Hecht and Miller-Day developed a substance abuse prevention program for adolescents, *keepin' it REAL (kiR)*. The program was recognized by the U.S. Surgeon General as one of the top three adolescent substance abuse prevention programs in the nation, and it's now offered in more than 50 countries around the world. Drs. Hecht and Miller-Day also established REAL Prevention, a company that disseminates *kiR* and other prevention programs.
Janice Krieger, PhD in Communication Arts & Sciences from The Pennsylvania State University	Dr. Krieger is the director of the STEM Translational Communication Center at the University of Florida. Her research focuses on increasing cancer screening and cancer clinical trial participation, and she has worked to establish strategic partnerships to develop and disseminate evidence-based communication interventions. She also participates in the National Cancer Institute's SPeeding Research-tested INTerventions (SPRINT) program, which trains scientists to expedite the transfer of cancer interventions into practice.
Rachael Record, PhD in Communication from the University of Kentucky	Dr. Record is a principal investigator with the Thirdhand Smoke Research Consortium. Funded by the California Tobacco-Related Disease Research Program, the consortium is a multi-institutional and interdisciplinary effort involving researchers from the disciplines of chemistry, biology, psychology, nursing, public health, global health, and communication. Together, they work to understand the risks of environmental tobacco exposure. Dr. Record's role is to oversee the translation and dissemination of consortium findings through educational materials and communication campaigns. These resources are available at thirdhandsmoke.org.
Kami Silk, PhD in Communication from the University of Georgia	Dr. Silk has engaged in extensive interdisciplinary research to develop advocacy and practice initiatives around environmental impacts on breast cancer. Part of this work involved creating continuing medical education training for pediatric healthcare workers that increased their knowledge and their efforts to spread prevention practices to young women in the pre-pubertal and pubertal windows of breast cancer susceptibility during well-child visits.
Arvind Singhal, PhD in Communication Theory and Research from the University of Southern California Annenberg School for Communication	Dr. Singhal's work integrates principles of diffusion of innovations, positive deviance (going against the norm in a good way), and entertainment-education to promote cost-effective and culturally appropriate interventions and to influence policy around human rights, health, and healthcare, as well as nutrition, STEM education, micro-lending, and agriculture. He has worked on communication development projects in numerous countries, including India, Thailand, Mexico, Brazil, and Kenya.
Elaine Wittenberg, PhD in Communication from the University of Oklahoma Joy Goldsmith, PhD in Communication from the University of Oklahoma	Drs. Wittenberg and Goldsmith led the development of the COMFORT Communication palliative care curriculum, which is the first theoretically grounded and evidence-based program for teaching healthcare providers how to deliver life-altering news, assess patient and family health literacy needs, practice mindful communication, acknowledge family caregivers, and address patient and family goals of care. Their work has reached healthcare providers from nearly all states in the nation.

Organization and Features of This Book

Now that you are familiar with health, healthcare, and health communication, let's familiarize you with the organization and features of this book. We've organized the book into six sections. The first section, *Understanding Health Communication Foundations*, includes this introductory chapter and a chapter covering discrimination and health communication. The second section, *Being a Patient*, contains chapters on patient–provider communication; patient experiences of uncertainty, decision making, coping, and health literacy; and health information seeking. The third section, *Caring for a Patient*, features chapters on healthcare provider roles and perspectives, social support and informal caregiving, and end-of-life communication. The fourth section, *Health Communication Challenges*, includes chapters on mental health, intercultural health communication, and ethical issues in health communication. The fifth section, *Societal Level Health Communication Concerns*, addresses health communication in the media, environmental health communication, and public health crises. The last section, *Looking Forward*, offers a chapter focused on practical information for students wishing to continue their studies in health communication, find a career in health communication, or become allies in efforts to end discrimination and promote patient empowerment. You might have noticed that we do not include a chapter on technology. This is because technology changes so rapidly and becomes out of date so quickly, a standalone chapter would soon become obsolete. So instead, we chose to infuse how technology is being used across health communication contexts in each chapter. We do the same thing with social media. Instead of having a specific section devoted to social media in the chapter on health communication in the media, we cover the topic across chapters where applicable. In addition, although we devote a chapter to discrimination in health and healthcare, we also include concerns of historically marginalized and disadvantaged communities in each chapter. This is because the pervasive discrimination in the healthcare system must be consistently recognized and challenged through communication and other efforts if the system is to work for everyone.

In reviewing the literature for each chapter, we strived to locate research studies that would reflect the breadth of the discipline. We also strived to emphasize the results and implications of research studies, while also highlighting relevant aspects of theory and method. Each chapter also offers pedagogical features to facilitate this book's use as a textbook. We have summary boxes to highlight main points of the chapter, and **key terms** are bolded throughout the text. Theory tables present theories described in the chapter, including a summary of their principles and a reference for further reading. Each chapter also offers suggestions for in-class activities and discussion questions. Online resources are available for students and instructors through the textbook's page on the Routledge website. And, of course, there is the Montgomery family narrative, the first installment of which you've already read. As several prominent health communication scholars have emphasized over the years, health is embodied in and experienced through narrative (Harter et al., 2022). We decided, therefore, to craft the story of Cheryl Montgomery and her family and friends to demonstrate in story form some of the principles we cover in each chapter. We hope you enjoy this aspect of the book and find it useful in aiding understanding and promoting discussion.

Conclusion

Our goal for this introductory chapter was to give you a sense of what a complex, vibrant, and exciting field health communication is. From its beginnings in the early 1970s until today, health communication has benefited from the research of scholars from communication and other social, behavioral, and health-related disciplines, all of whom have made extensive contributions to our knowledge of health communication across a multitude of contexts. Scholars have learned so much about the experiences and perspectives of being a patient and caring for patients. They have enhanced understanding of the challenges and complexities that people encounter in health promotion and disease prevention, including systemic discrimination. And they have advanced knowledge of societal-level concerns regarding the mass media, environmental health communication, and public health crises. Yet there is so much more to learn.

As health communication scholars continue their work, knowledge will be enriched through multidisciplinary and interdisciplinary research, and when that research is translated into practice, the potential to improve the health and well-being of society will be monumental. Furthermore, visionary efforts to build systems and infrastructures to advance health at national and global levels hold promise for a healthier tomorrow. Although all of us have been or inevitably will be participants in some form of healthcare, our hope is that the knowledge gained and shared by health communication scholars will help everyone manage these experiences skillfully and effectively to achieve the best possible outcomes.

And because we are told that laughter is the best medicine, we'll leave you with one more health communication joke:

> A patient goes to the doctor and says, "Doctor, I have this problem with passing gas. It really doesn't bother me too much, though. It never smells, and it's always silent. In fact, I've passed gas at least 20 times since I've been here in your office, and you didn't know because it doesn't smell and it's silent." "I see," the doctor says. "Take these pills and come back to see me next week." The next week, the patient goes back and says, "Doctor, I don't know what you gave me, but now my gas… although it's still silent, it stinks terribly." "Good," the doctor said. "And now that we've cleared up your sinuses, we'll start to work on your hearing."

References

Adebayo, C. T., Parcell, E. S., Mkandawire-Valhmu, L., & Olukotun, O. (2022). African American women's maternal healthcare experiences: A critical race theory perspective. *Health Communication, 37*(9), 1135–1146.

Caughlin, J. P. (2010). A multiple goals theory of personal relationships: Conceptual integration and program overview. *Journal of Social and Personal Relationships, 27*(6), 824–848.

Dutta, M. J., & Zoller, H. M. (2008). Theoretical foundations: Interpretive, critical, and cultural approaches to health communication. In H. M. Zoller & M. J. Dutta (Eds.), *Emerging perspectives in health communication: Meaning, culture, and power* (pp. 1–27). Routledge.

Fishbein, M., & Ajzen, I. (2010). *Predicting and changing behavior: The reasoned action approach.* Psychology Press.

Harrington, N. G., Scott, A. M., & Spencer, E. A. (2020). Working toward evidence-based guidelines for cost-of-care conversations between patients and physicians: A systematic review of the literature. *Social Science & Medicine, 258,* 113084.

Harter, L. M., Yamasaki, J., & Kerr, A. M. (2022). Narrative features, forms, and functions: Telling stories to foster well-being, humanize healthcare, and catalyze change. In T. L. Thompson & N. G. Harrington (Eds.), *The Routledge handbook of health communication* (3rd ed., pp. 47–60). Routledge.

Himmelstein, D. U., Lawless, R. M., Thorne, D., Foohey, P., & Woodhandler, S. (2019). Medical bankruptcy: Still common despite the Affordable Care Act. *American Journal of Public Health, 109*(3), 431–433.

Kaiser Health News. (2018–present). *Bill of the month.* Podcast. https://khn.org/news/tag/bill-of-the-month/

Kashian, N., & Jacobson, S. (2020). Factors of engagement and patient-reported outcomes in a Stage IV breast cancer Facebook group. *Health Communication, 35*(1), 75–82.

Kim, Y.-C., & Ball-Rokeach, S. J. (2006). Civic engagement from a communication infrastructure perspective. *Communication Theory, 16*(2), 173–197.

Kreps, G. L., Sharf, B., Harrington, N. G., & Thompson, T. L. (2022). The ICA health communication division. In E. Y. Ho, C. L. Bylund, & J. C. M. Van Weert (Eds.), *The international encyclopedia of health communication*. Wiley Blackwell.

Littlejohn, S. (2001). *Theories of human communication* (7th ed.). Wadsworth.

National Center for Complementary and Integrative Health. (2021). *Whole person health: What you need to know*. https://www.nccih.nih.gov/health/whole-person-health-what-you-need-to-know

National Communication Association. (n.d.). *What is communication?* https://www.natcom.org/about-nca/what-communication

Office of Disease Prevention and Health Promotion. (2021). *History of Healthy People*. https://health.gov/our-work/national-health-initiatives/healthy-people/about-healthy-people/history-healthy-people

Parrott, R., & Kreuter, M. W. (2011). Multidisciplinary, interdisciplinary, and transdisciplinary approaches to health communication: Where do we draw the line? In T. L. Thompson, R. Parrott, & J. Nussbaum (Eds.), *The Routledge handbook of health communication* (pp. 3–17). New York: Routledge.

Reid, T. R. (2010). *The healing of America: A global quest for better, cheaper, and fairer health care*. Penguin Books.

Rogers, E. M. (2001). The digital divide. *Convergence, 7*(4), 96–111.

Rosenstock, I. M. (1974). Historical origins of the health belief model. *Health Education & Behavior, 2*(4), 328–335.

Rosenstock, I. M., Strecher, V. J., & Becker, M. H. (1988). Social learning theory and the health belief model. *Health Education Quarterly, 15*(2), 175–183.

Schramm, W. (1997). *The beginnings of communication study in America: A personal memoir*. Sage.

Scott, A. M. (2022). A longitudinal examination of enacted goal attention in end-of-life communication in families. *Communication Research*. Advance online publication. doi: 10.1177/00936502211058040

Scott, A. M., & Caughlin, J. P. (2014). Enacted goal attention in family conversations about end-of-life health decisions. *Communication Monographs, 81*(3), 261–284.

Scott, A. M., & Van Scoy, L. J. (2020). What counts as "good" clinical communication in the coronavirus disease 2019 era and beyond? Ditching checklists for juggling communication goals. *CHEST, 158*(3), 879–880.

United Nations. (n.d.a). *The 17 goals*. https://sdgs.un.org/goals

United Nations. (n.d.b). *Transforming our world: The 2030 agenda for sustainable development*. https://sdgs.un.org/2030agenda

United Nations. (2022). *SDG good practices: A compilation of success stories and lessons learned in SDG implementation*. United Nations.

U.S. Public Health Service. (1979). *Healthy People: The Surgeon General's report on health promotion and disease prevention* (chapter 1). https://profiles.nlm.nih.gov/spotlight/nn/catalog/nlm:nlmuid-101584932X94-doc

van Dijk, J. A. G. M. (2013). A theory of the digital divide. In M. Ragnedda & G. W. Muschert (Eds.), *The digital divide: The internet and social inequality in international perspective* (29–51). Routledge.

Van Scoy, L. J., Reading, J. M., Scott, A. M., Green, M. J., & Levi, B. H. (2016). Conversation game effectively engages groups of individuals in discussions about death and dying: A feasibility study. *Journal of Palliative Medicine, 19*(6), 661–667.

Van Scoy, L. J., Scott, A. M., Green, M. J., Witt, P. D., Wasserman, E., Chinchilli, V. M., & Levi, B. H. (2022). Communication Quality Analysis: A user-friendly observational measure of patient-clinician communication. *Communication Methods and Measures, 16*(3), 215–235.

Van Scoy, L. J., Scott, A. M., Reading, J. M., Chuang, C., Chinchilli, V. M., Levi, B. L., & Green, M. J. (2017). From theory to practice: Measuring end-of-life communication quality using multiple goals theory. *Patient Education and Counseling, 100*(5), 909–918.

Whole Health Institute. (n.d.). *Our purpose*. https://www.wholehealth.org/about-the-whole-health-institute

Wilkin, H. A., Moran, M. B., Ball-Rokeach, S. J., Gonzalez, C., & Kim, Y.-C. (2010). Applications of communication infrastructure theory. *Health Communication, 25*(6–7), 611–612.

World Health Organization. (1948). *Definition of health*. http://apps.who.int/gb/bd/PDF/bd47/EN/constitution-en.pdf

Zhou, S., Villalobos, J. P., Munoz, A., & Bull, S. (2022). Ethnic minorities' perceptions of COVID-19 vaccines and challenges in the pandemic: A qualitative study to inform COVID-19 prevention interventions. *Health Communication, 37*(12), 1476–1487.

In-class Activities

1. In *Healthy People 2030*, there are eight core objectives, nine developmental objectives, and two research objectives related to health communication. Some are focused on information technology and electronic health records, whereas others are related to health communication in general or in specific contexts. Divide students into small groups and have them visit the *Healthy People 2030* website to explore these objectives. Have each group pick one (no overlap, please) and report back to the class describing the objective and its current status. https://health.gov/healthypeople/objectives-and-data/browse-objectives/health-communication

2. Put the students in small groups. Have each student share a story of how health communication has affected their lives in some way. It could be a particularly memorable conversation with a healthcare provider, something they saw on television that made a strong impact, or a new communication technology they're using to promote their health. Have each group pick one story to share with the rest of the class. Throughout the rest of the term, keep these stories in mind to see if the research presented in the forthcoming chapters sheds light on any of them.

Discussion Questions

1. Health is more than a product of a person's individual decisions and behaviors. Instead, it's influenced by the decisions and behaviors of other people in social networks. The chapter demonstrated this with examples of vaccination and smoking. What are other examples of how individual decisions can influence the health of others?

2. The leading cause of lung cancer, the most preventable form of cancer, is tobacco use. How might a team of all nurses seek to study and reduce rates of lung cancer? How about a team of all pediatricians? Or a team of all psychologists? Or a team of all communication scholars? Now, how might an interdisciplinary team with a nurse, pediatrician, psychologist, and communication scholar seek to study and reduce rates of lung cancer?

3. Translational research is important for taking what is learned in research studies and implementing that knowledge to positively impact the health of the public. Consider the exemplar studies described in the section on paradigmatic perspectives. What are some ways that these studies' results could be translated to improve people's health?

The First Year of College Scaries

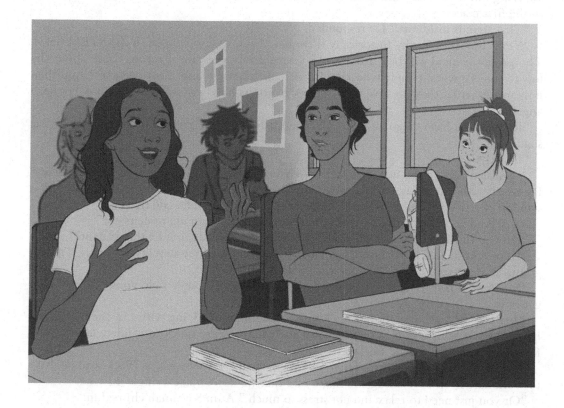

Cheryl's first year of college was off to a great start. She'd settled into her dorm room, and her roommate, Liz, a young lady with red hair, freckles, and a friendly disposition, was terrific. Cheryl was comfortably managing her pre-med coursework, but it was one of her electives, a sociology course on discrimination, that was giving her some concern. She was learning about types of discrimination in multiple forms and contexts and all the negative repercussions that came from it. The latest lecture on stereotype threat was really bothering her. After class, Cheryl met up with Liz at the library, feeling despondent. Liz noticed right away.

"What's wrong, Cher?" Liz asked.

"All of it," Cheryl replied, slumping in her chair.

"What do you mean?"

Cheryl heaved a sigh. "You know my sociology of discrimination class, right? And how we've been covering all these types of discrimination that are just everywhere."

DOI: 10.4324/9781003214458-4

"Yeah," Liz acknowledged. "I can't believe some of the things you're learning in that class. The latest stuff about ableism? I'd never really thought about how society is still so stacked against people with disabilities."

"Well, you're not going to believe this, either," Cheryl stated. "The professor today was talking about this concept called stereotype threat. It's when people in groups that have been stereotyped as performing poorly at something actually do perform worse when they're reminded of that stereotype. Like the ridiculous notion that Black students aren't as smart as white students, or girls aren't as smart as boys in science or math." Cheryl shook her head. "And the professor talked about how these threats are so subtle, but they have real effects and actually become self-fulfilling prophecies, with people just self-selecting out of certain education or career paths because they believe they can't succeed in the first place."

"That sounds insidious," Liz responded.

"Yeah. I mean, it's why historically there have been so few women in the STEM fields. The professor cited all these studies. And what really gets me, I mean, think about the loss to society when people who could make contributions just don't even try? And then how much harder they do have to try if they're gonna have a shot." Cheryl shook her head angrily.

"It's like you have to go above and beyond before people give you a second look," Liz stated.

"Exactly!"

A puzzled look came across Liz's face. "You know what I'm just now remembering? Remember the first day in bio, when the professor stood there and said half the class wouldn't be able to pass? I swear, he looked right at me when he said that."

"Yes! And he did it again last week, with midterms coming up, remember?"

"Do you think he did it on purpose?" Liz asked. "I mean, can it be that blatant?"

"I don't know," Cheryl said. "But now that I know about stereotype threat, I'm not gonna let it get to me, and I'm gonna ace that test."

"Me, too!" Liz searched through her backpack and pulled out her bio book. "We'd better get busy."

After Cheryl got home from three hours in the library studying with Liz, she hopped on her family's weekly Zoom where Michael and Monica were quick to validate how Cheryl felt about what she learned in class.

"Yes, that is completely infuriating," Monica stated. "It's why we, as Black women, have to work harder on everything and make sure that we don't make a single mistake."

"Or you just need to relax and not stress so much," Aunt Savannah chimed in.

Everyone on the call rolled their eyes at Savannah. It was no surprise that she was downplaying the fact that some people had it harder than others because of bigotry—that's just what she always did. Sometimes Cheryl wondered why they ever gave her the password to the family Zoom. Although Monica and Michael made Cheryl feel better, she still felt anger and despair because it seemed like marginalized communities always had it worse.

The next week in her communication class, Cheryl had an opportunity to think through these disparities a bit more. Liz happened to be in that class with her, too.

"Still feeling good about your 98% on the bio midterm?" Liz asked Cheryl, taking a seat one spot away from her so there'd be room to spread out.

"As good as you're feeling about your 97%," Cheryl replied, grinning.

"You two talking about the history midterm?" asked a voice from behind them. Cheryl turned around to find herself sitting in front of a very handsome boy with hazel green eyes.

"Uh, yeah, no. Hi. Biology actually. So, you had a history midterm?" Cheryl asked, trying to be polite and hide the fact that she found herself a bit nervous.

"Yeah," the boy smiled back. "It was not fun. But I bet bio wasn't fun either."

"NOPE!" Liz shouted, "But we nailed it!" Cheryl was so focused on the boy that she'd missed the fact that Liz had also turned around to see who belonged to the voice.

"By the way, I'm Cheryl. This is Liz."

"Nathian. Nice to meet you both. Hey, mind if I, uh…" Without another word, Nathian moved to take the spot between Cheryl and Liz. "So, what do you think of this class?"

"Good so far," Liz replied, leaning back a bit to shoot Cheryl a '*Wow, he's cute*' look as Nathian glanced down at his phone. "Although I still don't quite understand how the instructor is so young," she added.

"Oh, she's a graduate student," Nathian explained. "She's getting a PhD in communication and is teaching this course as part of her graduate program."

"How do you know that?" Cheryl asked, a bit surprised by how much he knew.

Nathian chuckled a little before replying, "Remember, she told us on the first day?"

"Oh!" Cheryl and Liz replied together. They did not remember.

"Yeah," Nathian continued. "She's doing her dissertation on health disparities looking at how communication interventions can help differently abled communities achieve better health outcomes," Nathian said. "It's pretty cool."

"Okay, that I actually remember," Cheryl replied. Cheryl also found herself remembering how much she enjoyed listening to the instructor talk about her work. The instructor was dedicating her career to trying to help underserved communities be healthy. Cheryl hoped her pre-med path would lead her in a similar direction.

After the week of midterms passed, Cheryl, Liz, and Nathian found themselves spending more time together. Before long, they were meeting weekly to study, have dinner, and watch movies. Over the next three years, Cheryl and Liz were able to take most of their classes together. And when an elective was needed, they always tried to take a class with Nathian. Liz and Nathian would be Cheryl's pillars not only for the next few years of college but for many years after.

Notes

Learn more about the negative impact of stereotype and identity threats on academic performance among racial minorities and women and how interventions can be designed to diminish the impact of these threats from the following resources:

- Cohen, G. L., Purdie-Vaughns, V., & Garcia, J. (2012). An identity threat perspective on intervention. In M. Inzlicht & T. Schmader (Eds.), *Stereotype threat: Theory, process, and application* (pp. 280–296). Oxford University Press.
- National Institutes of Health. (2017). *Stereotype threat.* https://diversity.nih.gov/sociocultural-factors/stereotype-threat

Transitioning to college is stressful. Drexel University provides some great tips for adjusting to the college lifestyle. These tips are sure to be helpful no matter what year in college you find yourself: https://drexel.edu/counselingandhealth/counseling-center/students/adjustment/.

2 Discrimination and Health Communication

As an author, activist, and founder of the digital media and education company *The Body Is Not An Apology*, Sonya Renee Taylor has dedicated her life to understanding and revealing how the inequity and injustice experienced in the world are based on relationships with bodies—our own and others'. Her thesis is that through societal structures, people are acculturated into a belief system that some bodies are better than others: male bodies are better than female bodies; white bodies are better than Black or Brown bodies; slender bodies are better than fat bodies; bodies that are attracted to the opposite sex are better than bodies attracted to the same sex; able bodies are better than disabled bodies; and so on, and so on, and so on. She calls this the "ladder of body hierarchy." Those at the top of the ladder want to stay there because of inherent privileges in society, while those on lower rungs must strive to climb higher (somehow) if they want to attain those privileges. But here's the thing: The ladder is an illusion. It only exists because people continue to perpetuate it through social systems.

Topics within the discipline of health communication cannot be comprehensively explored without considering the societal and cultural systems within which they reside because health is inherently a product of those systems. Ethical health communication practices seek to be anti-discriminatory by (a) recognizing the complexities and influences of healthcare systems, (b) contextualizing individual health experiences and decision making within the constraints of societal and cultural experiences, and (c) actively recognizing instances and implications of systemic barriers on health. To that end, this chapter presents an overview of discriminatory practices, their implications for health, and research approaches to studying and reducing discrimination. Discriminatory practices will be exemplified by considering their actions against race, sex, gender, and disability in healthcare. As part of that discussion, we'll present anti-discrimination efforts being implemented through various organizations and initiatives. Finally, we'll explore discrimination as evidenced through media representation. First, however, we'll introduce discrimination and its impact on health.

Introduction to Discrimination and Health

Discrimination is the prejudicial treatment of others based on their personal characteristics, such as race, age, gender, sex, or disability (American Psychological Association [APA], 2019). It is perpetuated not only by people who engage in discriminatory behaviors at the individual level but also by societal systems and structures that marginalize and disenfranchise persons on the basis of differences. Experiencing discrimination can negatively affect people's health. In a meta-analysis of 134 research studies examining the relationship between discrimination and health, Elizabeth Pascoe and Laura Smart Richman (2009) found that experiencing discrimination negatively influenced mental and physical health,

DOI: 10.4324/9781003214458-5

including increased risks of anxiety, depression, obesity, high blood pressure, and substance abuse. Tien Dong and colleagues (2022) showed that such outcomes occur because experiencing discrimination has negative biological impacts, including "alterations of brain networks related to emotion, cognition and self-perception, and structural and functional changes in the gut microbiome" (n.p.). Moreover, APA (2019) argues that discrimination can be harmful to health "even if you haven't been the target of overt acts of bias" (n.p.). They go on to explain how:

> Regardless of your personal experiences, it can be stressful just being a member of a group that is often discriminated against, such as racial minorities or individuals who identify as lesbian, gay, bisexual or transgender (LGBT). The anticipation of discrimination creates its own chronic stress. People might even avoid situations where they expect they could be treated poorly, possibly missing out on educational and job opportunities.

Although people may think of discrimination as blatant acts, that's not always the case. Indeed, there are subtler forms of discrimination called microaggressions that also do substantial damage.

Discrimination

Discrimination is the prejudicial treatment of others based on their personal characteristics (e.g., race, gender). Discrimination can occur interpersonally (i.e., one person discriminating against another) or structurally (i.e., policies that discriminate against particular groups). Acts of discrimination can be both overt and subtle.

Microaggressions

Microaggressions are "everyday verbal, nonverbal, and environmental slights, snubs, or insults, whether intentional or unintentional, that communicate hostile, derogatory, or negative messages to target persons based solely upon their marginalized group membership" (Sue, 2010, p. 3). In a review of 32 published taxonomies for organizing microaggressions, Monnica Williams and colleagues (2021) identified 16 distinct categories of microaggressions committed against people of color. Table 2.1 presents these categories with descriptions of what they look like in action. Repeatedly receiving one or more of these microaggressions can negatively impact health.

For example, research consistently shows that exposure to microaggressions leads to poor mental health outcomes (Nadal et al., 2014), particularly among Black (Gómez, 2015), disabled (Kattari, 2020), and transgender (Nadal et al., 2011) communities. Research also shows that microaggressions can negatively affect physical health. For example, Kelley Sittner and colleagues (2018) surveyed American Indian adults about their experiences with microaggressions and healthcare. They found that experiencing microaggressions increased diabetes distress, which in turn reduced diabetes self-care, such as following a recommended diet and exercising.

Clearly, microaggressions are very damaging at the individual level, as "people on the receiving end of day-to-day discrimination often feel they're in a state of constant vigilance, on the lookout for being a target of discrimination" (APA, 2019, n.p.). So, we all certainly should strive to combat microaggressions whenever we encounter them. It's the structural

Table 2.1 Microaggressions Against People of Color (POC)

Category of Microaggressions	Description
Not a true citizen	Suggesting a POC is not a real citizen or a meaningful part of society
Racial categorization and sameness	Compelling a POC to disclose their racial identity; assumption that all people from a group are alike
Assumptions about intelligence, competence, or status	Behaviors or statements derived from racial stereotypes
False color blindness	Expressing that a POC's racial or ethnic identity should not be acknowledged
Criminality or dangerousness	Demonstrating belief in stereotypes that POC are dangerous, untrustworthy, and likely to commit crimes or cause bodily harm
Denial of individual racism	Trying to make a case that one is not biased to deflect perceived scrutiny of their own biased behaviors
Myth of meritocracy	Deeming success as being rooted in personal efforts and denial of existence of racism/white privilege
Reverse-racism hostility	Expressions of jealousy or hostility surrounding the notion that POC get unfair advantages and benefits
Pathologizing minority culture or appearance	Criticizing based on perceived or real cultural differences in appearance, traditions, behaviors, or preferences
Second-class citizen	Treating POC with less respect, consideration, or care than is normally expected or customary
Tokenism	Including a POC to promote the illusion of inclusivity; expecting one individual to understand or speak for a whole ethnic group
Connecting via stereotypes	Trying to communicate or connect with a POC through stereotyped speech or behaviors
Exoticization and eroticization	Stereotypically sexualizing a POC or paying attention to differences characterized as exotic
Avoidance and distancing	Avoiding POC or taking measures to prevent physical contact or close proximity
Environmental exclusion	Minimizing someone's racial identity by excluding decorations, literature, or depictions of a racial group
Environmental attacks	Decorations that pose a known affront or insult to a cultural group, history, or heritage

Note. From Williams et al. (2021).

factors promoting discrimination, though, that if effectively redressed can have profound, systemic effects for reducing discrimination. This is where social determinants of health come into play.

Social Determinants of Health

Social determinants of health are often referred to as the "causes of the causes" of poor health (Braveman & Gottlieb, 2014). The Centers for Disease Control and Prevention (CDC; 2021) describe them as the "nonmedical factors that influence health outcomes. They're the conditions in which people are born, grow, work, live, and age, and the wider set of forces and systems shaping the conditions of daily life" (para. 1). One of the most profound demonstrations of the impact of social determinants of health occurred at the 2012 *American Public Health Association* (APHA) conference. Conference attendees were greeted by three large billboards from the nonprofit California Endowment's *Health Happens Here* campaign. Each billboard presented a picture of a child with their age, zip code, and life expectancy, along with the statement "Your Zip Code shouldn't predict how long you'll live." The campaign was making the point that neighborhood-level social and

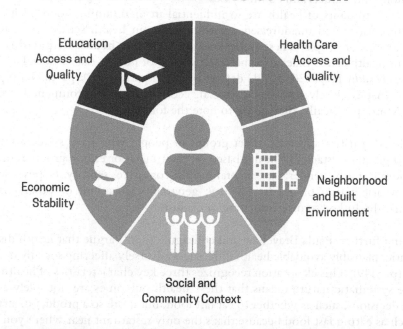

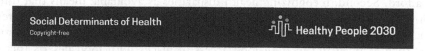

Figure 2.1 Social Determinants of Health.
Source: U.S. Department of Health and Human Services (n.d.).

environmental factors played an enormous role in determining longevity. Nobody gets to choose where they're born and raised, so to have that be such a major influence on health hardly seems just.

The *Healthy People 2030* report organizes social determinants of health into five categories (see Figure 2.1). Across these categories, numerous social and structural factors exist that influence the status of an individual's health, including race/ethnicity, socioeconomic status, employment, education, healthcare access/quality, neighborhood safety, transportation, and air/water quality. To this list, communication scholar Vish Viswanath adds communication inequalities.

Communication inequalities are defined as "the differences among social groups in their ability to generate, disseminate, and use information at the macro level and to access, process, and act on information at the individual level" (Viswanath, 2006, p. 222). For example, there are differences in rates of subscribing to cable/satellite television and the internet based on socioeconomic status, with poorer, less educated people being less likely to subscribe. The same is true for newspaper readership. When you consider the vital role of information in promoting health and preventing disease (as we'll explore in Chapter 5), it's easy to think of ways that communication inequalities affect health outcomes. For example, Morgan Philbin and colleagues (2019) explored the relationships between U.S. women's internet use and perceived quality of life. They found that women who had access to daily internet use reported high levels of health-related quality of life. For health communication

researchers, then, recognizing and understanding the influence of communication inequalities on health is essential for enacting communication strategies that promote healthy
living among individuals and communities.

Social determinants of health are so influential in maintaining good health that when
they go unnoticed and unaddressed, vast differences in health status can result between
different groups of people. These differences are known as **health disparities**, or the differences in health status that occur between groups of people due to social and structural
influences. *Healthy People 2030* (n.d.) defines health disparities as "a particular type of health
difference that is closely linked with social, economic, or environmental disadvantage"
(para 6). More specifically, they go on to note the following:

> Health disparities adversely affect groups of people who have systematically experi-
> enced greater obstacles to health based on their racial or ethnic group; religion; socio-
> economic status; gender; age; mental health; cognitive, sensory, or physical disability;
> sexual orientation or gender identity; geographic location; or other characteristics
> historically linked to discrimination or exclusion.

Elaborating further, Paula Braveman and colleagues (2011) argue that health disparities are
"systematic, plausibly avoidable health differences adversely affecting socially disadvantaged
groups" (p. S149). This elaboration recognizes three key characteristics of health disparities.
First, the systematic nature means that these health outcomes are not solely a product of
personal decisions, such as whether to eat fast food, but more so a product of structural systems, such as eating fast food because that's the only restaurant near where you live or that
you can afford. Second, recognizing health disparities as avoidable means that differences
in health status between groups are preventable and changeable. Most often, preventing
and reducing health disparities requires revisiting and redistributing social and structural
resources, such as investing in fresh food access in places with food deserts (places with
limited healthy food options). Finally, the definition calls attention to the fact that health
disparities are most commonly experienced by communities with the least amount of social
and political power. This lack of power perpetuates the challenge of changing the distribution of resources that would reduce or eliminate health disparities.

For decades, researchers have compiled ongoing evidence of the prevalence of health disparities. For example, the CDC's (2013) *Health Disparities and Inequalities Report* found that (a)
African American adults were at least 50% more likely to prematurely die of heart disease or
stroke than their white counterparts, (b) the prevalence of diabetes was higher among adults
without a college degree, those with lower household incomes, and those who identify as Hispanic, African American, or mixed race, (c) the infant mortality rate for African Americans
was more than double the rate for non-Hispanic whites, and (d) suicide rates were highest
among American Indians/Alaska Natives and non-Hispanic whites. Such group differences
become starker when you consider the ways in which individuals can be members of multiple
underserved groups and communities, a concept known as intersectionality.

Intersectionality

Think about all the characteristics that make you who you are. There's your race, your
sex, and your gender. There's also your age. And what about your nationality? How would
you characterize your socioeconomic status? Maybe you have a physical or intellectual
disability. All these characteristics (and more) comprise your identity. The fact that you are
many things all at once—not just female or male, not just gay or straight, not just Asian or
Black—captures the concept of intersectionality.

Lisa Bowleg (2012) writes that **intersectionality** involves the study of how "multiple social identities such as race, gender, sexual orientation, socioeconomic status, and disability intersect at the micro level of individual experience to reflect interlocking systems of privilege and oppression (i.e., racism, sexism, heterosexism, classism) at the macro social-structural level" (p. 1267). In other words, depending on their intersectional identities, individuals will encounter varying degrees of social opportunity and discrimination. Further, having multiple marginalized identities leads to having more experiences with systemic barriers. In the context of health, this manifests as experiencing more health disparities.

Health disparities that are well-documented between groups based on race, sex, and socioeconomic status alone are exacerbated when people have membership in multiple marginalized groups (Viswanath et al., 2022). For instance, in an analysis of health disparities among Black women, Juanita Chinn and colleagues (2021) revealed that although 14% of all women live in poverty, 24% of all Black women live in poverty. Further, whereas the maternal mortality rate among all women is 17.4 per 100,000, it is 37.1 per 100,000 among Black women, and pregnancy mortality is 16.9 versus 42.4 per 100,000 respectively. Additional disparities were demonstrated for life expectancy, rates of obesity, and prevalence of cardiovascular disease. These are but a few examples for one group (Black women) of the relationship between intersectionality and health disparities.

A great deal of research has also demonstrated the unique experiences of different intersectional identities. For instance, Ashley Lacombe-Duncan (2016) explored the systemic ways in which transgender women experience less access to HIV-related healthcare than cisgender individuals. In another example, Thi Vinh Nguyen and colleagues (2021) conducted interviews with Vietnamese women with a physical disability to explore their pregnancy experiences, finding that the intersectionality of the women's identity had profound influence on their pregnancy experience, including negative community views, inaccessible environments, and poverty. These studies demonstrate the importance of considering intersectionality when attempting to draw conclusions about health status and developing interventions to reduce health disparities.

Intersectionality

Intersectionality recognizes that individuals have multiple social identities reflecting a variety of distinct characteristics, such as race, sex, age, gender, (dis)ability, and socioeconomic status. These combinations create power dynamics that influence social relations across diverse societies, as well as individual experiences in everyday life.

Reducing Health Disparities and Increasing Health Equity

Communication research plays a vital role in developing interventions to reduce health disparities by reducing communication inequalities or targeting other social determinants of health. Table 2.2 offers a few of the theoretical frameworks that have been used in health communication research to examine discrimination. Communication research to identify and reduce health disparities covers a wide range of topics and involves efforts on two fronts. **Understanding-focused efforts** investigate and document individuals' lived experiences with health disparities. Examples of such efforts include interviewing public health officials to explore competing tensions between influencing policy and reducing health disparities

Table 2.2 Theoretical Frameworks in Discrimination and Health Communication

Theory/Model	Brief Summary	Citation
Communication Theory of Identity	Social experiences are internalized by individuals as identities that, in turn, influence social behaviors. There are four levels of identity: personal, enacted, relational, and communal.	Hecht (1993)
Critical Race Theory	The study and critical questioning of the relationship among race, racism, and power in society.	Bell (2004)
Feminist Standpoint Theory	Circumstances of an individual's life will affect perceptions and constructions of their social world.	Hartsock (1983)

Note. See *Supplemental Online Theory Table* for additional theories/models.

(Grier & Schaller, 2020), examining perceptions of community health workers who support women experiencing health disparities (Vardeman-Winter, 2017), and identifying challenges for health communication interventions seeking to reduce reproductive health disparities (Matsaganis & Golden, 2015). Such efforts highlight experiences with health disparities, drawing attention to their negative impacts on communities.

Solution-focused efforts use communication strategies to reduce health disparities. Examples of these efforts include taking a culture-centered approach to build community-based solutions to disparities (Dutta, 2018), integrating interpersonal communication skills into HIV prevention interventions (Rimal et al., 2013), and implementing internet and health literacy skills training programs, such as the *Click to Connect* project, in underserved communities (Nagler et al., 2013). Such efforts contribute to attempts to eliminate health disparities, which is a tall task. Tall, but not impossible.

Today, a primary strategy for reaching and educating the public with health promotion efforts to reduce health disparities is through eHealth interventions. Eng (2001) defined **eHealth** as "the use of emerging information and communication technology, especially the Internet, to improve or enable health and health care" (p. 1). Today, such interventions are ubiquitous. Lee and colleagues (2022) describe how researchers have used **eHealth interventions** in multiple ways: "researchers have piloted and designed web portals to specifically aid health-information seeking among different populations, encouraged the use of patient portals for health care management, and developed smartphone apps and wearables to improve health monitoring" (p. 2). Following an analysis of lessons learned from a series of eHealth interventions, Lee et al. propose five principles for creating and implementing eHealth interventions that effectively reduce health disparities (pp. 5–6):

1. Develop a strategic road map to address communication inequalities
2. Engage multiple stakeholders from the beginning for the long haul
3. Design with usability in mind, enhancing readability and navigability
4. Build privacy safeguards into eHealth interventions and communicate privacy–utility tradeoffs that come with simplicity
5. Strive for an optimal balance between open science aspirations and protection of underserved groups

Whether through increasing understanding of the challenges surrounding health disparities or engaging in applied efforts to reduce health disparities, all of this research ultimately seeks to reduce health disparities through supporting equitable health solutions.

The *Healthy People 2030* (n.d.) report defines **health equity** as

> the attainment of the highest level of health for all people. Achieving health equity requires valuing everyone equally with focused and ongoing societal efforts to address avoidable inequalities, historical and contemporary injustices, and the elimination of health and health care disparities.
>
> (para. 5)

Equitable solutions to health disparities recognize that providing *equal resources* does not always produce *equal health outcomes*. For example, consider the popular image of three kids of differing heights trying to look over a tall wood fence to watch a baseball game. An *equal solution* would be to give each child a box of the same height to stand on. In this scenario, although the box allows the tallest kid to look over the fence, the second tallest still needs to stand on their tiptoes to see, and the shortest still cannot see over the fence. An *equitable solution* would give each child the size box they need to see over the fence, recognizing that some kids don't need much at all, but some kids need a lot because they have different starting points. In this case, the shortest kid would receive the tallest box and the tallest kid would receive the shortest box. Although the distribution of resources seems unequal, the result is that everyone has an equal chance to see over the fence. Thus, equitable solutions are focused on equality as the end goal. Applying this example to efforts to reduce health disparities, equitable solutions focus on distributing resources as needed for people to have equal access to healthcare, equal high quality of healthcare, and equal opportunity to live a healthy life.

We'd like to make two points about equitable solutions before we move to the next section. First, the "box" solution to see over the fence distributes resources to people based on need, so it is a solution that has to be replicated for each individual. In this example, that would mean continuing to invest in and distribute boxes of various sizes to kids everywhere. A structural solution would obviate the need to target individuals by making macro-level policy or legislative changes that affect everyone in one fell swoop. For instance, imagine if the fence were chain link instead of wood or if it were removed altogether. Then all kids could see regardless of their height, and no one would need any boxes. This type of solution is called *justice*. Second, some people believe that addressing discrimination so that traditionally marginalized people have equitable access to the resources they need (healthcare and otherwise) means that other people will be cheated out of what they "deserve." But in the words of poet and civil rights activist Maya Angelou (1997), "a society is only as healthy as its sickest citizen and only as wealthy as its most deprived" (p. 108). Thus, if we don't provide equitable resources to promote equal healthcare opportunities, we'll never reach the healthiest potential of our society. To achieve such a lofty goal, we, as a society, must first confront and correct all forms of discrimination. To fully understand what that means for health communication, we now turn our attention to a review of "isms."

Health Communication and Isms

Isms, sometimes called phobias (e.g., homophobia, Islamophobia), represent a distinctive practice, system, philosophy, or ideology that centers on "negative attitudes and beliefs about groups of individuals who embody characteristics that differ from the 'norm' of our society" (Liu et al., 2021, p. viii). Isms are typically motivated by stereotypes, fear, and ignorance. Common isms, and the four we'll review in the coming paragraphs, are racism, sexism, homophobia, and ablism. Ibram X. Kendi (2019) explains that society's inability to overcome isms is partially due to the perception that isms are all-or-nothing labels such that people either are or are not racist, sexist, and so on. But in reality, any person or any policy is capable of supporting, promoting, or perpetuating any ism at any given time. For instance, a person might not see themselves as racist, but if they're unable to recognize or acknowledge systemic policies that keep particular races in poverty, that's a racist perception. Kendi's argument is that if people can't acknowledge when they're engaging in an ism, then the ism will continue to exist in society. Further, most isms are propagated by individuals who don't consciously realize that they're promoting them. This is known as implicit bias.

The National Institutes of Health (NIH; 2022) defines **implicit bias** as "a form of bias that occurs automatically and unintentionally, that nevertheless affects judgments, decisions, and behaviors" (n.p.). Implicit bias can impact health in a variety of ways, especially during the patient–provider interaction. In 2001, the Institute of Medicine (IOM; 2003) released its report *Unequal Treatment: Confronting Racial and Ethnic Disparities in Health Care*, which was commissioned by Congress to assess the extent of differences in the quality of healthcare received by patients of different races and ethnicities. The report concluded that implicit bias was not only prevalent during medical visits but also a causal factor in perpetuating U.S. health disparities. More than a decade later, in a review of 42 studies examining implicit bias among healthcare professionals, Chloë FitzGerald and Samia Hurst (2017) concluded that healthcare professionals continue to exhibit problematic levels of implicit bias during their interactions with patients, noting that in some circumstances, biases were likely to influence diagnosis, treatment decisions, and levels of care. For example, some of the studies noted that providers asked fewer questions and provided fewer treatment options to members of marginalized groups. Because implicit bias is, by definition, something people do subconsciously, it can be hard to address. Hard, but not impossible.

Project Implicit (n.d.) is a nonprofit organization founded in 1998 that conducts research and offers training and consulting on how to reduce implicit bias. Although education sessions are offered at the organizational level, individuals can assess their implicit biases toward various groups by visiting the Project Implicit website (www.projectimplicit.net). Beyond such self-assessment, Elizabeth Chapman and colleagues (2013) argue that if providers simply acknowledged that they carry their own implicit biases and actively worked to check their preexisting assumptions, health disparities stemming from their implicit biases (e.g., dismissive treatment, misdiagnosis) could be decreased. Interestingly, active self-awareness and critical self-reflection are not just recommendations to help medical providers reduce their implicit biases. Active self-awareness and critical self-reflection can help *everyone* identify and correct moments of implicit bias. For example, the next time you find yourself making assumptions about someone based on their identity, think of examples of individuals who break the social stereotypes (Blair et al., 2001). Or take a second to imagine what it would be like to be a person who experiences constant social judgment of their ability and skills because of their identity (Galinsky & Moskowitz, 2000). These strategies may seem simple, but studies show these reflections can catch and reduce moments of implicit bias. Even for members of marginalized communities, Kendi (2019) argues that all people have some form of implicit biases, and everyone can benefit from recognizing and addressing their own biases.

Implicit Bias

Implicit bias is a form of bias that occurs automatically and unintentionally. Although implicit, it still affects judgments, decisions, and behaviors. Project Implicit is a nonprofit organization founded in 1998 that conducts research and offers training and consulting on how to reduce implicit bias. You can learn more about the project here: www.projectimplicit.net.

Now that we've reviewed isms and implicit bias, the following paragraphs will address four common forms of discrimination: race, sex, gender, and disability. Of course, you know from our review of intersectionality that these characteristics do not occur independent of one another. We're addressing each on its own to clearly emphasize the characteristic. For each form of discrimination, we explore implications for health, as well as health communication efforts to understand and reduce the perpetuation of the ism.

Race and Racism

Race is a socially constructed term based on the inappropriate classification of people grouped by common descent or origin and on their biologically-based characteristics, such as bone density, skin color, or hair texture despite the fact that "under the skin, there is no true biological race" (DiAngelo, 2018, p. 15). As a social construct, race remains a powerful influence. Discrimination based on race is known as **racism**, or the collection of policies and ideas reflecting the alleged superiority or inferiority of particular racial groups that produces, reproduces, and normalizes inequalities based on race (Kendi, 2019). You might have seen a lot of media coverage using the terms institutional, structural, or systemic racism. These terms are another way of referencing racist policies or practices. Whether people want to admit it or not, racism continues to persist in our society. The question is how to encourage people to not engage in racist behaviors. Enter antiracism.

Antiracism is the effort to correct policies or ideas to provide equitable experiences across races (Kendi, 2019). It's defined as "a state of mind, feeling, political commitment and action to eradicate racial oppression and transform unequal social relations between black and white people to egalitarian ones" (Dominelli, 2008, p. 28). Like an ism, the term anti-racist is not a personality characteristic. To be antiracist requires a constant and dedicated commitment to see racial inequalities in policies and ideas, as well as to actively fight against them. The Smithsonian (n.d.) exhibit on *Talking about Race* emphasizes the role of personal choice in enacting antiracist behaviors (para. 7):

> Being antiracist results from a conscious decision to make frequent, consistent, equitable choices daily. These choices require ongoing self-awareness and self-reflection as we move through life. In the absence of making antiracist choices, we (un)consciously uphold aspects of white supremacy, white-dominant culture, and unequal institutions and society. Being racist or antiracist is not about who you are; it is about what you do. … No one is born racist or antiracist; these result from the choices we make.

Antiracist efforts are essential because

> racial and ethnic minorities are burdened with higher rates of disease, disability, and death, and tend to receive a lower quality of health care than non-minorities, even when access-related factors, such as insurance status and income, are taken into account.
> (Anderson et al., 2003, p. 68)

Research also shows that racial minorities and persons with low socioeconomic status receive poorer quality of care than whites and persons with higher socioeconomic status (IOM, 2003). During the COVID-19 pandemic, racial health disparities were perpetuated further, with Black patients diagnosed with, and dying from, the virus at significantly higher rates than white patients (Williamson et al., 2020). Thus, addressing and eliminating racism is an important public health initiative (Ford & Airhihenbuwa, 2010), one that can be promoted through antiracist communication.

For instance, the 2015–2016 APHA president, Camara Jones (2018), launched a National Campaign Against Racism. To be part of this campaign, Jones called on everyone to (a) name racism, recognizing that it exists and calling it out when you see it, (b) critically reflect, asking yourself "how is racism operating here," and (c) organize and strategize to eliminate racism, refusing to accept any presence of racism. These antiracist goals and practices can also be seen in the grassroot efforts of healthcare professionals.

For example, in 2015, a group of medical students began a working group, White Coats for Black Lives (WC4BL), that has grown into an activist movement among medical professionals. In the October 2016 special issue of the *American Journal of Public Health*, members of WC4BL detailed how the movement was born in response to the senseless murder of young Black individuals, including Michael Brown and Eric Garner (Garvey, Woode, et al., 2016). Dr. Ashley Paige White-Stern recalled being moved to join WC4BL by the silence she didn't expect in her classrooms:

> I thought, "surely there will be outrage here in the classroom around senseless death." And initially there really wasn't. It was medical students organizing that showed our professors, schools, and hospitals that the erasure of a young body of color was a heinous crime.
>
> (Garvey, Gomez, et al., 2016, p. 1753)

The nationwide spread of WC4BL has brought together more than 3,000 medical students from more than 80 medical schools (Charles et al., 2015). Although this initiative is still relatively new, this type of activism is setting the tone for the intolerance of racism in healthcare.

To effectively address racism in healthcare systems, the extent to which patients experience it must be systematically accounted for. One way in which healthcare organizations can account for patient experiences is through patient satisfaction surveys, the results of which influence how much money hospitals get paid by insurers (Bichell, 2022). Rae Ellen Bichell (2022), however, suggests that such surveys are failing to account for the experiences of people of color. In a report on hospital customer satisfaction surveys following medical stays, she notes that patients are not asked about whether they experienced discrimination during their stay or whether they received culturally competent care. Without this data, the extent to which hospitals are fully caring for diverse groups of patients is unknown.

Sex and Sexism

The term **sex** seems straightforward given that it is "assigned at birth and refers to the underlying biological aspects of being male or female" (van Diemen et al., 2021, p. 2990). Furthermore, students are taught in biology class that a person's sex is determined by X and Y chromosomes. If you have an XX pair, you're a girl; if you have an XY pair, you're a boy. Easy peasy, right? Not exactly. A fascinating series of episodes on the podcast RadioLab, called *Radiolab Presents: Gonads* (Webster, 2018), delved into the incredible complexities involved in sex determination. The series revealed that the simple XX versus XY distinction is not so simple. In short, every single human starts out as inherently female *and* male, and microscopic genetic expressions along the way result in diversity far beyond "girl" and "boy."

Even with such underlying diversity, our society approaches sex as binary and holds stereotypical assumptions about men and women. This is known as **sexism**, or discrimination based on one's sex. According to Patricia Homan (2019, p. 489), both men's and women's health can be negatively affected by sexism because "patriarchal social systems foster a toxic culture" that is harmful to everyone. Let's take a quick look at a few studies to see what this means.

Women have been traditionally seen through the lens of their reproductive biology, first and foremost as "baby makers." Although childbearing is essential to the survival of humanity, essential to the survival of women is the acknowledgment that they are fully functional human beings who have hearts, lungs, and livers in addition to reproductive organs. However, women get short shrift in the diagnosis and treatment of disease. For example, women historically have been underrepresented in medical studies (Dusenbery, 2019). This has led to a medical system where disease, including diagnosis and treatment, is best understood as it affects male bodies. A prime example is cardiovascular disease (CVD). CVD is the leading killer of both men and women in the United States (CDC, 2022). However, in an editorial on sex differences in CVD treatment and mortality, Noel Bairey Merz and colleagues (2015) draw attention to the fact that healthcare systems do not consider the "differences in metabolism, hormones, and the autonomic nervous system" that can lead to different symptoms of CVD for women that are "not detected by male pattern diagnostics" (p. 1958). They also point to sociocultural sex differences and implicit biases that suggest that physicians assess CVD in women based on "objectified appearance/body weight rather than validated risk factors" (p. 1959). Such individual and structural bias lead to under- and misdiagnosis of CVD in women.

Of course, men also face negative health consequences from sexism. One overarching effect is that because of masculinity norms, which require men to be strong, independent, and resilient at all costs, men are more likely than women to avoid healthcare (e.g., Novak et al., 2019) while also being more likely to engage in risky, unhealthy behaviors (e.g., Helme et al., 2020). These influences may, in part, be responsible for men's overall greater mortality and morbidity relative to women. As a more specific example, although breast cancer is perceived as a disease that affects only women, men do have breast tissue and can develop breast cancer, especially men who carry the BRCA-1 or BRCA-2 genetic mutation. Yet men do not perceive themselves as at risk of this cancer, and even men who know they are at risk for breast cancer because of family history tend not to discuss it as such (e.g., they refer to cancer in their "chest") and have considerable difficulty coming to terms with the need to engage in screening mammography (Skop et al., 2018). Unfortunately, such perceptions can lead to later-stage diagnosis of breast cancer in men, which makes treatment more difficult and survival less likely.

Sexism in healthcare needs to be addressed to ensure that women and men alike receive care guided by evidence-based medicine, not biased perceptions. For instance, to reduce disparities in CVD diagnosis and treatment among women, the nonprofit organization Women's Heart Alliance (n.d.) was established to advocate for sex equity in research on heart disease and in its prevention and treatment. The organization also works to raise awareness among patients and providers and enact policy change to promote women's heart health. Similarly, to increase awareness of male breast cancer, the nonprofit organization Male Breast Cancer Happens (n.d.) was established to highlight the real stories of men with breast cancer. Their efforts seek to normalize the idea that men can get breast cancer, ideally increasing the willingness of men to screen for and talk about breast cancer.

Gender and Homophobia

Unlike sex, whose definition is based on biological characteristics (even with all the noted complications), **gender** is socially constructed following assumptions, beliefs, and perceived norms around what people believe to be male/masculine or female/feminine. As such, gender varies across cultures, can change over time, and is understood to be on a spectrum

(World Health Organization [WHO], 2023a). Within discussions of gender, one's preference for a romantic partner, called sexuality, is often considered. Sexuality includes terms such as heterosexual (preferring a romantic partner of a different sex), homosexual (preferring a romantic partner of the same sex), and bisexual (not have a sex preference for a romantic partner). There are numerous terms that reflect various gender or sexual identifications. The most common are lesbian, gay, bisexual, transgender, and queer (LGBTQ+ or LGBTQQIA, which includes questioning, intersex, and asexual).

Discrimination on the basis of gender or sexuality is called **homophobia**. The term is broadly used to describe individuals and systems advocating against any non–heterosexual, non–cisgender lifestyle. Efforts to address and eliminate gender-based discrimination are called **gender-inclusive**. These efforts seek to promote the acceptance of all individuals regardless of gender identification. More so, they reject the notion that gender is a choice and accept the potential for gender identification to change.

The historical presence of homophobic rhetoric has perpetuated the stigmatization of members of the queer community. This stigmatization has had significant negative effects on the health of members of this community. In the 2010 IOM report, *The Health of Lesbian, Gay, Bisexual, and Transgender People: Building a Foundation for Better Understanding*, the committee found that HIV/AIDS disproportionately affected men who have sex with men; LGB youth were at increased risk for depression and suicidal ideation and attempts; LGBT youth reported experiencing more violence, victimization, and harassment than heterosexual and nongender-variant youth; and LGBT individuals experienced elevated stigma, discrimination, and violence. Unchecked gender discrimination will only continue to perpetuate such health disparities. Interventions are clearly needed to promote gender-inclusive healthcare practices.

Such interventions will require a common language to discuss gender issues, yet many people struggle to engage in conversations about gender, including patients and providers. To provide a resource for individuals looking to talk about and reduce gender discrimination, the Human Rights Campaign (n.d.) maintains an active glossary of gender-related terms. They explicitly state that the purpose of the glossary is to "help give people the words and meanings to help make conversations easier and more comfortable" (para. 1). Such tools assist in communication efforts to promote awareness of and discourage gender-based discrimination. They may also be helpful in health professions training. Indeed, in a survey of more than 1,000 medical, dental, and nursing students, Greene et al. (2018) found that most students felt they were inadequately trained to provide care for the LGBTQ population; this perception was higher for students who identified as members of the LGBTQ community. Part of providing competent care, of course, includes having a vocabulary to discuss gender-related concerns. The Human Rights Campaign glossary can help.

Disabilities and Ableism

Presently, 12.7% of the U.S. population reports some form of **disability**, defined as visual, hearing, ambulatory, cognitive, self-care, or independent living disability (Erickson et al., 2022). That's more than 41 million people in the United States who have one or more of these disabilities. Worldwide, that figure jumps to 15%, or more than 1 billion people (WHO, 2023b). People with disabilities face more challenges than just their physical or intellectual disability because of systems of **ableism**, or "ideas, practices, institutions and social relations that presume ablebodiedness, and by so doing, construct persons with disabilities as marginalized" (Chouinard, 1997, p. 380).

Lisa Iezzoni and colleagues (2021) cite multiple studies documenting how people with disabilities face disparities in "screening and preventive services, cancer diagnosis and treatment, reproductive and pregnancy care, communication with health care profession-als, and satisfaction with care" (p. 297). Furthermore, in a survey of 32 countries from 2002 to 2014, Carla Branco and colleagues (2019) found that individuals who experienced discrimination based on a disability reported lower assessments of health and well-being than people who faced discrimination based on sexism and ageism. These poorer out-comes for people with disabilities are likely due to not receiving the care they need either because they don't have access or because they report being dissatisfied with inadequate care (Gibson & O'Connor, 2010; WHO, 2023b).

Many factors play into inadequate care for persons with disabilities, and biased attitudes among some physicians may be one of them. Iezzoni et al. (2021) conducted a national sur-vey of 741 U.S. physicians to investigate their perceptions of people with disabilities. Their results showed that only 40.7% of physicians reported being very confident that they could provide the same quality of care to their patients with disabilities as their non-disabled patients, and only 56.5% strongly agreed that they would welcome patients with disabilities into their practices. Furthermore, 82.4% believed that the quality of life of people with disabilities was worse than that of non-disabled people, a belief that is not accurate but that may bias their treatment of patients (Health Affairs Blog, 2021). In addition to physician bias, one study found nurse educators exhibited strong implicit bias against people with disabilities (Aaberg, 2012). Such attitudes are troubling because with an adequate built environment, adequate support, and unbiased attitudes, disabilities would not be so dis-abling. Some groups are already working to make these goals a reality.

The National Center for Disability, Equity, and Intersectionality is an interdisciplinary co-alition that was created expressly "to identify and reduce life-limiting healthcare inequities faced by people with intellectual and developmental (ID/DD) disabilities" (National Center for Disability, Equity, and Intersectionality, 2023, n.p.). It has four aims, which we quote here:

1. Increase understanding of gaps in existing policies and guidelines related to medical discrimination
2. Increase access to anti-discrimination guidelines co-created by clinicians, profession-als, self-advocates, and family members
3. Increase informational access on barriers to healthcare and the value of improved life outcomes for people with ID/DD
4. Increase support for families and individuals with ID/DD to defend against healthcare discrimination

Such work is crucial in light of the challenges that people with disabilities face in the healthcare environment.

We've spent a lot of time reviewing discrimination in the healthcare environment and its impact on health. We've also considered how health communication strategies can reduce some of these isms. To wrap up the chapter, we're going to shift gears and consider how the media perpetuate discrimination in society through biased representation of marginalized groups.

Media Representation

Traditional media channels, such as television, have historically misrepresented the preva-lence and experiences of minority communities, including those based on race, sex, gender, and disability. Because media is an important tool for social learning, how minority groups are represented affects not only how non-members perceive the marginalized group but also how members of the marginalized group perceive themselves and their role in society.

Accurate media representation is an important factor in acceptance of others and self (see Behm-Morawitz & Ortiz, 2013). Although recent years have seen improvements in media representation, production still has a long way to go to accurately represent the demographic composition and experiences of marginalized groups.

Regarding race and ethnicity, Darnell Hunt and Ana-Christina Ramón published two reports (one on film and one on television) on diversity in Hollywood media productions that were released in 2018 and 2019. Regarding film, they note that despite major gains in media representation, "people of color remained underrepresented on every industry employment front" (Hunt & Ramón, 2020a, p. 3). Specifically, although people of color make up more than 40% of the U.S. population, the authors' data analysis found minorities made up 27.6% of lead roles, 15.1% of film directors, 13.9% of film writers, 9% of studio heads, and 32.7% of all actors. Similarly, regarding scripted television leads, they found minorities made up 24% of broadcast, 35% of cable, and 24.1% of digital scripted leads (Hunt & Ramón, 2020b). Underrepresentation in television was also found among broadcast, cable, and digital show creators (10.7%, 14.5%, and 10.3%, respectively), episodes directed (24.3%, 22.9%, and 18.2%, respectively), and writers (23.4%, 22.8%, and 8%, respectively).

Hunt and Ramón's analysis found similar underrepresentation of women in film and television. Although women make up more than half of the U.S. population, they made up 44.1% of lead roles, 15.1% of film directors, 17.4% of film writers, 18% of studio heads, and 40.2% of all actors (Hunt & Ramón, 2020a). Similarly, women were underrepresented on television in broadcast, cable, and digital scripted leads (41.3%, 44.8%, and 49.4%, respectively), as show creators (28.1%, 22.4%, and 28.6%, respectively), in episodes directed (29.3%, 29.7%, and 29.1%, respectively), and as writers (39.4%, 40.9%, and 42.4%, respectively; Hunt & Ramón, 2020b).

Regarding gender identification, representation has been noticeably missing from most media, including in film and television. For example, Stacy Smith and colleagues (2019) analyzed the representation of LGBTQ individuals in film. In 2018, they found that only two of the 100 top-grossing films featured a protagonist from the LGBTQ community. Worse yet, they found only one transgender character was depicted as a protagonist from the 100 top-grossing films in the five-year span of 2014–2018. These low estimates of representation were also found surrounding characters with a disability. Across the 4,445 characters they coded for, only 1.6% were depicted with a disability. To make matters worse, unlike race, sex, and gender, which appear to be slowly increasing in their representation, Smith et al. (2019) noted that disability representation was moving backward at almost all points, including having any character with a disability, women with a disability, and racially diverse characters with disabilities.

Although including characters is important, *how* characters are included is equally as important. Simply having a token minority character on the screen is not sufficient to represent the unique and diverse experiences of these communities. For example, when LGBTQ characters are included in media, they are often depicted in ways acceptable to heterosexual audiences (see Avila-Saavedra, 2009), such as living a single, child-free life. This aligns with the finding from Smith et al. (2019) that only six LGB characters across the 100 top films of 2018 were shown as parents, playing into the discriminatory perspective that children should be raised in households with one female and one male parent. How characters are included is important not only for breaking stereotypes but also for how members of those communities see themselves. Lauren McInroy and Shelley Craig (2017) interviewed LGBTQ-identifying youth to discuss perceptions of media representation. They found that traditional media "continues to represent LGBTQ people as one-dimensional and stereotypical, ignoring many LGBTQ sub-groups, limiting LGBTQ young people's perceptions of their future trajectories, and offering no opportunities for critique" (p. 32). Although their conclusion applied explicitly to the LGBTQ community, their findings encompass the general importance of representation that can be seen among all marginalized groups.

One of the primary challenges of achieving representation in the media is discriminatory push-back from the public. On a podcast episode of *Morning Edition* for National Public Radio (NPR), A Martinez (2022) interviewed NPR TV critic Eric Deggans about the online backlash following a wave of forthcoming diverse characters in film and television, including Ariel from *The Little Mermaid*, dwarves in a *Lord of the Rings* series, and elves in a *Game of Thrones* series. Deggans explained that the backlash stems from the changes playing "into one of the great myths of racist thought, which is that people of color want to replace white people at the top of society, rather than trying to get equality and seek an end to racism" (n.p.). There is possibly no clearer example of implicit bias than claiming the anger expressed over the skin tone of fictional characters has nothing to do with race (as many outraged individuals claimed). As Deggans put it, "enshrining beloved characters as forever white is kind of the definition of white privilege" (n.p.).

Conclusion

We have covered a lot of information in this chapter, and you may be feeling a little overwhelmed right now and reeling from learning about all the unnecessary hurt in this world that's brought about through discrimination based on race, sex, gender, and disability. We know that talking about these issues makes some people uncomfortable, but because discrimination has such negative impacts on healthcare and the health communication experience of patients and providers, we believe that such talk is essential.

At the beginning of this chapter, we mentioned the work of Sonya Renee Taylor, who studies how discrimination is perpetuated through societal structures that acculturate people to believe that some bodies are not as good as others because they are "different." Taylor (2021) argues that such beliefs stem from an evolutionary in-group out-group perspective, where humans see differences associated with the out-group as dangerous. She also observes that when something is different, humans don't understand it and therefore conclude it must be wrong. And calling differences wrong is what creates systems of discrimination based on different races, sexes, genders, and disabilities, among others. But all is not lost. Taylor suggests that the problem is not actually the differences between people but people's approach to dealing with those differences. Instead of not understanding the differences, concluding they are wrong, and discriminating based on them, we all must grapple with our differences, try to understand them, and not let them come between us. And when that happens, our society will be one step closer to "the opportunity for every human, no matter their body, to have unobstructed access to their highest self" (Taylor, 2021, p. 130).

References

Aaberg, V. A. (2012). A path to greater inclusivity through understanding implicit attitudes toward disability. *Journal of Nursing Education, 51*(9), 505–510.

American Psychological Association. (2019). *Discrimination: What it is, and how to cope*. https://www.apa.org/topics/racism-bias-discrimination/types-stress

Anderson, L. M., Scrimshaw, S. C., Fullilove, M. T., Fielding, J. E., Normand, J., & Task Force on Community Preventive Services. (2003). Culturally competent healthcare systems: A systematic review. *American Journal of Preventive Medicine, 24*(3), 68–79.

Anderson, M. J. [@MarciaJAnderson]. (2017, December 13). *From now on instead of "vulnerable people" I'm going to use the phrase "people we oppress through policy choices and*. [Tweet]. Twitter. https://twitter.com/marciajanderson/status/940945441042116608?lang=en

Angelou, M. (1997). *Even the stars look lonesome*. Random House, Inc.

Avila-Saavedra, G. (2009). Nothing queer about queer television: Televized construction of gay masculinities. *Media, Culture & Society, 31*(1), 5–21.

Behm-Morawitz, E., & Ortiz, M. (2013). Race, ethnicity, and the media. In K. E. Dill (Ed.), *The Oxford handbook of media psychology* (pp. 252–266). Oxford University Press.

Bell, D. (2004). *Race, racism, and American law.* Aspen Pub.

Bichell, R. E. (2022, September 8). Patient satisfaction surveys fail to track how well hospitals treat people of color. *National Public Radio.* https://www.npr.org/sections/health-shots/2022/09/08/1121647094/patient-satisfaction-surveys-fail-to-track-how-well-hospitals-treat-people-of-co

Blair, I. V., Ma, J. E., & Lenton, A. P. (2001). Imagining stereotypes away: The moderation of implicit stereotypes through mental imagery. *Journal of Personality and Social Psychology, 81*(5), 828–841.

Bowleg, L. (2012). The problem with the phrase women and minorities: Intersectionality—An important theoretical framework for public health. *American Journal of Public Health, 102*(7), 1267–1273.

Branco, C., Ramos, M. R., & Hewstone, M. (2019). The association of group-based discrimination with health and well-being: A comparison of ableism with other "isms". *Journal of Social Issues, 75*(3), 814–846.

Braveman, P., & Gottlieb, L. (2014). The social determinants of health: It's time to consider the causes of the causes. *Public Health Reports, 129*(Suppl. 2), 19–31.

Braveman, P. A., Kumanyika, S., Fielding, J., LaVeist, T., Borrell, L. N., Manderscheid, R., & Troutman, A. (2011). Health disparities and health equity: The issue is justice. *American Journal of Public Health, 101*(S1), S149–S155.

Centers for Disease Control and Prevention. (2013). CDC health disparities and inequalities report—United States, 2013. *Morbidity and Mortality Weekly Report Supplement, 62*(3), 1–189.

Centers for Disease Control and Prevention. (2021). *Social determinants of health: Know what affects health.* https://www.cdc.gov/socialdeterminants/index.htm

Centers for Disease Control and Prevention. (2022). *About heart disease.* https://www.cdc.gov/heartdisease/about.htm

Chapman, E. N., Kaatz, A., & Carnes, M. (2013). Physicians and implicit bias: How doctors may unwittingly perpetuate health care disparities. *Journal of General Internal Medicine, 28*(11), 1504–1510.

Charles, D., Himmelstein, K., Keenan, W., & Barcelo, N. (2015). White coats for black lives: Medical students responding to racism and police brutality. *Journal of Urban Health, 92*(6), 1007–1010.

Chinn, J. J., Martin, I. K., & Redmond, N. (2021). Health equity among Black women in the United States. *Journal of Women's Health, 30*(2), 212–219.

Chouinard, V. (1997). Making space for disabling differences: Challenging ableist geographies. *Environment and Planning D: Society and Space, 15*, 379–387.

DiAngelo, R. (2018). *White fragility: Why it's so hard for white people to talk about racism.* Beacon Press books.

Dominelli, L. (2008). *Anti-racist social work* (3rd ed.). Palgrave Macmillan.

Dong, T. S., Gee, G. C., Beltran-Sanchez, H., Wang, M., Osadchiy, V., Kilpatrick, L. A., Chen, Z., Subramanyam, V., Zhang, Y., Guo, Y., Labus, J. S., Naliboff, B., Cole, S., Zhang, X., Mayer, E. A., & Gupta, A. (2022). How discrimination gets under the skin: Biological determinants of discrimination associated with dysregulation of the brain-gut microbiome system and psychological symptoms. *Biological Psychiatry.* https://doi.org/10.1016/j.biopsych.2022.10.011

Dusenbery, M. (2019). *Doing harm: The truth about how bad medicine and lazy science leave women dismissed, misdiagnosed, and sick.* Harper Collins.

Dutta, M. J. (2018). Culture-centered approach in addressing health disparities: Communication infrastructures for subaltern voices. *Communication Methods & Measures, 12*(4), 239–259.

Eng, T. R. (2001). *The eHealth landscape: A terrain map of emerging information and communication technologies in health and health care.* Robert Wood Johnson Foundation.

Erickson, W., Lee, C., & von Schrader, S. (2022). *2019 disability status report: United States.* Cornell University Yang Tan Institute on Employment and Disability.

FitzGerald, C., & Hurst, S. (2017). Implicit bias in healthcare professionals: A systematic review. *BMC Medical Ethics, 18*, Article 19.

Ford, C. L., & Airhihenbuwa, C. O. (2010). Critical race theory, race equity, and public health: Toward antiracism praxis. *American Journal of Public Health, 100*(S1), S30–S35.

Galinsky, A. D., & Moskowitz, G. B. (2000). Perspective-taking: Decreasing stereotype expression, stereotype accessibility, and in-group favoritism. *Journal of Personality and Social Psychology, 78*(4), 708.

Garvey, A., Gomez, J., Pottinger, S., White-Stern, A. P., & White Coats for Black Lives National Working Group. (2016). White Coats for Black Lives: Young voices within medicine. *American Journal of Public Health, 106*(10), 1752–1753.

Garvey, A., Woode, D. R., Austin, C. S., & White Coats for Black Lives National Working Group. (2016). Reclaiming the White Coat for Black Lives. *American Journal of Public Health, 106*(10), 1749–1751.

Gibson, J. C., & O'Connor, R. J. (2010). Access to health care for disabled people: A systematic review. *Social Care and Neurodisability, 1*(3), 21–31.

Gómez, J. M. (2015). Microaggressions and the enduring mental health disparity: Black Americans at risk for institutional betrayal. *Journal of Black Psychology, 41*(2), 121–143.

Greene, M. Z., France, K., Kreider, E. F., Wolfe-Roubatis, E., Chen, K. D., Wu, A., & Yehia, B. R. (2018). Comparing medical, dental, and nursing students' preparedness to address lesbian, gay, bisexual, transgender, and queer health. *PLoS One, 13*(9), e0204104.

Grier, S. A., & Schaller, T. K. (2020). Operating in a constricted space: Policy actor perceptions of targeting to address U.S. health disparities. *Journal of Public Policy & Marketing, 39*(1), 31–47.

Hartsock, N. C. M. (1983). *Money, sex, and power: Toward a feminist historical materialism.* Northeastern University Press.

Health Affairs Blog. (2021). *Misperceptions of people with disabilities lead to low-quality care: How policy makers can counter the harm and injustice.* https://www.healthaffairs.org/do/10.1377/forefront.20210325.480382/

Healthy People. (n.d.). *Disparities.* https://health.gov/healthypeople/priority-areas/health-equity-healthy-people-2030

Hecht, M. L. (1993). 2002-A research odyssey: Toward the development of a communication theory of identity. *Communication Monographs, 60*(1), 76–82.

Helme, D. W., Morris, E., de la Serna, A., Zelaya, C., Oser, C., & Knudsen, H. K. (2020). "Country boys spit and dip": Masculinity and rural adolescent smokeless tobacco use. *Journal of Men's Studies, 29*(2), 213–234.

Homan, P. (2019). Structural sexism and health in the United States: A new perspective on health inequality and the gender system. *American Sociological Review, 84*(3), 486–516.

Human Rights Campaign. (n.d.). *Glossary of terms.* https://www.hrc.org/resources/glossary-of-terms

Hunt, D., & Ramón, A. (2020a). *Hollywood diversity report 2020: A tale of two Hollywoods, part 1: film.* https://socialsciences.ucla.edu/wp-content/uploads/2020/02/UCLA-Hollywood-Diversity-Report-2020-Film-2-6-2020.pdf

Hunt, D., & Ramón, A. (2020b). *Hollywood diversity report 2020: A tale of two Hollywoods, part 2: Television.* https://socialsciences.ucla.edu/wp-content/uploads/2020/10/UCLA-Hollywood-Diversity-Report-2020-Television-10-22-2020.pdf

Iezzoni, L. I., Rao, S. R., Ressalam, J., Bolcic-Jankovic, D., Agaronnik, N. D., Donelan, K., Lagu, T., & Campbell, E. G. (2021). Physicians' perceptions of people with disability and their health care. *Health Affairs, 40*(2), 297–306.

Institute of Medicine. (2003). *Unequal treatment: Confronting racial and ethnic disparities in health care.* National Academies Press.

Institute of Medicine. (2010). *The health of lesbian, gay, bisexual, and transgender people: Building a foundation for better understanding.* National Academies Press.

Jones, C. P. (2018). Toward the science and practice of anti-racism: Launching a national campaign against racism. *Ethnicity & Disease, 28*(Suppl. 1), 231–234.

Kattari, S. K. (2020). Ableist microaggressions and the mental health of disabled adults. *Community Mental Health Journal, 56*(6), 1170–1179.

Kendi, I. X. (2019). *How to be an antiracist.* One World, Penguin Random House LLC.

Lacombe-Duncan, A. (2016). An intersectional perspective on access to HIV-related healthcare for transgender women. *Transgender Health, 1*(1), 137–141.

Lee, E. W., McCloud, R. F., & Viswanath, K. (2022). Designing effective eHealth interventions for underserved groups: Five lessons from a decade of eHealth intervention design and deployment. *Journal of Medical Internet Research, 24*(1), e25419.

Liu, D., Burston, B., Mulligan, H. H., & Stewart, S. C. (2021). *Isms in health care human resources: A concise guide to workplace discrimination.* Jones & Bartlett Publishers.

Male Breast Cancer Happens. (n.d.). *Home.* https://malebreastcancerhappens.org/

Martinez, A. (Host). (2022, September 18). Why black characters in "Rings of Power" and "Little Mermaid" make fantasy better [Audio podcast episode]. In *Morning Edition: Culture*. National Public Radio. https://www.npr.org/transcripts/1122073064

Matsaganis, M. D., & Golden, A. G. (2015). Interventions to address reproductive health disparities among African-American women in a small urban community: The communicative construction of a "field of health action." *Journal of Applied Communication Research, 43*(2), 163–184.

McInroy, L. B., & Craig, S. L. (2017). Perspectives of LGBTQ emerging adults on the depiction and impact of LGBTQ media representation. *Journal of Youth Studies, 20*(1), 32–46.

Merz, C. N. B., Andersen, H. S., & Shufelt, C. L. (2015). Gender, cardiovascular disease, and the sexism of obesity. *Journal of the American College of Cardiology, 66*(18), 1958–1960.

Nadal, K. L., Griffin, K. E., Wong, Y., Hamit, S., & Rasmus, M. (2014). The impact of racial microaggressions on mental health: Counseling implications for clients of color. *Journal of Counseling & Development, 92*(1), 57–66.

Nadal, K. L., Wong, Y., Issa, M. A., Meterko, V., Leon, J., & Wideman, M. (2011). Sexual orientation microaggressions: Processes and coping mechanisms for lesbian, gay, and bisexual individuals. *Journal of LGBT Issues in Counseling, 5*(1), 21–46.

Nagler, R. H., Ramanadhan, S., Minsky, S., & Viswanath, K. (2013). Recruitment and retention for community-based eHealth interventions with populations of low socioeconomic position: Strategies and challenges. *Journal of Communication, 63*(1), 201–220.

National Center for Disability, Equity, and Intersectionality. (2023). *What we do*. https://thinkequitable.com/what-we-do/

National Institutes of Health. (2022). *Implicit bias*. https://diversity.nih.gov/sociocultural-factors/implicit-bias

Nguyen, T. V., King, J., Edwards, N., & Dunne, M. P. (2021). "Under great anxiety": Pregnancy experiences of Vietnamese women with physical disabilities seen through an intersectional lens. *Social Science & Medicine, 284*, 114231.

Novak, J. R., Peak, T., Gast, J., & Arnell, M. (2019). Associations between masculine norms and healthcare utilization in highly religious, heterosexual men. *American Journal of Men's Health, 13*(3), Article 1557988319856739.

Pascoe, E. A., & Richman, L. S. (2009). Perceived discrimination and health: A meta-analytic review. *Psychological Bulletin, 135*(4), 531–554.

Philbin, M. M., Parish, C., Pereyra, M., Feaster, D. J., Cohen, M., Wingood, G., Konkle-Parker, D., Adedimeji, A., Wilson, T. E., Cohen, J., Goparaju, L., Adimora, A. A., Golub, E. T., & Metsch, L. R. (2019). Health disparities and the digital divide: The relationship between communication inequalities and quality of life among women in a nationwide prospective cohort study in the United States. *Journal of Health Communication, 24*(4), 405–412.

Project Implicit. (n.d.). https://www.projectimplicit.net/

Rimal, R. N., Limaye, R. J., Roberts, P., Brown, J., & Mkandawire, G. (2013). The role of interpersonal communication in reducing structural disparities and psychosocial deficiencies: Experience from the Malawi BRIDGE Project. *Journal of Communication, 63*(1), 51–71.

Sittner, K. J., Greenfield, B. L., & Walls, M. L. (2018). Microaggressions, diabetes distress, and self-care behaviors in a sample of American Indian adults with type 2 diabetes. *Journal of Behavioral Medicine, 41*(1), 122–129.

Skop, M., Lorentz, J., Jassi, M., Vesprini, D., & Einstein, G. (2018). "Guys don't have breasts": The lived experience of men who have BRCA gene mutations and are at risk for male breast cancer. *American Journal of Men's Health, 12*(4), 961–972.

Smith, S. L., Choueiti, M., Choi, A., Piper, K., & Moutier, C. (2019). *Inequality in 1,200 popular films: Examining portrayals of gender, race/ethnicity, LGBTQ & disability from 2007 to 2018*. USC Annenberg Inclusion Initiative and American Foundation for Suicide Prevention. https://assets.uscannenberg.org/docs/aii-inequality-report-2019-09-03.pdf

Smithsonian. (n.d.). *Talking about race*. https://nmaahc.si.edu/learn/talking-about-race/topics/being-antiracist

Sue, D. W. (2010). Microaggressions, marginality, and oppression: An introduction. In D. Sue (Ed.), *Microaggressions and marginality: Manifestation, dynamics, and impact* (pp. 3–25). Wiley.

Taylor, S. R. (2021). *The body is not an apology: The power of radical self-love* (2nd ed.). Berrett-Koehler Publishers, Inc.

U.S. Department of Health and Human Services. (n.d.). *Healthy People 2030: Social determinants of health.* https://health.gov/healthypeople/objectives-and-data/social-determinants-health

van Diemen, J., Verdonk, P., Chieffo, A., Regar, E., Mauri, F., Kunadian, V., Sharma, G., Mehran, R., & Appelman, Y. (2021). The importance of achieving sex-and gender-based equity in clinical trials: A call to action. *European Heart Journal, 42*(31), 2990–2994.

Vardeman-Winter, J. (2017). The framing of women and health disparities: A critical look at race, gender, and class from the perspectives of grassroots health communicators. *Health Communication, 32*(5), 629–638.

Viswanath, K. (2006). Public communications and its role in reducing and eliminating health disparities. In G. E. Thomson, F. Mitchell, & M. B. Williams (Eds.), *Examining the health disparities research plan of the National Institutes of Health: Unfinished business* (pp. 215–253). Institute of Medicine.

Viswanath, K., McCloud, R. F., & Bekalu, M. A. (2022). Communication, health, and equity: Structural influences. In T. L. Thompson & N. G. Harrington (Eds.), *The Routledge handbook of health communication* (pp. 426–440). Routledge.

Webster, M. (Host). (2018, June 30). Gonads: X & Y. [Audio podcast episode]. In *Radiolab*. WNYC Studios. https://radiolab.org/episodes/gonads-xy

Williams, M. T., Skinta, M. D., & Martin-Willett, R. (2021). After Pierce and Sue: A revised racial microaggressions taxonomy. *Perspectives on Psychological Science, 16*(5), 991–1007.

Williamson, E. J., Walker, A. J., Bhaskaran, K., Bacon, S., Bates, C., Morton, C. E., Curtis, H. J., Mehrkar, A., Evans, D., Inglesby, P., Cockburn, J., McDonald, H. I., MacKenna, B., Tomlinson, L., Douglas, I. J., Rentsch, C. T., Mathur, R., Wong, A. Y. S., Grieve, R., Harrison, D., ... & Goldacre, B. (2020). Factors associated with COVID-19-related death using OpenSAFELY. *Nature, 584*(7821), 430–436.

Women's Heart Alliance. (n.d.). *About.* https://womensheartalliance.org/about/

World Health Organization. (2023a). *Gender and health.* https://www.who.int/health-topics/gender#tab=tab_1

World Health Organization. (2023b). *Disability.* https://www.who.int/health-topics/disability#tab=tab_1

In-class Activities

1. Have students complete one or more of the Harvard Implicit Bias Tests (https://implicit.harvard.edu/implicit/takeatest.html). There are 15 tests available (e.g., race, disability, religion, weight, age, sexuality). During class, have them share what they learned about their own biases, how they compare with others' (based on the summary distribution scores presented with their test results), and how they think this information will help them communicate more inclusively moving forward, especially in healthcare settings.

2. Have students watch season 14, episode 11 of Grey's Anatomy, *Don't Fear The Reaper* (or watch the YouTube clips available in the online resources). After, discuss Dr. Bailey's communication with the attending physician.

Discussion Questions

1. Dr. Marcia J. Anderson (2017) tweeted, "From now on instead of 'vulnerable people' I'm going to use the phrase 'people we oppress through policy choices and discourses of racial inferiority.' It's a bit longer but I think will help us focus on where the problems actually lie." In thinking about the numerous social and political infrastructures that perpetuate discrimination (e.g., laws, policies, normative practices), to what extent is the discrimination reflected and perpetuated through communication messages, language choices, and mediated channel selection?

2. Beyond television and film, to what extent do you feel that minority representation is accurate in other media, such as podcasts, social media, digital platforms, etc.?

3. You have been hired to develop a communication intervention to reduce one of the isms plaguing society. What communication strategies do you employ and why do you expect your plan to be effective? (Note: Isms not discussed in the chapter are encouraged!)

Unit II
Being a Patient

There's No Getting Around Going to the Doctor

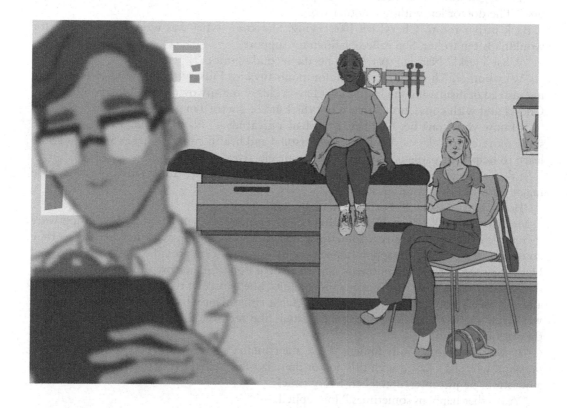

It was a little over a year later, and Cheryl was about halfway through the last semester of her sophomore year. And like most of her peers, she was feeling overwhelmed. To make matters worse, she woke up Monday morning and immediately felt the soreness in her throat. As she tried to sit up, her head started to throb, and her body felt achy.

"Oh, no," she said out loud and then winced at the pain. She dragged herself into the bathroom and took her temperature, shaking her head when she saw 103. She gingerly felt the glands in her neck. They felt swollen. "Not this again," she sighed. After texting Liz to ask her to tell their professor that Cheryl was sick and needed to see a doctor, Cheryl Googled the student health clinic in hopes of getting an appointment that day. Luckily, she was able to get a walk-in appointment.

A few hours later, she was sitting on the exam table waiting for the doctor. Finally, a doctor entered the room, staring at an iPad. He didn't even look at Cheryl as he asked, "So, what seems to be the problem?"

DOI: 10.4324/9781003214458-7

"I have mono," Cheryl said, offering her diagnosis with confidence based on the last time she had it.

"No, that can't be," the doctor said, still looking at the iPad. "Your chart says you had it two years ago. People rarely get it twice."

"But I have the exact same symptoms as last time," Cheryl tried. "I have a fever and a sore throat. Everything aches, and I'm exhausted. Even my lymph nodes are swollen."

The doctor finally looked up at her and smiled. "I'm sure it's just the bug that's going around. Always happens at the end of a semester when students burn themselves out. Go home, drink plenty of fluids, take ibuprofen, and rest."

"Can we do a blood test to be sure?" Cheryl tried.

"The registration desk might have samples of ibuprofen if you want to check on your way out." The doctor left without another word.

Back in her room, Cheryl felt like crying. She knew what was wrong, but the doctor wouldn't listen to her. She called Nathian for support.

"What a jerk!" Nathian spat. "You need a second opinion."

"Why bother. There's no treatment for mono anyway. I just wish he would've listened to me instead of dismissing me like I didn't have a clue about my own body. I tell you, Nathe," Cheryl said with conviction, "that is not the kind of doctor I'm going to be."

"I know you won't be. And hey, I just had a great idea," Nathian said. "You could take some more comm classes! We have interpersonal and health comm. There's a lot you could learn to help your patients. You still need some electives, right?"

"I do," Cheryl replied. "But you know what? I have time. I think I'm going to double major with health communication."

"Bold. And awesome!" Nathian excitedly replied.

Meanwhile, back home, Helen hadn't been her energetic self lately. Sally and Joe were secretly starting to worry that something serious was going on with her health, so they convinced her to make an appointment with her primary care provider. Sally accompanied Helen to the doctor's appointment, just like she'd done for her own mother. Sally knew that doctors often were dismissive of older adults. She hadn't let that happen with her mom, and she wasn't going to let it happen with Helen either. But what she saw from this doctor was far worse than anything she'd anticipated. She recounted the experience to Joe after they got home.

"It was just unreal," Sally fumed. "First, she couldn't get a word in edgewise. I don't understand why she's stayed with this doctor these last few years. Every time she'd start to ask a question, he just interrupted her. Every time!"

"Yeah, that happens sometimes," Joe replied.

"And your mother didn't say anything!" Sally continued without missing a beat.

"Were you surprised about that?" Joe asked. "I mean it's awful, yes. But you know Ma. She doesn't talk over people in positions of authority. I bet she just nodded and agreed."

"She did," Sally said. "But I didn't. I didn't want to upset your mom, but I finally shut him down when he interrupted her *again*, and I said, "Let's let Mrs. Montgomery finish her thought." Sally huffed. "He'd been calling her Helen. Jerk."

Joe laughed. He loved seeing Sally's passion come out in defense of the people she loved. "Ignorance emerges in crazy ways, sweets."

"And his tone was so patronizing," Sally continued. "And he was dismissive. I swear, he was ready to just attribute her symptoms to age, but I wouldn't stand for that."

"Ma's lucky to have you," Joe said, approaching Sally to give her a hug. "And so am I."

"We have a follow-up appointment scheduled for her lab work," Sally said into Joe's shoulder, "but it's not till next month. Stupid scheduling."

"It'll be okay, sweets," Joe told her, hoping he was right.

3   Patient–Provider Communication

When you need medical care beyond what you can do for yourself, such as having to remove a fishhook from your arm after an unfortunate casting incident (true story), you'll need to see a healthcare provider. And when you do, you'll experience what has attracted the scholarly attention of a myriad of social science researchers around the globe: patient–provider communication. **Patient–provider communication** involves the exchange of information and the creation of shared meaning and understanding between a healthcare provider and a patient. Why has this topic attracted so much attention? One reason is because patient–provider is so pervasive. Nearly every person on the planet will see some kind of healthcare provider at some point in their lives, and so it's a common experience that everyone shares. Another reason is because communication between patients and providers is essential to having good patient health outcomes. And who doesn't want that?

We begin this chapter with a discussion of how communication is linked to health outcomes. Then we discuss patient-centered medicine, the leading model for patient care, and the importance of patient-centered communication in promoting patient-centered care. In this section, we pay particular attention to the influence of individual differences between patients and of technology on patient-centered communication. Because excellent communicators are made, not born, we then cover approaches to patient and provider communication skills training. Finally, we introduce the concept of multiple conversational goals in healthcare and review four types of difficult patient–provider conversations where good communication skills are essential to good health outcomes. We hope this chapter helps to make you aware of the central role that high-quality communication plays in promoting patient health and well-being and gives you some tools to be a more prepared patient the next time you get a fishhook caught in your arm.

Communication and Health Outcomes

You might have heard the quote, "If you haven't got your health, you haven't got anything." Count Rugen tells this to Prince Humperdinck in the classic film *The Princess Bride*, but plenty of other people have been saying this for, well, maybe forever. The importance of health is part of what makes the health sciences so fascinating: how medical, pharmaceutical, and surgical interventions can treat and cure injury and disease, getting people back on their feet. But did you know that communication has that power, as well? It's true. As a social science, our discipline may not seem like an obvious player on Team Healthcare, but let us assure you that we play a vital role. To demonstrate this point, Rick Street and his colleagues wrote an essay to explicitly address how communication heals.

In their essay, Street et al. (2009) presented a model that identified multiple paths along which verbal and nonverbal communication have an impact on health (see Figure 3.1). First, they listed six functions that communication serves in healthcare encounters: exchanging

DOI: 10.4324/9781003214458-8

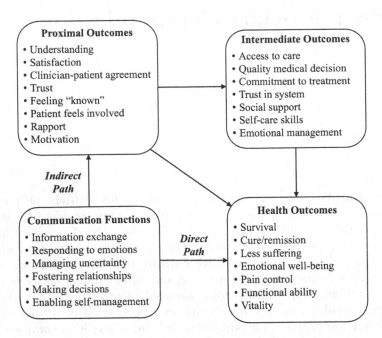

Figure 3.1 Direct and Indirect Pathways from Communication to Health Outcomes.
Source: Street et al. (2009).

information, responding to emotions, managing uncertainty, fostering relationships, making decisions, and enabling self-management. Then they described how communication can affect health both directly and indirectly through proximal (near or short term) and intermediate outcomes. Proximal outcomes include variables like patient understanding and satisfaction, patient–provider agreement, and trust and rapport. Intermediate outcomes include things like access to care, self-care skills, commitment to treatment, and social support. Finally, acknowledging the multidimensional nature of health, the researchers identified physical (survival, cure/remission, pain control, and functional ability) and socio-emotional (less suffering, emotional well-being, and vitality) outcomes for health.

As an example of how communication influences these different outcomes, let's consider high blood pressure, a condition known as the "silent killer" because it usually doesn't have symptoms and it can be deadly. One way communication can heal high blood pressure is indirectly. The healthcare provider *shares* the diagnosis with the patient and *explains* how serious high blood pressure is (communication function); the patient develops an *understanding* of their condition (proximal outcome); they *commit to treatment*, which means taking daily blood pressure medication (intermediate outcome); and then their *blood pressure is lowered* (health outcome). Another way communication can heal is directly. For example, research has shown that touch, which is a type of nonverbal communication, can temporarily lower blood pressure. It can also lower respiratory rate, improve sleep, and decrease pain (Papathanassoglou & Mpouzika, 2012). To benefit from the positive effects of touch on blood pressure, the patient may look into massage therapy as a complementary treatment option as part of an overall lifestyle change. Although the research is clear that communication is an important factor in promoting positive health outcomes, there are still many questions surrounding the ways in which communication affects health outcomes in different contexts.

Table 3.1 Theoretical Frameworks in Patient–Provider Communication

Theory/Model	Brief Summary	Citation
Communication Pathways to Improved Health Outcomes	Communication behaviors have an impact on health outcomes either directly or indirectly through proximal and intermediate outcomes.	Street et al. (2009)
Extended Ecological Model of Communication in Medical Encounters	Patient–provider communication is influenced by multiple contextual factors, including organizational, media, cultural, political–legal, and everyday interpersonal communication about health.	Head and Bute (2018)
Multiple Goals Theory	Conversations involve task, identity, and relational goals, and these goals sometimes conflict. Messages that resolve conflicting goals are more competent than those that prioritize one goal at the expense of others.	Caughlin (2010)

Note. See *Supplemental Online Theory Table* for additional theories/models.

Indeed, there is much more we need to know about how communication directly and indirectly affects health outcomes. To fill these gaps in knowledge, Street (2013) argues that researchers need to be more systematic in their approach to how all these variables relate to each other in ways that lead to improved health outcomes and in conceptualizing and measuring the communication variables of interest. He presents four steps to accomplish this research goal (Street, 2013, p. 287, Table 1):

Step 1: Identify the health outcome and the mechanism for improved health
Step 2: Model the pathway through which communication leads to improved health
Step 3: Select appropriate measures for communication variables, proximal outcomes, and intermediate outcomes
Step 4: Develop interventions to target communication processes to activate that mechanism

As researchers follow these steps, they need **theory-driven explanations** of *why* communication variables would have an impact on proximal, intermediate, or health outcomes, not just *that* they do. Unfortunately, scholars have noted a decidedly *atheoretical* streak in patient–provider communication research (Shen et al., 2018; Thompson & Schulz, 2021), so this need is especially pressing. There is also a need for multivariate, multilevel models that capture how patient–provider communication is influenced by multiple contextual factors, including organizational, media, cultural, political–legal, and everyday interpersonal communication about health (Head & Bute, 2018). Researchers also need to conduct longitudinal studies that can account for changes in health outcomes over time, not just one-shot cross-sectional studies. If you decide to pursue a career in health communication research, we hope you'll keep these goals in mind. To give you a start, Table 3.1 presents three theoretical frameworks that can inform patient–provider research.

Patient-Centered Medicine

Not too long ago (and sometimes still today), the medical community followed what was called a **biomedical model of healthcare**. This model privileged the physical manifestation of a disease, and it pretty much snubbed psychological and sociological influences such as stress, mental health, and family dynamics on the patient's illness experience. Recognizing the deficiencies in the biomedical model for providing adequate patient care, psychiatrist George Engel (1977) proposed a **biopsychosocial model of healthcare**, which added psychological and sociological dimensions to how healthcare should be conceptualized. The biopsychosocial model promotes a **systems approach** to the practice of medicine, recognizing multiple levels of influence on health and the importance of the whole person in the experience of both disease and illness. It prompts healthcare providers to explore multilevel influences on health, not only biological-level influences but also psychological, relational, community, and societal-level influences. This model emphasizes how social and psychological characteristics interact with biological factors to influence health experiences and outcomes. Acknowledging that and using that information to inform diagnosis and treatment marked important progress for Western medicine.

A related evolution in Western medicine was the shift from physician-centered, or paternalistic, medicine to patient-centered medicine. In **physician-centered medicine**, the provider has all the knowledge, power, and decision-making authority. Patients are expected to do what they're told. This may be ideal for a busy doctor who just wants to treat "the tumor in room 12," but it's hardly appropriate for Mrs. Helen Montgomery, a 68-year-old grandmother who is reluctant to question a provider and only made an appointment following her sons' insistence. What Mrs. Montgomery needs is patient-centered medicine.

What exactly is **patient-centered medicine**? Moira Stewart and her colleagues (2014) present the four components of this influential model of clinical care. First, providers need to *explore the concepts of health, disease, and illness* with the patient. What does health (or being healthy) mean to the patient? To a college student, it may mean being able to run three flights of stairs between classes without getting winded. To an elderly person with diabetes and heart disease, it may mean being able to walk to the mailbox without falling. The distinction between disease and illness also is important. **Disease** is the physical manifestation of the health condition. **Illness** is the individual patient's experience of the health condition. Although a particular disease may be identical across patients, the illness experiences can be profoundly different. COVID-19 provides a good example (that's about all it's good for). The virus killed millions of people and debilitated millions more. Others who caught the virus, however, either had minor symptoms or no symptoms at all. Beyond that, some people had access to plenty of resources and support. Others did not. Same disease; vastly different illness. The patient-centered approach recognizes these differences in health, disease, and illness and takes them into consideration for diagnosis and treatment.

Second, patient-centered medicine requires that healthcare providers work to *understand the patient as a whole person*. This means learning about patients as unique individuals, exploring their life histories, and eliciting their health beliefs and values. It also means understanding the contexts in which they live, from their family to their career to their community and their culture. You can readily imagine the multiple ways in which people differ and how that may influence their health and healthcare experience. Has a person rarely been ill, or have they had a chronic illness since childhood? Do they live alone in a crowded, polluted city where they work two jobs, or are they a member of a large family that has resources and lives on multiple acres in a wooded suburb? Are they atheist, or do they practice a religion that rejects some, most, or all aspects of modern medicine? Factors such as these play into both health and healthcare, and so it's essential to patient-centered care that they be considered.

Third, patient-centered medicine encourages healthcare providers and patients to *find common ground* on several issues. Both should come to an agreement on what the health problems are and what should be prioritized. Sometimes, that's easy. A deep gash from a rusty barbed wire (another true story) needs stitches, antibiotics, and a tetanus shot. Pretty straightforward. But sometimes it's not easy at all. A patient with multiple, chronic health conditions will need a complex plan of care. That plan of care will consider specific goals, such as what can and should be treated and whether the condition can be cured or must be managed. There also needs to be agreement on the roles of the patient and provider. Perhaps the patient wants their provider to just tell them what to do to get better, but perhaps the provider believes that the patient must be an active participant in their medical decision making. In cases with diverging role perspectives, the opportunity for optimal care may not be as likely as in cases where both parties see eye-to-eye. That is why the patient-centered approach to healthcare encourages practitioners to elicit patient perspectives and meet their needs as much as possible.

Finally, patient-centered medicine emphasizes the importance of *enhancing the patient– provider relationship*. Compassion, empathy, respect, and trust are essential qualities for patient-centered care. Even in the briefest visit, and even when patients and providers have not met before, there is an opportunity for providers to be respectful of patients and show them compassion. Patients will vary in how much they tend to trust healthcare providers, especially patients from marginalized populations that have faced inequitable treatment (Institute of Medicine, 2003). For the best healthcare outcomes, all patients need to be able to trust that their providers will take their health concerns seriously, tailor treatment decisions to their needs, actually care about them as human beings, and not shame or blame them when they self-disclosure potentially stigmatizing health behaviors.

The Four Components of Patient-Centered Medicine

There are four components to patient-centered medicine:

- Explore the concepts of health, disease, and illness
- Understand the patient as a whole person
- Find common ground between the patient and provider
- Enhance the patient–provider relationship

Patient-Centered Communication

For all these components of patient-centered medicine to come together into quality patient-centered care, there needs to be **patient-centered communication**. Street (2019) presents an analysis of how various communication behaviors map onto conceptual components of patient-centered medicine. Instead of using Stewart et al.'s (2014) four-component conceptualization, he uses a more recent conceptualization based on how patient-centeredness was defined across 80 empirical studies (Langberg et al., 2019), but the specific communication behaviors apply to patient-centered care no matter how you slice it. For example, Street states that providers need to ask about patients' health beliefs and concerns, elicit their perspectives on health, and clarify patients' values as related to health. They need to work toward building a partnership with the patient and set an agenda for each visit that considers both patient and provider perspectives. They need to present information clearly and check for patient understanding. They need to be supportive, to listen, and to show respect for the patient. Importantly, the patient must do their part, as well, by being a partner in the relationship (to the extent they feel comfortable), by asking questions when they don't understand, by listening and showing respect to the provider, and by sharing their beliefs, concerns, perspectives, and values. All these patient-centered communication behaviors act in concert to promote more effective, quality healthcare. Let's look at a few studies that show the positive health outcomes that can result from patient-centered communication.

One example comes from Lila Finney Rutten and colleagues (2016), who found that the more patients with chronic conditions experienced patient-centered communication, the higher their levels of self-efficacy for managing their conditions. This association was stronger the more chronic conditions a person had. Another example comes from Jelena Zwingmann and colleagues (2017). These researchers were interested in the role of patient-centered communication during the delivery of a cancer diagnosis. Through an experimental video simulation, they found that an enhanced patient-centered communication style that emphasized empathy was associated with less self-reported patient anxiety and greater patient trust in the physician than a low patient-centered communication style that was nonempathic. Other studies have shown that patient-centered communication has an indirect effect on health outcomes. For example, in a longitudinal study of patient–provider interactions in China, Shaohai Jiang (2019) found that patient-centered communication significantly improved patient satisfaction and patient trust, which in turn improved perceived emotional and physical health.

The **patient–provider relationship** is at the core of the latest evolution in thinking about patient-centered communication: recognizing the centrality of mutual persuasion between the patient and the provider. Freytag and Street (2022) argue that inherent in any communication that produces patient-centered care is a process of **mutual persuasion** between the patient and provider. This perspective elevates the status of the patient, highlighting how they are not simply at the center of patient-centered care but how they are actually on par with providers as each tries to influence the other's thinking, emotions, and behaviors. For example, while a clinician is sharing information about the benefits of exercise, trying to boost the patient's self-confidence, and encouraging them to start a fitness routine, the patient may be replying with information about their family and work situation and how they've tried and failed several times to fit exercise into their daily schedule. In other words, each participant in the conversation is trying to persuade the other about the extent to which exercise is or is not reasonable in the patient's life.

Freytag and Street (2022) use the lens of mutual persuasion to discuss shared decision making and relational autonomy as two important outcomes of patient-centered communication. **Shared decision making** happens when the patient and provider work together to make a high-quality decision that is based on the best current clinical evidence and the patient's values and preferences, as well as being feasible (e.g., a medication the patient can afford). Providers, of course, bring their medical expertise to the conversation, but patients have their own expertise based on their lived experience and any health information seeking they may have done (see Chapter 5 for health information seeking).

Importantly, Freytag and Street (2022) emphasize how

> patients as communicators have the opportunity, *if chosen*, to actively advocate for desired courses of treatment, assert their goals or wishes for their care, or even tailor or withhold information so that they may receive a desired diagnosis, procedure, or treatment.
>
> (p. 166, emphasis added)

In other words, to be competent participants in patient-centered communication and their own healthcare, patients need to recognize and be mindful of their persuasive power in clinical encounters. Thus, patient-centered communication doesn't merely mean that patients are at the center of healthcare, it means they are central to the process.

Patient-Centered Communication and Individual Differences

Patient-centered communication should apply to all patients equally. Yet, you know from Chapter 2 that the U.S. healthcare system is rife with inequalities and disparities based on certain individual differences. So it's important to look at the literature that explores the influence of demographics on the practice of patient-centered communication The question is whether there are disparities in patient-centered communication as experienced by different groups. The short answer is "yes, there are." Let's take a closer look at some of the research to see what's been found.

Megan Johnson Shen and her colleagues (2018) conducted a systematic review of the literature on race and **racial concordance** (whether patients and providers are the same race) in patient–physician communication. They included 40 articles in their review and coded them along several communication variables. They found that Black patients experienced significantly lower quality of communication, less participatory decision-making, and less patient information giving and participation than white patients. There were mixed results across studies in terms of patient satisfaction, partnership building, and length of visit, with studies tending either to show worse outcomes for Black patients or to show no differences. Interestingly, however, when studies looked at whether there was racial concordance and whether that had an influence on communication, there were better outcomes across all the variables except for quality of communication. In other words, Black patients tended to have better experiences when their physicians were Black, and white patients tended to have better experiences when their physicians were white. Similar research has been conducted to explore differing experiences based on sex.

Debra Roter and her colleagues (2002) conducted a meta-analysis of the literature on the influence of patient and physician sex on patient-centered communication. They included 29 articles in their analysis and coded them along several aspects of information giving and seeking, partnership building, socioemotional behavior, and visit length. They found that female physicians engaged in more psychosocial information giving and information seeking, more partnership building, and more positive talk than male physicians. They also found that visits with female physicians were about two minutes longer than visits with male physicians. Only two of the 29 articles considered sex concordance. Both found that there were better communication outcomes for female concordant visits than any other combination. A later study conducted by Klea Bertakis and Rahman Azari (2012) also looked at the influence of patient and physician sex on patient-centered communication. Like Roter et al.'s meta-analysis, they found that female physicians provided greater patient-centered care than male physicians and that female concordant visits had the greatest amount of patient-centered communication. But what about the intersectionality of race and sex on patient-centered care?

A study by Jamie Mitchell and Ramona Perry (2020) looked at the intersection of race and sex when the authors analyzed data from 3,082 white, Black, and Latino males on their experiences with patient-centered communication during medical visits. The measures assessed how often healthcare providers gave their male patients easily understandable information, listened to them carefully, showed them respect, and spent enough time with them. Results showed differences based on race across all questions. On average, white patients reported receiving more patient-centered communication than Black and Latino patients, and Black patients reported receiving more patient-centered communication than Latino patients. In addition, experiencing discrimination and not having health insurance were associated with receiving less patient-centered communication for Black men, whereas not having a usual healthcare provider was associated with receiving less patient-centered communication for Latino men. This study did not consider race or sex concordance, so we cannot be sure about potential concordance effects.

Patient-centered communication is especially important for patients whose intersectional identities are particularly marginalized. For example, in a study looking at the intersection of gender and ableness, Cara Miller and colleagues (2019) were interested in LGBTQ-identifying deaf adults' likelihood of disclosing their sexual orientation to healthcare providers. Historically, the LGBTQ community has experienced barriers related to such disclosure, such as stigma, denial of care, and substandard care. These barriers are likely elevated for deaf patients whose disclosure to providers would also involve disclosure to a translator. The lack of disclosure is concerning because providers "may be unaware of patients' specific risk factors, medical contraindications, and healthcare needs. Omission of such information may result in under- or mis-diagnoses of conditions and missed opportunities for patient education on risky behaviors or risk susceptibilities" (p. 196). In a survey of 313 LGBTQ deaf adults, Miller et al. found patient-centered communication to be significantly related to patient likelihood of disclosing their sexual orientation to their provider. In other words, patient-centered communication increased the opportunity for deaf LGBTQ adults to receive relevant, comprehensive care.

What conclusions should be drawn from these studies that investigate the influence of race and sex on patient-centered communication? First, providers need to be aware that patient demographics can produce different patient–provider experiences. It is only through this awareness that providers can self-reflect on their own communication behaviors that may be perpetuating these disparities and make the appropriate changes in their communication to engage in equitable patient-centered care. Second, patients who are discouraged by past negative patient–provider experiences can look to these findings for strategies to elicit more positive encounters in future medical visits, such as seeking racial concordance, engaging more intentionally in decision making, or requesting additional information. It is important to remember that disparities, by definition, are a product of systemic injustices. The U.S. healthcare system has taken generations to build and is filled with disparities. It is not, however, immutable. It can be changed and improved, even though it will take time and effort.

Patient–Centered Communication and Technology

Think about the last time you had a medical appointment. When your healthcare provider entered the exam room, they probably brought with them a tablet through which they accessed your **electronic health record (EHR)**. The EHR is a digital version of patients' medical records. It allows patient information to be shared by multiple healthcare providers, labs, pharmacies, hospitals, and insurance companies. The goal, ideally, is to promote efficient, effective, and safe healthcare. When the system works properly, patient information is available instantly and "follows the patient" from appointment to appointment. And, depending on the system being used, patients may have access to their EHRs via patient portals, which can also be used to make appointments, access test results, and communicate with healthcare providers through email, direct messaging, or video chat.

This is all well and good, but there is some concern that having a computer involved in the medical visit may inadvertently compromise patient-centered communication or damage the patient–provider relationship. Street and his colleagues (2014) designed a study to investigate this very question. They involved 23 primary care providers from four Veterans Administration clinics, recruiting up to six patients per provider (total $n = 125$). The researchers used video recordings so they could document how much time the providers spent looking at the computer screen and how much of the visit was spent in conversational silence. They had independent observers code the video recordings for patient-centered communication and patient involvement (e.g., whether the patient asked for explanations, whether they expressed concerns). Results showed that the average visit length was a little more than 30 minutes. Of that time, providers spent nearly 40% of the visit looking at the computer screen, and a little more than 30% was spent in silence. Perhaps unsurprising, the more time providers spent looking at the computer screen and the more silence there was, the lower the ratings of patient-centeredness. Although higher patient involvement scores were associated with higher ratings of patient-centeredness, patient involvement can be compromised if a provider is staring at a screen in silence. These findings paint a rather bleak picture of the impact of EHRs on patient-centered communication, but there's more to the story.

Cheryl Rathert and colleagues (2017) did a systematic review of the literature on patient–provider communication and EHRs. They included 41 studies in their analysis, and they organized their findings on how the use of EHRs during medical visits influenced the six functions of communication from Street et al.'s (2009) model. They found that every study had implications for at least one, if not more, of the communication functions: 31 studies had implications for fostering relationships, 29 for exchanging information, nine for making decisions, six for enabling self-management, five for managing uncertainty, and four for responding to emotions. Let's take a closer look at findings across all six functions. We'll organize the review by positive and negative communication implications, starting with the negatives.

In terms of fostering relationships, Rathert et al.'s (2017) review found that studies showed the vital importance of eye contact and how it can be undermined if a provider spends too much time focusing their attention on the computer screen and too little time engaging the patient. For information exchange, although the exchange of biomedical information may be facilitated by having access to the EHR, there was concern that the exchange of psychosocial information may be hampered. Another negative implication was that too great a focus on the EHR may compromise a healthcare provider's ability to recognize and respond to patient emotions. (It's a little difficult to notice fear or worry in a patient's eyes if you're focused on a computer screen.) In terms of uncertainty, there were both positive and negative implications. Although patients who studied their health records gained knowledge and confidence, they had a lot of uncertainty about the privacy of their health information, such as who could access it and whether it was secure. Finally, in terms of making decisions and enabling patient self-management, the positive implications of EHRs appear to win. Especially for those systems that allow patients to access their own records and to message their providers with questions and concerns, EHRs can lead to more informed decisions and greater patient involvement and management in their own care.

Now let's look a little closer at how EHRs can promote patient involvement by allowing them to communicate electronically with their providers and whether that communication can be characterized as patient-centered. Jordan Alpert and colleagues (2017) designed a study to investigate the nature of messages that patients sent to their providers via online portals and the extent to which provider responses were patient-centered. They worked with a large healthcare system that had recently instituted the EpicCare system, which includes MyChart, a portal that allows patients to access their records, make appointments, and communicate with their providers. The researchers targeted a one-week period and collected all message threads that were initiated by a patient who was at least 21 years old and had at least one provider response. This resulted in 58 threads, which they content analyzed for the topic of discussion that the patient initiated and the extent to which providers responded in a way that involved partnership building (working to understand patient preferences and encouraging or praising a patient's positive health behavior) or supportive talk (working to make a connection with the patient and ease their concerns or distress).

Patient messages fell into two categories: to seek solutions and to make administrative requests. In terms of seeking solutions, patients asked about things like follow-up appointments and what test results meant. They also asked about symptoms that concerned them or expressed concerns about prescription medications (e.g., cost, side effects). In terms of administrative requests, patient messages ran the gamut from asking for help with paperwork and insurance forms to asking for help with appointment scheduling and confirming medical record accuracy.

When you consider both categories combined, provider responses to patient messages contained patient-centered responses about half the time. Partnership building was evident in 36.2% of responses, and supportive talk was evident in 22.4% of responses. Both types of patient-centered communication were present in 12.1% of responses. Although there was some evidence of patient-centeredness in some provider responses, the authors characterized the responses as coming up short: "In general, provider messages were succinct and to-the-point; they did not reciprocate the patients' rapport-building attempts. Providers did not usually reference their relationship or experience with that particular patient, limiting their responses strictly to the information or feedback requested" (Alpert et al., 2017, p. 1855).

We find these results discouraging and a little depressing. As communication scholars and students, we all understand the power of communication to either make or break a relationship. And frankly, we know that it doesn't take much effort at all to show just a little patient-centeredness—and a little can go a long way. To make our point, we'll shift our attention briefly to a StoryCorps story (Fadel, 2022). The story shows the profound impact that healthcare providers can have on people's lives when they go just a small step out of their way.

The storyteller was Robert Corolla. His younger brother, John, had died from cancer during adolescence. John's physician, Dr. Doan, had written a letter of condolence to the family, which they received about six weeks after John died. Robert said his parents were overwhelmed by Dr. Doan's thoughtfulness. They read the letter multiple times and would share it with friends who would visit. Robert went on to become a physician himself. He hadn't met Dr. Doan during his brother's illness, but he serendipitously encountered him during medical school. Dr. Doan saw Robert's nametag and remembered his name—after all those years. Robert vowed to become the kind of physician Dr. Doan was. And he did. To find out how and to learn the rest of this touching story, including a twist at the end, we encourage you to take two minutes to listen to it in the online supplemental materials.

The StoryCorps story (Fadel, 2022) demonstrates the value of developing relationships with patients and families and how even in times of tragedy, making just a little effort to show care and concern can make all the difference in the world. Healthcare providers who do *not* choose to be even minimally patient-centered in their responses to patient messages are missing a ready opportunity to strengthen the patient–provider relationship. If they're worried that being patient-centered will "open a can of worms," encouraging patients to go on at length and monopolize their time, they needn't be. The average length of a patient message in the Alpert et al. (2017) study was 85 words. This paragraph has 115 words.

So, what can researchers do to encourage providers not to let an EHR computer get in the way of a patient-centered visit and take advantage of the system to send patient-centered replies to their patients' inquiries? Pamela Duke and colleagues (2013) have some advice and offer tips to help healthcare providers "optimize use of the EHR in the examination room while maintaining rapport with the patient and building the patient–provider relationship" (p. 359). One tip is to realize that the presence of a computer turns the dyadic patient–provider relationship into a triadic patient–provider–computer relationship, and so interaction with the computer must be navigated competently while still making the patient the focus of the interaction. Another tip is for providers to explain to patients what they're doing on the computer (e.g., "I'm just gonna update your chart based on what you just told me") and even ask permission or apologize if they need to focus their attention on the computer (e.g., "Excuse me for a moment while I type this into your record"). They can also increase patient involvement by showing them what's on the screen and reviewing patient data together (of course, it's important to assess the patient's health literacy before doing so, as we'll discuss further in Chapter 4). But when patients want the healthcare provider's attention, they need to focus on the patient, facing them, making eye contact, and even possibly pushing the computer away to optimize patient-centered communication. Duke et al. (2013) didn't offer any tips for getting providers to be more patient-centered in their electronic messaging, but that can be helped with communication skills training.

Communication Skills Training

With the challenges inherent in patient-centered communication, you might be thinking it would be a good idea to have communication skills training available to patients and healthcare providers. Well, you're in luck because there is such training available. In this section, we're going to present information on a patient communication skills training program called PACE. We're also going to present information on provider communication skills training, looking briefly at competencies that have been identified for nurses and physicians by professional accrediting bodies and a communication skills intervention called Teach-back Training.

Patient Communication Skills Training

How did you learn to communicate with your healthcare providers? Did you take a class in elementary, middle, or high school? Or did you just observe the way your parents or guardians communicated with your pediatrician and then modeled that behavior moving forward? If you're like the rest of us, you did the latter. That said, and with all due respect to everyone's family members, we suspect that there's room for improvement in your patient–provider communication skills. Lucky for you, health communication researcher Don Cegala developed a program to help patients communicate more effectively with their physicians.

Called **PACE**, this program involves teaching patients how to *present* information about their health concern, *ask* questions about the diagnosis and treatment, *check* their understanding of information the provider gives, and *express* any concerns they might have about the treatment. In their studies, Cegala and colleagues have shown that PACE can have positive effects on communication and health behavior outcome variables.

One study (Cegala, McClure, et al., 2000) involved 25 family physicians and 150 patients. The patients were randomly assigned to three groups. Patients in the *trained group* received a PACE booklet in the mail a few days before their doctor's visit. The booklet included space for them to make notes and answer questions about their health condition. It also provided examples of questions they might ask their doctor. Patients were asked to review the booklet and fill it out in preparation for their visit. You can think of patients in this trained group as getting the biggest "dose" of PACE. Patients in the *informed group* did not receive the booklet in advance. Instead, they received a brief written summary of PACE while they were in the waiting room just before their visit. So, they learned about PACE but didn't have any time to really digest it. The *untrained group* didn't receive any information about PACE. Results of this experiment showed that trained patients were better at seeking and obtaining information from their doctors, better at giving their doctors more information about their health condition, and more likely to summarize and verify the information their doctors gave them than the informed or untrained patients. So, PACE worked but only when patients had enough time to process the material and really prepare for the visit.

Patient Participation in the PACE System

Patient participation has four components:

- Information seeking: When patients ask medically related questions and attempt to verify information the doctor has provided
- Assertive utterances: When patients state an opinion, preference, suggestion, recommendation, disagreement, or request
- Information provision: When patients respond to questions from the doctor or volunteer medically related information
- Expression of concern: When patients express fear, anxiety, or worry about their medical condition

---

In this same study, the researchers also explored the impact of PACE on patient versus physician "control" during the medical visit. They looked at questions asked by patients and physicians and answers obtained in response. The greater the ratio of patient questions/doctor replies to doctor questions/patient replies in an interaction, the more the patient was in control. The data analysis showed that visits involving PACE-trained patients were more patient controlled than visits with informed or untrained patients (Cegala, McClure, et al., 2000). So once again, we're seeing a positive impact of patient training through PACE.

In another study of PACE, there was evidence that PACE-trained patients were more likely to comply with their doctor's recommendations for behavioral treatments (e.g., diet, exercise, quitting smoking) and for follow-up appointments and referrals than informed or untrained patients (Cegala, Marinelli, & Post, 2000). Compliance with, or adherence to, treatment recommendations and follow-up care is associated with better healthcare outcomes on the whole, so this was an important finding.

The PACE system has been used by various healthcare organizations across the globe to help empower patients and improve their communication skills with their physicians. For example, the system is available through the American Heart Association, the Amputee Coalition, and the Patient Voices Network in Canada. This makes it an excellent example of translational research (see Chapter 1). It also has inspired other scholars to investigate the application of PACE principles in different contexts. For example, Nancy Harrington and colleagues (2007) developed *PACE for Parents* and *PACE for Physicians* to help improve parent-pediatrician communication about prescribing antibiotics for children. The PACE acronym for parents mirrors that for patients from Cegala's work. For physicians, though, there were modifications: *present* treatment options in a *positive* manner; *acknowledge* parents' feelings, concerns, and expectations; *create* a partnership; and *encourage* questions.

The researchers tested the impact of their intervention in a study of four pediatricians and 81 parents (Harrington et al., 2007). This study design involved just two experimental conditions: *trained* and *untrained*. Before the four participating pediatricians received PACE training, baseline data was collected for visits with 42 untrained parents. In other words, neither parents nor pediatricians had any training. After these visits, pediatricians received their PACE training in 45-minute sessions, and then experimental treatment data was collected for visits with 39 PACE-trained parents. Training for parents this time involved a research assistant meeting with the parents in the waiting room before their child's visit and reviewing the PACE booklet and principles in detail for about 15 minutes, allowing time for questions, and encouraging the parents to follow the guidelines. Results of the study showed that parents who received PACE training were more likely to give information, verify information, and express concerns than parents who weren't trained. Results also showed that pediatricians were more likely to encourage questions from parents, spend more time addressing treatment options, and spend more time creating a partnership with parents after they received PACE training than before. The *PACE for Parents* and *PACE for Physicians* programs are available online through the Kentucky Antibiotic Awareness campaign. If you're interested in improving your own patient–provider communication skills, we provide a copy of PACE in the final chapter of this book (see Table 15.3).

Provider Communication Skills Training

Accrediting bodies for nursing and medicine include communication skills as an essential competency. For example, the American Association of Colleges of Nursing (2021) includes establishing a caring relationship and communicating effectively with patients as part of providing "person-centered care." The Association of American Medical Colleges (2005), which applies to undergraduate medical education, identifies communication skills as a component of "specific clinical skills" and includes aspects such as building the doctor–patient relationship, understanding the patient's perspective, and engaging in shared, informed decision making and informed consent. And the Accreditation Council for Graduate Medical Education (2021), which applies to residency programs, includes "interpersonal and communication skills that result in the effective exchange of information and collaboration with patients, their families, and health professionals" (p. 178) as a core competency.

Communication skills training extends beyond nursing and medical education, of course. This is where continuing education opportunities come into play. To stay up to date in their practice areas and maintain licensure, healthcare providers are required to earn **continuing education credits** on an ongoing basis. Taking courses on communication skills counts toward those credits. These courses are available through numerous organizations, such as the Academy of Communication in Healthcare and the Centers for Disease Control and Prevention. Here, we focus on one such training program, Teach-back.

The Institute for Healthcare Advancement (2022) describes **Teach-back Training** as "a research-based health literacy intervention that promotes adherence, quality, and patient safety" (n.p.). Teach-back training is based on the principle that patient understanding is essential to achieving optimal healthcare outcomes. If patients don't understand their conditions or treatment plans, the chance of them doing what they need to do to effectively treat or manage their health condition is reduced. Thus, the goal of Teach-back is to ensure patient understanding.

How is this achieved? After healthcare providers explain to the patient what their condition is and how to treat or manage it, they ask them to describe *in their own words* what has been explained. Providers are supposed to frame this request as being a way to make sure they presented the information clearly, not to "test" or shame the patient. Listening to the patient "teach back" the information in their own words gives providers the opportunity to check for understanding and, if necessary, explain the information again and then check for understanding again.

There are 10 components to using Teach-back effectively. They include using a caring tone of voice and attitude, using plain language, and using non-shaming, open-ended questions (see Table 3.2). You can visit the Teach-back Training website (www.teachbacktraining.org) and go through an interactive Teach-back learning module to learn more about this technique. You can also watch video testimonials from a physician who learned to use Teach-back and a woman who inadvertently overdosed a family member because the doctor had not used teach-back techniques to ensure her accurate understanding of how to administer the medication (don't worry, the family member was not seriously harmed by the overdose).

Table 3.2 10 Elements of Competence for Using Teach-back Effectively

---

1. Use a caring tone of voice and attitude.
2. Display comfortable body language and make eye contact.
3. Use plain language.
4. Ask the patient to explain back, using their own words.
5. Use non-shaming, open-ended questions.
6. Avoid asking questions that can be answered with a simple yes or no.
7. Emphasize that the responsibility to explain clearly is on you, the provider.
8. If the patient is not able to teach back correctly, explain again and re-check.
9. Use reader-friendly print materials to support learning.
10. Document use of and patient response to teach-back.

Note. From Institute for Healthcare Advancement (2022).

Difficult Conversations in Healthcare

If you've taken an interpersonal communication course, you may have encountered **multiple goals theory** (see Table 3.1). Central to the theory is the concept of **multiple conversational goals**. The idea is that every conversation involves three goals: task, identity, and relational. *Task goals* are what you are trying to accomplish in the conversation, such as telling your doctor you have a headache or getting a prescription refill. *Identity goals* have to do with how you want to be perceived as an individual, such as a doctor seeing you as being responsible and knowledgeable about your health, and how you perceive them, such as being kind and competent. *Relational goals* get at establishing and maintaining your doctor–patient relationship, which can range from warm and egalitarian to cold and hierarchical. The salience of these goals will vary across conversations, but they're always present. Sometimes you can accomplish all three goals without much trouble, but in more complex, difficult situations, the goals might conflict. In those cases, some people may pursue one goal at the expense of the others. John Caughlin (2010) has argued that people who craft their messages to address task, identity, and relational goals have higher quality communication than those who do not.

Allison M. Scott is one of our discipline's leading scholars on difficult conversations in healthcare. She has identified four types of difficult patient–provider conversations: sensitive disclosures, challenging health contexts, high-stakes decisions, and charged topics (Scott, 2022). Scott notes that these types of conversations are difficult in part because they tend to involve conflicting task, identity, and relational goals, and they also involve dealing with negative emotions, such as sadness, fear, and embarrassment. Let's take a closer look at each type of conversation.

Four Types of Difficult Conversations in Healthcare

Allison M. Scott has described four types of difficult healthcare conversations:

- Sensitive disclosures: bad news delivery, medical errors
- Challenging health contexts: end-of-life planning, pregnancy
- High-stakes decisions: genetic testing, complicated treatment decisions, participation in clinical trials
- Charged topics: obesity and weight management, sexuality and sexual behavior, religiosity or spirituality, substance use, disability, mental health

---

Scott (2022) describes *sensitive disclosures* as involving information that "someone does not want to hear" or that "renders someone vulnerable to negative evaluation or action" (p. 180). The first instance relates directly to bad news delivery. Healthcare providers must share bad news, such as a diagnosis of heart disease, diabetes, or cancer, with patients regularly. What is routine for providers, however, is often life changing for patients, who may go from "healthy" to "sick" in an instant. Such disclosures can cause strong emotional reactions that make continuing the conversation difficult, and they also have consequences for identity and relational goals, such as possibly stripping independence from a patient or damaging the patient–provider relationship if the provider delivers the news poorly. Protocols for delivering bad news, such as the well-known SPIKES protocol (Baile et al., 2000), coupled with attention to multiple conversational goals can help improve bad news delivery. The second instance could involve providers disclosing when they've made some kind of medical mistake, such as misdiagnosing a condition or operating on the wrong limb during surgery. Such errors may have serious consequences, including patient death. We'll have more to say about medical mistakes in Chapter 12 when we discuss ethics in health communication. For now, suffice it to say that such disclosures can have profound implications for provider identity as a competent, caring practitioner and for patient trust.

The second kind of difficult conversation involves dealing with *challenging contexts*. Some health contexts, by their very nature, are inherently more challenging than others. Scott (2022) identifies end-of-life and pregnancy as two particularly challenging contexts. She notes how end-of-life conversations involve several competing goals, such as being truthful about a terminal diagnosis (task) while trying to maintain patient hope (identity), respecting patient autonomy (identity) when the provider disagrees with patient wishes (task and relational), and providing adequate support (task) while remaining professional (identity). (Note that we cover end-of-life communication extensively in Chapter 8.) Patients who are pregnant may face challenges such as miscarriages, fetal abnormalities, premature birth, and abortion needs. Such conversations are difficult under normal circumstances, but the Supreme Court decision overturning Roe v. Wade raised the stakes even more. The implications for patient autonomy and trust in the provider, not to mention patient health outcomes, are profound.

Difficult conversations involving *high-stakes decisions* include topics like genetic testing, complicated treatment decisions, and whether to enroll in a clinical trial. Part of what makes these conversations difficult is the inherent uncertainty involved, such as whether changing a treatment plan will lead to better outcomes. But there can be added complications when patient and provider opinions differ. For example, take the issue of vaccination. Although the scientific literature on vaccinations clearly establishes their efficacy (see World Health Organization, 2021), some patients and surrogate decision makers (e.g., parents) have concerns, and so conversations about vaccination have the potential to be difficult. In these cases, there clearly are multiple conflicting goals. The provider task of persuading to vaccinate conflicts with the patient task of resisting vaccination. In terms of identity, the provider who wants to be perceived as competent may be perceived by the patient as unsupportive, and the patient who wants to be perceived as informed may be perceived by the provider as irresponsible. And if the conversation is not handled well, the goal of maintaining a trusting patient–provider relationship may be scuttled.

Like making sensitive disclosures, having discussions about *charged topics* also involves disclosing sensitive information, but in this case, the information relates specifically to identity concerns of the patient. Scott (2022) identifies the following topics as being especially charged: obesity and weight management, sexuality and sexual behavior, religiosity or spirituality, substance use, disability, and mental health. These issues involve potential embarrassment, stigma, or shame, which is threatening to patients' identities and therefore makes conversations about them difficult. Of course, patients sometimes choose to not disclose certain behaviors to simply avoid having these conversations. For example, patients may lie about a history of substance use or risky sexual behavior. Although lying may achieve their goal of maintaining an identity as a "responsible" patient, it certainly risks the task goal of promoting patient health and, depending on how the provider would have responded, the relational goal of developing a trusting patient–provider relationship.

In summary, although many healthcare conversations may be relatively easy, some are decidedly not, especially those involving sensitive disclosures, challenging health contexts, high-stakes decisions, and charged topics. The more that patients and providers can be aware of and manage the likely conflicting task, identity, and relational goals in these conversations, the greater the potential for more competent, patient-centered conversations and improved health outcomes.

Conclusion

In this chapter, we have addressed one of the major areas of health communication research and practice: patient–provider communication. We established at the outset that communication can have both direct and indirect influence on health outcomes. We reviewed models of patient care, including patient-centered medicine, which emphasizes the importance of exploring the concepts of health, disease, and illness; understanding the patient as a whole person; finding common ground between the patient and provider; and enhancing the patient–provider relationship. We reviewed some of the research showing how race and sex, as well as technology, can complicate patient-centered communication. We reviewed how communication skills training has the potential to remediate and overcome such complications. And we presented four types of difficult conversations in healthcare that are best navigated by paying attention to multiple communication goals as a way to promote patient centeredness.

Is patient-centered communication a tall order? You bet it is. As we discussed in the first two chapters, there are powerful forces that present incredible barriers to adequate care in the U.S. healthcare system. And as we'll discuss in subsequent chapters, patients and providers alike face terrible burdens and stressors in their roles. Being patient centered under these conditions takes effort. But it is possible, and, most importantly, it is worth it. We encourage you to do your part and try.

References

Accreditation Council for Graduate Medical Education. (2021). *The program director guide to the common program requirements (residency)*. https://www.acgme.org/globalassets/pdfs/program-director-guide---residency.pdf

Alpert, J. M., Dyer, K. E., & Lafata, J. E. (2017). Patient-centered communication in digital medical encounters. *Patient Education and Counseling, 100*(10), 1852–1858.

American Association of Colleges of Nursing. (2021). *The essentials: Core competencies for professional nursing education*. https://www.aacnnursing.org/Portals/42/AcademicNursing/pdf/Essentials-2021.pdf

Association of American Medical Colleges. (2005). *Recommendations for clinical skills curricula for undergraduate medical education*. https://store.aamc.org/downloadable/download/sample/sample_id/174/

Baile, W. F., Buckman, R., Lenzi, R., Glober, G., Beale, E. A., & Kudelka, A. P. (2000). SPIKES—A six-step protocol for delivering bad news: Application to the patient with cancer. *The Oncologist, 5,* 302–311.

Bertakis, K. D., & Azari, R. (2012). Patient-centered care: The influence of patient and resident physician gender and gender concordance in primary care. *Journal of Women's Health, 21*(3), 326–333.

Caughlin, J. P. (2010). A multiple goals theory of personal relationships: Conceptual integration and program overview. *Journal of Social and Personal Relationships, 27*(6), 824–848.

Cegala, D. J., Marinelli, T. M., & Post, D. M. (2000). The effects of patient communication skills training on compliance. *Archives of Family Medicine, 9*(1), 57–64.

Cegala, D. J., McClure, L., Marinelli, T. M., & Post, D. M. (2000). The effects of communication skills training on patients' participation during medical interviews. *Patient Education and Counseling, 41*(2), 209–222.

Duke, P., Frankel, R. M., & Reis, S. (2013). How to integrate the electronic health record and patient-centered communication into the medical visit: A skills-based approach. *Teaching and Learning in Medicine, 25*(4), 358–365.

Engel, G. L. (1977). The need for a new medical model: A challenge for biomedicine. *Science, 196*(4286), 129–136.

Fadel, L. (Host). (2022, July 8). A doctor's condolence letter was much more than a piece of paper [Audio podcast episode]. In *StoryCorps*. National Public Radio. https://www.npr.org/2022/07/08/1110435821/a-doctors-condolence-letter-was-much-more-than-a-piece-of-paper

Finney Rutten, L. J., Hesse, B. W., St. Sauver, J. L., Wilson, P., Chawla, N., Hartigan, D. B., Moser, R. P., Taplin, S., Glasgow, R., & Arora, N. K. (2016). Health self-efficacy among populations with multiple chronic conditions: The value of patient-centered communication. *Advances in Therapy, 33*(8), 1440–1451.

Freytag, J., & Street, R. L., Jr. (2022). Mutual persuasion as patient-centered communication. In T. L. Thompson & N. G. Harrington (Eds.), *The Routledge handbook of health communication* (3rd ed., pp. 165–178). Routledge.

Harrington, N. G., Norling, G. R., Witte, F., Taylor, J. A., & Andrews, J. (2007). The effects of communication skills training on pediatricians' and parents' communication during "sick child" visits. *Health Communication, 21*(2), 105–114.

Head, K. J., & Bute, J. J. (2018). The influence of everyday interpersonal communication on the medical encounter: An extension of Street's ecological model. *Health Communication, 33*(6), 786–792.

Institute for Healthcare Advancement. (2022). *Always use Teach-back!* http://www.teachbacktraining.org

Institute of Medicine (US) Committee on Understanding and Eliminating Racial and Ethnic Disparities in Health Care, Smedley, B. D., Stith, A. Y., & Nelson, A. R. (Eds.). (2003). *Unequal treatment: Confronting racial and ethnic disparities in health care*. National Academies Press (US).

Jiang, S. (2019). Pathways linking patient-centered communication to health improvement: A longitudinal study in China. *Journal of Health Communication, 24*(2), 156–164.

Langberg, E. M., Dyhr, L., & Davidsen, A. S. (2019). Development of the concept of patient-centredness—A systematic review. *Patient Education and Counseling, 102*(7), 1228–1236.

Miller, C. A., Biskupiak, A., & Kushalnagar, P. (2019). Deaf LGBTQ patients' disclosure of sexual orientation and gender identity to health care providers. *Psychology of Sexual Orientation and Gender Diversity, 6*(2), 194–203.

Mitchell, J. A., & Perry, R. (2020). Disparities in patient-centered communication for Black and Latino men in the U.S.: Cross-sectional results from the 2010 health and retirement study. *PLoS ONE, 15*(9), e0238356.

Papathanassoglou, E. D., & Mpouzika, M. D. (2012). Interpersonal touch: Physiological effects in critical care. *Biological Research for Nursing, 14*(4), 431–443.

Rathert, C., Mittler, J. N., Banerjee, S., & McDaniel, J. (2017). Patient-centered communication in the era of electronic health records: What does the evidence say? *Patient Education and Counseling, 100*(1), 50–64.

Roter, D. L., Hall, J. A., & Aoki, Y. (2002). Physician gender effects in medical education. *JAMA, 288*(6), 756–764.

Scott, A. M. (2022). Difficult conversations between healthcare providers and patients. In T. L. Thompson & N. G. Harrington (Eds.), *The Routledge handbook of health communication* (pp. 179–193). Routledge.

Shen, M. J., Peterson, E. B., Costas-Muniz, R., Hernandez, M. H., Jewell, S. T., Matsoukas, K., & Bylund, C. L. (2018). The effects of race and racial concordance on patient-physician communication: A systematic review of the literature. *Journal of Racial and Ethnic Health Disparities, 5*(1), 117–140.

Stewart, M., Brown, J. B., Weston, W. W., McWhinney, I. R., McWilliam, C. L., & Freeman, T. R. (2014). *Patient-centered medicine: Transforming the clinical method* (4th ed.). CRC Press.

Street, R. L., Jr. (2013). How clinician–patient communication contributes to health improvement: Modeling pathways from talk to outcome. *Patient Education and Counseling, 92*(3), 286–291.

Street, R. L., Jr. (2019). Mapping diverse measures of patient-centered communication onto the conceptual domains of patient-centered care. *Patient Education and Counseling, 102*(7), 1225–1227.

Street, R. L., Jr., Liu, L., Farber, N. J., Chen, Y., Calvitti, A., Zuest, D., Gabuzda, M. T., Bell, K., Gray, B., Rick, S., Ashfaq, S., & Agha, Z. (2014). Provider interaction with the electronic health record: The effects on patient-centered communication in medical encounters. *Patient Education and Counseling, 96*(3), 315–319.

Street, R. L., Jr., Makoul, G., Arora, N. K., & Epstein, R. M. (2009). How does communication heal? Pathways linking clinician-patient communication to health outcomes. *Patient Education and Counseling, 74*(3), 295–301.

Thompson, T. L., & Schulz, P. J. (2021). *Health communication theory.* Wiley Blackwell.

World Health Organization. (2021, July 14). *Vaccine efficacy, effectiveness, and protection.* https://www.who.int/news-room/feature-stories/detail/vaccine-efficacy-effectiveness-and-protection

Zwingmann, J., Baile, W. F., Schmier, J. W., Bernhard, J., & Keller, M. (2017). Effects of patient-centered communication on anxiety, negative affect, and trust in the physician in delivering a cancer diagnosis: A randomized, experimental study. *Cancer, 123*(16), 3167–3175.

In-class Activities

1. Have students complete the interactive Teach-back Training module outside of class (45 minutes: http://www.teachbacktraining.org/interactive-teach-back-learning-module). Then in class, do role plays, having one pair of students engage in a non-teach-back interaction and a second pair engage in a teach-back-driven interaction. The "provider" should come up with a medical condition for the "patient."

2. Drawing on Baile et al. (2000), review the four objectives of bad news delivery and the six-step SPIKES protocol for delivering bad news. Then watch the following videos on two different bad news delivery scenarios, and in small groups, have students discuss why, based on Baile et al. (2000) and any other observations, the excellent encounter was excellent and the other encounter was not.

Delivering bad news: What not to do. https://www.youtube.com/watch?v=HWAZnhCuAeE
Delivering bad news: An excellent encounter. https://www.youtube.com/watch?v=_uOS7hfKkVI

Discussion Questions

1. If you were to design a study of how communication affects health outcomes, what would you want to study? Use Street et al.'s (2009) model (communication functions, proximal outcomes, intermediate outcomes, health outcomes) to guide your answer.

2. How do patient-centered communication skills lead to the enactment of patient-centered medicine?

3. One of the types of difficult conversations Allison Scott (2022) identified was "charged topics." What other charged topics can you think of beyond those listed in the text? How might you navigate a conversation with a healthcare provider if you needed to bring up a charged topic? Think in terms of task, identity, and relational goals.

Life Is Complicated for the Montgomery Family

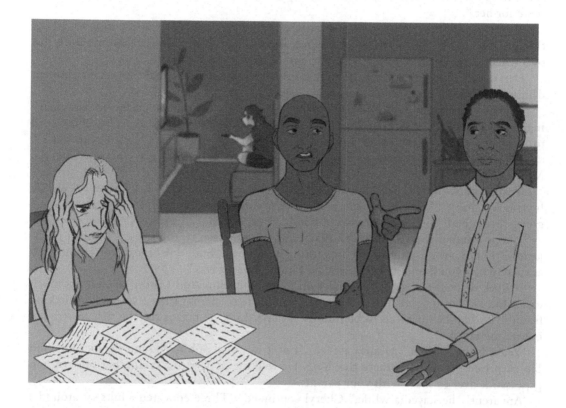

Uncertain is certainly the best word to describe how the Montgomery family was feeling over the next several months. Following a long-awaited diagnosis, which unfortunately turned out to be breast cancer, Helen was in the midst of a variety of medical appointments and waiting for a final treatment plan. To make matters worse, Samuel was starting to show signs of teenage mood swings, snapping at his parents and not wanting to participate in school activities anymore, especially ones related to sports. Cheryl knew that her family was starting to feel overwhelmed. Carrying her family's emotional stress plus the stress from her double major in pre-med and health comm was starting to add up. Whenever Cheryl started feeling this way, her first call (or in this case, Zoom) was always to Monica, who was starting her third year as an ER nurse.

"Have you heard anything from anyone today about how Grams is doing?" Cheryl asked Monica once she'd logged in.

DOI: 10.4324/9781003214458-9

"I think as well as can be expected, all things considered," Monica replied. "I do know she's been going to that breast cancer support group through the hospital. I think it's helping. She's dealing with so much now, and not just the cancer. I think she's feeling lost because she's always been our matriarch, and now that she's sick, it's like she's losing that role."

"But that's not true," Cheryl protested.

"It doesn't matter if it's true or not if that's how she feels. And all the information about breast cancer and the different treatment options. It's really overwhelming for her. I mean, I'm trying to help as best I can, but sometimes it just gets to be too much."

"Mom's helping, though, right?"

"Oh, yes. Your mom's taking Grams to all the support group meetings and doctor appointments. She's been invaluable. I really think she's helping Grams cope, just being there for her."

"She's the best. I do wish Grams was more comfortable joining an online support group, though. There'd be less driving her around. But I think all the different online tools just overwhelm her," Cheryl mused. "Is there any news on treatment yet?"

"Dad called yesterday and said he thought the doctors would be making some treatment decisions soon, but he couldn't give me any specifics."

"Do you know whether the doctors are involving Grams or your dad in the decision making?" Cheryl asked. "It's important for them to be involved, if they want to be. They need to know what choices they have. I read that it helps when patients can feel empowered."

"I'm not sure. It just seems to be taking so long. I'm starting to get worried, Cheryl," Monica shared.

"Yeah, I know. Me, too. Samuel texted me a picture yesterday," Cheryl shared. "While he was watching TV last night, our parents apparently sat at the table for over three hours going through all Grams' paperwork and bills. Everyone looked stressed. And worried."

"I hope Samuel was on his best behavior and not adding to the stress," Monica interjected. "I know he's having a hard time fitting in at school, but I don't recall you being quite as fussy when you found school hard, and I know I never was."

"I think he read the room and didn't make it about him. And I think school was much easier for us than it is for him. He seems to be having a harder time than we did making friends. It's like he's nervous to be himself. I don't think he means to take that frustration out on the family."

"Yeah, I can see that," Monica agreed. "But it was nice of him to send the picture. And I'm surprised my dad was there that long. He told me he was just taking her prescription paperwork over to share with your parents."

"Apparently he stayed a while," Cheryl continued. "Three educated adults sat around a table and struggled to organize and process a bunch of standard healthcare paperwork for one patient. Wild that it was that hard and stressful."

"Not at all," Monica stated. "Our healthcare system is a hot mess. The bureaucracy is ridiculous. Insurance companies can actually get in the way of treatment decisions that doctors and patients want to make. That had better not happen with Grams."

"No wonder everybody's so stressed."

Both women paused. Neither had anything comforting to say.

"Yes, well, one step at a time, I suppose," Monica said, finally breaking the silence. "Besides, *you* are finally starting to organize your med school applications. And all HBCUs, which I love for you. So you see, there are still reasons to be happy and hopeful."

"True. I'm excited. I can't believe I'm finally going to apply to medical school. If I actually get in, I might mail that awful counselor from high school a copy of my application as proof of how wrong she was," Cheryl joked.

"Ha! You should!" Monica laughed. "And you'll get in. I know it."

Through all the medical uncertainty and pending decisions facing the Montgomery family, Cheryl and Monica had found an essential support system in each other. They didn't yet realize just how important that support system was going to be. Almost a year from now, they would find themselves navigating even more uncertainty.

Notes

The term HBCU refers to Historically Black Colleges and Universities. There are 107 HBCUs in the United States. For a complete list of these schools, see here: http://www.thehundred-seven.org/hbculist.html

Managing the paperwork affiliated with medical care can feel overwhelming, particularly forms related to insurance. The podcast series *An Arm and a Leg*, a show about the outrageous cost of healthcare in the United States, featured this video to help explain complex insurance terms: https://armandalegshow.com/episode/brian-david-gilbert/. It's both entertaining and informative.

4   The Patient Experience

Heidi Ferrer was a Hollywood screenwriter, wife, and mother who was so vibrant and loving that her husband called her "sunshine in a dress" (Güthe, 2022, para. 5). In April 2020, Heidi contracted COVID-19. It was mostly asymptomatic at first, but then it turned into long COVID. Given her diagnosis early in the pandemic, substantial amounts of uncertainty surrounded her symptoms, treatment, and recovery. As her health declined over the next several months, Heidi experienced neurological tremors, extreme fatigue, and debilitating nerve pain, among many other horrible symptoms. By May 2021, she was bedridden. Her husband said, "Watching long Covid systematically take her apart, organ system by organ system, was the most terrifying deterioration of a human being I have ever witnessed" (Güthe, 2022, para 7). Struggling to cope with her situation, and with no end to her suffering in sight, Heidi committed suicide.

Long COVID affects millions of people (Centers for Disease Control and Prevention [CDC], 2022; University of Oxford, 2021). Although not all of them suffer to the extent that Heidi did, they do face profound uncertainty about their health. In addition, given the lack of medical knowledge about long COVID (Tufekci, 2022), patients are often ill-equipped to make treatment decisions, and they almost certainly are at a loss as to how to effectively cope. Although long COVID could be the poster child for challenges related to illness uncertainty, decision making, and coping, these concepts are encountered to some degree by anyone who faces an illness. Also coming into play is the concept of health literacy, or the extent to which people have the knowledge and skills needed to navigate their illness. These concepts are at the core of the patient experience and will be the focus of this chapter.

In this chapter, we'll explore health communication research on uncertainty, decision making, coping, and health literacy. Within each topic area, we'll cover how it has been conceptualized, its defining characteristics, and recent research findings. In addition, we'll review theoretical frameworks that have been applied to uncertainty, decision making, and coping, with Table 4.1 presenting summaries of the theories and models we chose to review.

Before we begin, we need to make two points. First, to say that there is a large body of literature on each of these topics is an understatement. We had to be quite selective in what we elected to include in the chapter. If you're interested in these topics, just know there is plenty more out there for you to learn. Also, although we are covering these topics separately for organizational purposes, they are all inextricably related and operate in concert to influence the patient experience. Keep that in mind as you read each section. All right, let's begin.

Uncertainty

Uncertainty is an inherent part of human existence, permeating all aspects of a person's life, from relationships with friends and family to interactions in educational settings and the workplace—and to the experience of health and illness. Communication scholar Dale

DOI: 10.4324/9781003214458-10

Table 4.1 Theoretical Frameworks for Patient Experiences

Theory/Model	Brief Summary	Citation
Communal Coping Framework	Stressful events are appraised and acted upon in the context of close relationships following one of four coping types: individual coping, support-seeking, parallelism, and communal.	Lyons et al. (1998)
Communication Privacy Management Theory	People "own" private information about themselves, and they follow implicit rules about what they share with whom and when. Other people who learn the private information become "co-owners" of it. If co-owners inappropriately share private information, the resulting "boundary turbulence" can harm the relationship.	Petronio (2002)
Health Disclosure Decision-making Model	The decision about whether to disclose personal health information involves three components: assessment of the health information, assessment of the receiver, and disclosure efficacy.	Greene (2009)
Social-contextual Model of Coping	Individuals, in connection with others, anticipate and cope with everyday life problems through one of four appraisal dimensions: isolated individual, parallel individual, indirect relational, and shared relational.	Berg et al. (1998)
Uncertainty in Illness Theory	Uncertainty results from the ambiguous, complex, and unpredictable nature of illness and is characterized by antecedents of uncertainty, appraisals, coping, self-organization, probabilistic thinking, and perspective.	Mishel (1988, 1990)
Uncertainty Management Theory	Uncertainty is a central part of human experience and interactions. The meaning of uncertainty varies by person and situation. People will try to reduce, maintain, or increase uncertainty depending on its meaning.	Brashers (2001)
Uncertainty Reduction Theory	Uncertainty is undesirable, and people will strive to reduce it so that their interactions with others will be more predictable.	Berger and Calabrese (1975)

Note. See *Supplemental Online Theory Table* for additional theories/models.

Brashers (2001), an expert on uncertainty in health, stated that "Uncertainty exists when details of situations are ambiguous, complex, or probabilistic; when information is unavailable or inconsistent; and when people feel insecure in their own state of knowledge in general" (p. 487). Think about the last time you were sick or when someone close to you was sick, and then think of all the uncertainty you had to deal with. There may have been questions about how you got sick in the first place, what treatment would entail, and how being sick would affect your life, among many other questions. Understanding the nature of uncertainty in illness and how people navigate that uncertainty helps researchers and practitioners provide recommendations and resources to improve the patient experience.

Broadly speaking, there are three types of health-related uncertainty: medical, personal, and social (Brashers et al., 2000; see also Babrow et al., 1998; Han et al., 2019). **Medical uncertainty** relates to several aspects of the clinical situation. The first is the nature of the disease and how information about it is communicated. Some diseases are quite straightforward, whereas others are incredibly complex. As you can imagine, communicating the meaning of a disease, including its etiology, diagnosis, prognosis, and treatment, becomes more complicated with increased disease complexity. Information characteristics such as *clarity, accuracy, completeness, amount,* and *ambiguity* can all influence the patient's uncertainty experience. A classic example is with clarity and how it's compromised when providers use medical jargon that patients simply do not understand. The second aspect of the clinical situation related to uncertainty is the state of scientific knowledge about the disease. This includes symptom patterns and whether symptoms are ambiguous, whether knowledge about the disease is advanced or rudimentary, probabilities surrounding disease progression and prognosis, and the efficacy and safety of treatment options. The third aspect is practical issues related to navigating the medical system. This includes *structures of care*, such as complex treatment regimens and complicated health insurance plans, and *processes of care*, such as the extent to which healthcare providers work together efficiently and whether they are fully competent (or perceived to be so by the patient). Together, these three situational aspects create uncertainty for patients about the medical facets of their illness. Patient uncertainty can also increase when providers, themselves, are navigating medically uncertain situations. In recent years, one of the most salient examples of this is the COVID-19 pandemic.

In an article about long COVID written for *The New York Times*, opinion columnist Zeynep Tufekci (2022) recounted how "Many clinicians who treat long Covid told me they just had to concoct treatment protocols themselves from experience and research and listening to the patients" and how "Primary care physicians are even less prepared. Patient after patient told me of even well-meaning doctors throwing up their hands because they simply didn't know where to begin" (n.p.). The medical uncertainty here is palpable, and it's not hard to see how physician uncertainty could increase uncertainty for patients. That's why Paul Han and colleagues (2019) argue that in addition to understanding the nature of patient uncertainty, how it originates, and how it affects patients, researchers also need to consider how uncertainty affects healthcare providers and stakeholders, and they need to understand *how* and *why* healthcare providers communicate uncertainty.

Personal uncertainty involves whether the illness will affect patient identity (e.g., active, independent) and roles (e.g., parent, breadwinner). It also involves unpredictable financial consequences faced by the patient because of their illness (e.g., potentially outrageous medical bills). Personal uncertainty can also be shaped by *lay epistemologies*, or a person's understanding of how the world works. Patients with different cultural perspectives likely have different lay epistemologies, which would influence their experience of illness uncertainty (Hsieh & Kramer, 2021). Furthermore, depending on the nature of the illness, existential concerns such as the meaning of life and death may characterize the personal uncertainty experience.

Finally, **social uncertainty** relates to unpredictable interpersonal reactions, such as encountering stigma, dealing with meddlesome or intrusive questions, and facing uncertain relationship implications. Some conditions or treatments are more likely to invite stigma, such as those that result in disfigurement (e.g., colostomies) or are perceived to be caused by unhealthy choices (e.g., lung cancer). Although social norms typically dictate that people

---

Definition and Types of Uncertainty

Uncertainty exists when details of situations are ambiguous, complex, or probabilistic; when information is unavailable or inconsistent; and when people feel insecure in their own state of knowledge in general.

The three broad types of health-related uncertainty are medical, personal, and social. Medical uncertainty relates to several aspects of the clinical situation. Personal uncertainty involves whether the illness will affect a patient's identity, roles, and finances and is influenced by their lay epistemologies. Social uncertainty relates to unpredictable interpersonal reactions in response to the patient's illness.

"mind their own business," patients inevitably face uncomfortable questions from people in their networks. How best to deal with those questions raises uncertainty. In addition, depending on the nature of the illness, even long-term relationships may face an uncertain future (Fugmann et al., 2022).

Brashers and colleagues (2000) originally identified the medical, personal, and social types of uncertainty in focus group interviews of people with HIV/AIDS, but these uncertainty types apply to any illness. For example, Lauren Perez and colleagues (2019) found that parents of children with type 1 diabetes experienced all three types of uncertainty. Importantly, their findings demonstrate how the nature of these uncertainties will vary across the illness trajectory. For instance, parents' medical uncertainty before diagnosis involved not understanding what type 1 diabetes was, but after diagnosis, it grew into concerns about having to manage daily care, such as monitoring insulin intake and blood sugar levels. Interestingly, these researchers found that personal uncertainty among parents primarily was defined in terms of financial uncertainty, which substantially increased after diagnosis. Dimensions of financial uncertainty included the exorbitant cost of diabetes treatment (thanks, Big Pharma and Congress!), whether costs would be covered by insurance, and how the children would manage costs once they reach adulthood. The uncertainty around finances was so pronounced that the authors argued financial uncertainty should be its own category. Finally, they found that "all participants experienced some form of social uncertainty with respect to not knowing how to deal with or interact with others about their child's illness" (Perez et al., 2019, p. 952). This uncertainty was reflected in worrying that disclosing their child's diagnosis might invite stigma and worrying that their child would never feel normal around other children and adults.

Beyond just classifying the three types of uncertainty, Perez et al. (2019) explored communication strategies used to manage uncertainty. The authors reported that most parents had appraised their uncertainty as negative and so sought strategies to reduce it. These strategies included seeking information from physicians, diabetes educators, and other sources to be able to better manage their child's diabetes; joining support groups; and using technology such as apps and medical devices to monitor their child's blood glucose levels. Some parents, however, preferred to maintain uncertainty, at least at first. These maintenance strategies involved temporarily deferring a diagnosis by rationalizing diabetes symptoms (e.g., hunger meant a growth spurt; thirst meant dehydration from too many outdoor sports). After diagnosis, maintaining uncertainty meant avoiding information that might cause stress and anxiety and temporarily putting the diagnosis out of mind. Examples of this behavior included avoiding online forums where parents saw other parents judging each other about the quality of care they were providing their children, which made them feel uncertain about the care they were providing to their own children. As you can tell, Perez et al. investigated several aspects of the uncertainty experience. In doing so, they had guidance from theory—uncertainty management theory, to be precise. It's to that theory, as well as some of the others that have been used to guide uncertainty research, that we turn our attention now.

Theorizing about Uncertainty

There are several theoretical approaches to studying uncertainty. The first came from Charles Berger and Richard Calabrese (1975), who developed **uncertainty reduction theory** to explain how strangers communicate during initial interactions. Their premise was that uncertainty was undesirable and that people would strive to reduce it so that their interactions with others would be more predictable. From there, interest in uncertainty burgeoned, with research leading to much more sophisticated conceptualizations of what uncertainty entails, the contexts in which it is experienced, and the strategies people use to manage it. Part of the advancements involved questioning basic assumptions such as whether all uncertainty is undesirable and whether people always strive to reduce it. As you saw with Perez et al.'s (2019) findings from parents of children with type 1 diabetes, for example, people do not always seek to reduce uncertainty. Merle Mishel's (1988, 1990) uncertainty in illness theory and Dale Brashers' (2001) uncertainty management theory are among those challenging these assumptions. Let's see how.

Uncertainty in illness theory suggests that uncertainty results from the "ambiguous, complex, and unpredictable" nature of illness, which makes it impossible for patients to "determine the meaning of illness-related events" (Clayton et al., 2018, p. 49). The original version of the theory (Mishel, 1988) focused on acute illness and described how *antecedents of uncertainty* influenced patients' cognitive *appraisals* of uncertainty as either a danger or an opportunity. Cognitive appraisals then affected how patients subsequently *coped* with uncertainty. Mishel (1990) later revised the theory to account for uncertainty in chronic illness, which had become more of a concern in patient populations, as well as to account for illnesses that might have a recurrence. The revised theory added the concepts of self-organization, probabilistic thinking, and the need to form a new life perspective and value system to deal with ongoing uncertainty (Clayton et al., 2018).

Uncertainty management theory focuses even more on the evaluative aspect of uncertainty and recognizes that in some situations, *maintaining* or even *increasing uncertainty* may be what is desired. This theory also emphasizes the role of communication in managing uncertainty:

> (a) information seeking can reduce uncertainty by allowing for better discrimination between or among alternatives; (b) information seeking can increase uncertainty by increasing the number of alternatives, or by blurring the distinction between or among alternatives; and (c) information avoidance can maintain uncertainty.
>
> (Brashers & Babrow, 1996, p. 246)

All these theories provide a slightly different perspective on uncertainty, but together, they provide a holistic understanding of what managing uncertainty entails.

To make these theories a little clearer, let's consider the situation of someone who has just been diagnosed with diabetes. Uncertainty reduction theory suggests that they would try to reduce the uncertainty around their diagnosis, such as by looking for additional information about diabetes. Uncertainty in illness theory, though, would suggest that such information seeking would not be done to reduce uncertainty but to help form a new life perspective on adapting to and living with a chronic illness that, by its very nature, will bring ongoing uncertainty. Finally, uncertainty management theory recognizes that the patient might want to maintain their current level of uncertainty or find new areas of uncertainty. They might do this because they aren't ready to process the diagnosis or feel unprepared to handle the treatment. How patients experience uncertainty and their response to it has implications for decision making, a topic we turn to next.

Decision Making

You'll remember that we discussed decision making in Chapter 3 in the context of patient-provider communication. Here, we focus on the patient's experience of the decision-making process. **Decision making** for patients begins with deciding whether to seek medical care in the first place (e.g., "Is this serious enough?") and, if so, when (e.g., "If this isn't better in a week, I'm calling Dr. Bombay"). When patients do decide to seek medical care, depending on the diagnosis (if there is one) there may be several treatment options or options may be limited. When there are options, the question becomes to what extent the patient is involved in the decision making. As a reminder, for many decades, physician-centered communication practices privileged the doctor in decision making and gave patients little say. Today, however, patient-centered communication and patient autonomy have become the norm, and patients can expect to be active participants in their own medical decision making. This process, called **shared decision making**, involves patients and their providers collaborating to reach a high-quality medical decision (Freytag & Street, 2022). But what exactly is involved in this process?

Jennifer Freytag and Rick Street (2022) list four components of shared decision making: (a) using the best clinical evidence, (b) considering the patient's values and preferences, (c) respecting the patient's desire to be involved in the decision-making process, and (d) assessing the feasibility of the decision. Let's consider each of these components briefly. First, sometimes clinical evidence is clear-cut. Other times, not much is known. Plus, medical knowledge is continually advancing, so best practices evolve over time. For example, there have been recent updates in recommendations regarding breast cancer screening, with different organizations (e.g., U.S. Preventive Services Task Force, American College of Radiology) supporting different recommendations (Lee et al., 2020). Developments like these can complicate patient decision making. Second, a patient's values and preferences should come into play at all decision points, especially when there are treatment options. Some women with breast cancer, for example, opt for full mastectomies even when less radical treatment is an option because they want to reduce the risk of recurrence as much as possible. Third, sometimes being patient-centered involves recognizing that the patient may prefer *not* to be involved in the decision-making process. The process can be taxing and intimidating, and some patients, especially those who are very ill, may prefer not to deal with such pressures. Even if patients are very involved during the decision-making process, they may defer the actual decision to the doctor. Finally, sometimes treatments just are not feasible in a particular situation. For example, a patient may want to participate in a clinical trial that's testing a promising new drug, but if the drug requires administration every other day by a physician, and the clinical trial is going on in a city two hours away from the patient's home, their participation may just not be possible. All four of these components need to be considered in medical decision making. Ultimately, the goal is to remember that decision making is, at heart, a communicative process that involves doctors and patients talking together to come to the "best" decision. Let's look at two systematic reviews to get a broader understanding of shared decision-making experiences among diverse populations.

The Four Components of Shared Decision Making

Four components go into shared decision making:

- Using the best clinical evidence
- Considering the patient's values and preferences
- Respecting the patient's desire to be involved in the decision-making process
- Assessing the feasibility of the decision

Victoria Basile and colleagues (2022) conducted a systematic review and meta-synthesis of 12 qualitative studies that investigated Australian, Canadian, and U.S. rural cancer patients' experiences with shared decision making. They identified four broad themes, the first of which they labeled, "Is there even a choice?" Disconcertingly, the authors determined that rural cancer patients were rarely given a choice in treatment decisions and often didn't even know there even was a choice. For those who did have a choice, the themes of personal factors, societal influences, and medical care came into play. In terms of *personal factors*, finances had to be considered both in terms of the actual cost of care at local versus metropolitan treatment centers and in terms of indirect costs that would be accrued with travel to urban settings, such as transportation and lodging costs. Availability of social support at different locations also was important, as was convenience, ease, and familiarity. *Societal influences* came in the form of cultural norms, which sometimes led to fatalistic views, skepticism, and ambivalence, as well as a desire to avoid disfiguring surgeries that would violate the sacredness of the body. Also at play were the opinions of family members and friends, who sometimes took an active role in decision making. Finally, in terms of *medical care*, patients invariably reported wanting to make "treatment decisions in line with receiving the best medical care possible" (p. 2699). A trusting patient-provider relationship with strong rapport also influenced decision making. For example, a patient in one of the studies stated that she would defer to her provider: "Whatever he decides for me, that's what I'm going to do" (p. 2699). The authors conclude that their results "illuminate the ongoing challenges facing rural cancer patients in treatment decision-making" and that the situation could be improved with the expansion of specialty rural treatment centers, social and financial support for patients who must travel to metropolitan clinics, and the expansion of telehealth options to reduce the need for travel.

In another systematic review, Antonio DeRosa and colleagues (2022) considered the literature on decision-making interventions for racial and ethnic minority breast or prostate cancer patients. One of their goals was to determine whether the interventions had an impact on patient quality of life outcomes. They identified 10 studies that met inclusion criteria, one of which was having at least 30% of the study population be racial or ethnic minorities. They found evidence of several positive outcomes from the interventions: Patients' decision-making self-efficacy increased; they felt more informed, supported, involved, and better able to communicate with healthcare providers; they understood their treatment options better and had less decisional conflict; and they were more likely to adhere to treatment, including chemotherapy. DeRosa et al.'s findings suggest that decision-making interventions targeting racial and ethnic minority communities can effectively support breast and prostate cancer patients with both decision making and improved patient outcomes. However, having found only 10 studies to review, they called for additional research in this area that would focus on "social determinants of health, social support outcomes, and clinical outcomes" (p. 1064).

Like communication skills, skills in making high-quality, informed decisions do not just come naturally. Instead, people often need some assistance. Fortunately, there are research-based tools available to help patients and physicians make informed decisions. These tools are called **decision aids**, and they "prepare people to participate in decisions that involve weighing benefits, harms, and scientific uncertainty" (Stacey et al., 2012, p. 2). Decision aids are especially helpful "when there is more than one reasonable option, when no option has a clear advantage in terms of health outcomes, and when each option has benefits and harms that patients may value differently" (Stacey et al., 2012, p. 4). There are numerous decision aids available from multiple sources, and they range from helping people make general to specific decisions. For example, the Ottawa Personal Decision Guide (n.d.) was designed for people making general health decisions. A two-page, interactive form, it asks questions to help people clarify their decisions; explore decision options in terms of knowledge, values, (un)certainty, and available support; identify decision-making needs across those same dimensions; and plan next steps based on their needs. Patients can fill this guide out on their own and use it to facilitate discussions about health decisions with family and providers. Other decision guides are meant to be used in consultation with healthcare providers. For example, the Mayo Clinic's Knowledge and Evaluation Research

Unit has as part of its mission to create decision aids (or what they call conversation tools) "for patients and clinicians to use together to make treatment choices in line with patient values and preferences" (Care That Fits, n.d., para. 3). They offer decision aids for numerous medical conditions, including treatment for chest pain, depression, diabetes, osteoporosis, and rheumatoid arthritis, among others. These tools are available in print or online. But do decision aids work?

In a review for the Cochrane Collaborative, Dawn Stacey and colleagues (2012) assessed the literature on the processes and outcomes of medical decisions made using decision aids. The researchers identified 86 studies involving more than 20,000 participants to include in their review. They considered *decision attributes* (knowledge, risk perception, and value-based choices) and *decision-making process attributes* (feeling informed and feeling clear about values). They found that decision aids increase knowledge, improve accurate risk perceptions, and result in decisions that are both informed and consistent with patients' values. They also found that decision aids improve physician–patient communication and, most importantly, increase patient involvement in decision making.

Theorizing about Decision Making

In addition to making decisions about their illness, patients must also make decisions about the communicative work of disclosing their diagnoses to other people. Sandra Petronio's (2002) **communication privacy management (CPM) theory** and Kathryn Greene's (2009) **health disclosure decision-making model (DD-MM)** lay groundwork for understanding this process. The key idea behind Petronio's CPM is that people believe that they "own" the private information about themselves and they have a right to control it in terms of what aspects they share, as well as when and with whom they share. People also have implicit rules for revealing or concealing their private information; the rules are shaped by culture, gender, motivation, context, and a risk-benefit ratio. Other people who learn the private information, either because they're told about it or happen to discover it somehow, become *co-owners* of the information, and with co-ownership come certain rights and responsibilities regarding what to share when and with whom (if at all). To avoid missteps, co-owners should negotiate how the information may or may not be shared with anyone else. If they don't and information is inappropriately shared, *boundary turbulence* results, which will lead to relationship troubles. Let's consider an example to make this all a little clearer.

Let's say that Marilyn gets the results of a pap smear through her electronic health record, and it shows she's tested positive for HPV. She doesn't know much about HPV, including what symptoms to expect, so she's scared and starts to cry. Just then, her roommate, Angie, comes home and asks what's wrong. Caught off guard by Angie's return, Marilyn hesitantly shares the diagnosis. Angie reassures Marilyn that everything will be okay. Weeks later, it gets back to Marilyn that Angie has told three of their friends about the diagnosis, and Marilyn is furious. She screams, "I told you that in confidence!" Angie gets defensive and snaps back, "Hey, you never said I couldn't tell anyone, and they're our friends anyway," to which Marilyn replies, "I shouldn't have to tell you to keep something like that quiet!" Can you see the communication problem here? Clearly, Marilyn and Angie were operating under different privacy management rules. Perhaps Marilyn should have given her decision to disclose her test results a little more thought. That's where Greene's DD-MM can help.

Greene (2009) realized that although CPM was extremely helpful in conceptualizing privacy management, what it didn't address were "the factors that people weigh in these disclosure decision processes" (p. 226). That's what her model does. Specifically, the DD-MM breaks down the disclosure decision-making process into three components. The first component is an *assessment of the health information* along five characteristics: stigma, preparation, prognosis, symptoms, and relevance to others. In Marilyn's case, she was dealing with a stigmatized diagnosis that she wasn't prepared for. She was unsure of the prognosis and what symptoms to expect. Therefore, she shared the diagnosis, which was not really relevant to Angie, without having thought things through. The second component is an *assessment of the receiver*, wherein relational quality and the receiver's anticipated response are considered. Marilyn and Angie were good friends and roommates, and Marilyn anticipated receiving emotional support from Angie upon disclosure, which in her mind, made it safe to disclose. Finally, the third component is *disclosure efficacy*. For disclosure efficacy, "Both confidence and skills are needed to share a difficult message such as a health diagnosis, although at times disclosers *do* share with trepidation, apprehension, and considerable uncertainty" (p. 242). In our example, Marilyn disclosed to Angie because she was surprised by Angie's return home. Marilyn's hesitation to tell Angie was an indication that maybe she wasn't ready to disclose just yet. Regardless of when or how someone ultimately discloses their health information, an important thing to keep in mind about this communicative work is that disclosure, especially with chronic disease, is not a one-and-done situation (Greene, 2009, p. 232):

> Rather, there is a continual disclosure process regarding treatment options, coping, and disease progression. People are constantly in a process where decisions have to be made about sharing updates, not simply the initial diagnosis. Thus, the process is complex, and people can simultaneously disclose some aspects yet avoid sharing other information.

To wrap up our review of decision making, we thought it might interest you to know that there is an **International Shared Decision Making Society (ISDM)**. The ISDM (2023) was founded in 2018 in Hamburg, Germany. They'd been hosting an international conference for several years and decided it was time to form an official society. Today, members represent a diverse group of academic researchers, healthcare practitioners, educators, patient partners, and others interested in promoting research, training, and practice in person-centered care and shared decision making in healthcare settings around the world. ISDM's website lists several resources, including decision aids, teaching materials, and evaluation measures. They also published a special issue of the journal *Health Expectations* based on one of their conferences (Barry et al., 2011). The issue contains articles that address basic issues of what defines a shared medical decision; how to implement patient decision aids, particularly considering the needs of special populations (underserved, chronically ill, multicultural); how to measure the effects of shared decision making; and how to teach shared decision-making skills to healthcare providers. The level of academic and professional interest in this topic is heartening and suggests how important shared decision making is to the patient experience. Whatever decisions patients reach, and by whatever means, they still have to cope with their illness and the challenges it brings to their lives.

Coping

Coping is defined as "ongoing cognitive and behavioral efforts to manage specific external and/or internal demands that are appraised as taxing or exceeding the resources of the person" (Lazarus, 1993, p. 237). Important in this definition is the concept of appraisal. We've mentioned this term a few times already, and now, in a big reveal, we're finally going to define it. An **appraisal** is a person's "cognitive evaluation of the nature and significance of a phenomenon or event" (American Psychological Association, 2023, n.p.). Just as two patients can have vastly different illness experiences from the same disease, so can they appraise their illness in different ways depending on a variety of individual, societal, cultural, and systemic factors. Although it's easy to see how illness appraisals would likely be quite negative, and rightly so, it is possible to make positive appraisals, as well. And the idea that people do have the capacity to control their attitudes and responses to external events is a powerful one.

There are numerous taxonomies of coping styles in the literature, and there's no agreement among researchers about what the core categories are (Stanislawski, 2019), but across the various taxonomies, five styles appear consistently (Berardi et al., 2019). A **problem-focused** coping style involves taking action to manage the illness as much as possible. For example, you might buy cold medicine if you think you have the flu. An **emotion-focused** coping style involves dealing with emotions in some capacity. This could be taking a walk to clear your head after being diagnosed with an unexpected disease. A **seeking-understanding** coping style involves trying to find meaning in the illness experience. For some patients, this could be deciding to enroll in a clinical trial and being comforted by knowing that the research findings might help someone in the future. A **seeking-help** coping style involves turning to others for social support (see Chapter 7). For example, patients commonly join support groups for people who share the same diagnosis. Finally, an **avoiding-the-problem** coping style involves attempting to ignore the illness. This could mean withholding the diagnosis from loved ones for as long as possible. Patients will adopt one or more of these styles in response to their illness and, within the styles, enact different strategies that can be more or less adaptive (helpful) or maladaptive (harmful). For example, health information seeking (which we explore next in Chapter 5) would be an example of adaptive problem-focused coping. Turning to alcohol or other drugs to "numb out" would be an example of maladaptive avoidance. Let's look at a study that examined using humor in blog posts as a means of adaptive coping.

Nick Iannarino (2018) conducted a thematic narrative analysis of three young adult cancer survivors' blogs to discover how these individuals used humor as a means of coping with their emotions. He noted that the National Cancer Institute identified young adults (aged 18–39 years) diagnosed with cancer as a "distinct group that experiences unique social, emotional, and transitional challenges from treatment through survivorship" (p. 1233). By examining the blogs of these three young adults, he hoped to learn more about how they "view themselves and make sense of their experience, gain and lose agency, make and justify health decisions, and navigate social relationships, particularly while using humor as a communicative tool to facilitate these ends" (p. 1233). In total, Iannarino analyzed 370 blog entries, each of which "focused on the narrator's daily experience with the condition (cancer)" (p. 1235). He found a rich trove of examples of humor being used to cope.

For example, one blogger named Matt used dark humor to create a character named Bob who was "evil incarnate" (Iannarino, 2018, p. 1236). (We'll spare you the gory details.) Matt made Bob be the one suffering from leukemia so Matt could distance himself and his wife from the experience. Matt also used sarcasm extensively, such as when, after discovering his type of cancer had been written into an episode of "Law & Order," he wrote, "This is the first time I can remember [being] 'part of' something dramatized on TV. And it had to be cancer. What the fuck? Why not 'Girls Gone Wild'? Or a documentary on the lives of lottery winners?" (p. 1236). Matt was not alone in his use of humor for coping.

A blogger named Megan, who nicknamed herself "shortcolon" because of her colon cancer surgery, endured multiple rounds of chemotherapy. In recounting what a rational brain might say about getting chemo, she wrote that her hindbrain screamed, "Nooooooooooooooo! No likey!" (Iannarino, 2018, p. 1237). As she neared the end of her treatment, she compared her anticipated joy to "the last few weeks of school where you know if you can make it through finals you'll have the WHOLE summer" (p. 1237). But when she found herself still harboring fear that the cancer may return once the chemo stopped, she concluded that she was experiencing "Chemo Stockholm Syndrome" (p. 1237).

Finally, a blogger named Kaylin had been diagnosed with Ewing's sarcoma, a rare bone cancer. As she tried to make sense of changes to her body due to chemo, she realized she looked like "Tank Girl, her favorite comic book character: 'I completely see it when I look in the mirror: Buzzed head; body scarred, bruised, bloodied, and bandaged from all of the blood draws…Enter Cancer Girl'" (pp. 1238–1239). Kaylin later started drawing a full-length comic featuring Cancer Girl. She said she wanted to give other cancer patients "something hilarious and uplifting to read while getting poison pumped into you" (p. 1239). These three young adult cancer survivors demonstrate how using humor helped them cope with the fear, uncertainty, and ravages of cancer treatment.

A universal experience we all have shared is having had to cope with the COVID-19 pandemic. Although there were countless coping mechanisms employed during the pandemic (some more successful than others), research suggests that technology was an especially vital tool for coping. This probably won't come as much of a surprise, but technology provided a means for filling important gaps in social support needs, such as through video conferencing, streaming live events, and engaging in online forums. Such services allowed many social activities, such as holiday gatherings, workouts, office parties, and religious services, to continue (Garfin, 2020). Although technology is not a perfect solution to all problems, it can serve as an important tool in the coping process.

Theorizing about Coping

Clearly, there is a lot to cope with when someone becomes ill. They don't have to go it alone, though. Many of the leading communication models about coping focus on coping as a social phenomenon. Indeed, a concept called **communal coping** speaks to this point. Renee Lyons and colleagues (1998) wrote, "Communal coping is a process in which a stressful event is substantively appraised and acted upon in the context of close relationships" (p. 583). The researchers classify coping along "appraisal" and "action" dimensions. The appraisal dimension answers the question, "Whose problem is this?" The action dimension answers the question, "Who's taking responsibility for the problem?" Answers to these questions reflect either an individual or shared orientation. Crossing the dimensions with the answers results in four possible coping types: individual coping ("It's my problem, and I'll take care of it"), support-seeking ("It's my problem, but will you help me?"), parallelism ("This is a problem for both of us, but I'm going to handle it"), and communal ("This affects both of us, so let's work together to deal with it"). Erin Basinger observed that evidence for all four styles of coping had been found in qualitative research, but they had never been validated quantitatively. So, she set out to evaluate this communal coping framework.

Basinger (2020) recruited 159 individuals with type 2 diabetes to participate in her study. She chose diabetes because although it affects individuals, it's managed in the context of family relationships, theoretically allowing all four coping styles to operate. Participants completed a questionnaire that included measures of the appraisal and action dimensions of communal coping, along with measures of family cohesion, self-care, adherence, and depressive symptoms. Participants were told to think about their family members when responding to the communal coping items, which included statements such as "I feel like I am the only one with ownership of my diabetes" (appraisal subscale item) and "My family members and I have joined together to deal with my diabetes" (action subscale item). Basinger's results showed that the data supported three coping styles, not four as predicted by the model. The three styles were individual coping, communal coping, and ambivalent coping. Individual and communal coping aligned with the original conceptualizations in the communal coping model. Ambivalent coping was characterized by moderate scores on the appraisal subscale items and low to moderate scores on the action subscale items, "indicating mixed feelings about who had ownership of the illness or who acted on it" (p. 590). Results showed that the ambivalent coping style was not related to any of the outcome measures. A communal coping style, however, was positively related to self-care (exercise), whereas an individual coping style was negatively related to self-care (exercise, blood glucose monitoring, and diet). Basinger concluded that "coping alongside one's family members is advantageous, whereas coping in isolation is detrimental" (p. 593).

Also exploring a communal approach to coping, Cynthia Berg and colleagues (1998) proposed a **social–contextual model of coping**. This model is similar to the communal coping framework in that it also includes four dimensions centered on the idea of coping as a social process experienced with others (called "social units"). It varies, however, in that it accounts for the fact that individuals can indirectly transfer their stress to another person. Through this lens, the four dimensions of appraisal are *isolated individual* (a stressor is perceived by one person, who is coping alone), *parallel individual* (a stressor is perceived by both individuals, who are coping separately), *indirect relational* (a stressor is leading one person to create new stress experienced by others), and *shared relational* (a stressor is perceived by both individuals who are coping together). The authors argue that "the social nature of many everyday problems and stressors is better captured by a formulation of stress, appraisal, and coping that recognises that stress may impact and be dealt with by social units as well as individuals" (Berg et al., 1998, p. 258). This model highlights the stressful impact of illness beyond the individual patient, a topic we'll explore further when we address caregivers in Chapter 7.

There are a lot of resources available on coping. The next time you find yourself in need of coping strategies, we recommend reading the tips provided by the CDC (2021). In addition to tips specifically for parents/caregivers, kids/teens, and school personnel, the CDC provides general coping strategies for anyone in need. These include taking breaks from media, making time to unwind, eating healthy, and recognizing when you need help. This is good advice whether you're coping with illness or coping with life in general. Let's all keep this in mind as we take a breath and move on to our final section in this chapter: health literacy.

Health Literacy

Think for a minute about everything you need to know to be able to manage your health effectively. If you're currently healthy, you need to have knowledge about how to stay healthy, such as following a specific diet or exercise plan and avoiding certain health risks. If you're sick, then you need to have knowledge about how to navigate the healthcare system so you can receive appropriate care, and then you need to be able to follow whatever care instructions you're given, such as filling and taking a prescription or making a lifestyle change. In other words, you need to be health literate. As noted by former U.S. Surgeon General Regina M. Benjamin (2010), numerous studies have shown that poor health literacy is related to poor health status and health disparities. Shockingly, however, 88% of Americans are not considered to be proficient in health literacy (Kutner et al., 2006). Fortunately, health literacy interventions have been shown to improve health literacy and health behavior (Walters et al., 2020). Therefore, understanding health literacy and ways to improve it is paramount to promoting global health. So what exactly is health literacy?

The term health literacy was coined by Scott Simonds (1974), a professor of health education who argued that "Minimum standards for 'health literacy' should be established for all grade levels K through 12" (p. 9). By the 1990s, the term had moved into the healthcare literature (Parnell, 2014) and quickly became a major focus of health research. Although many definitions were offered by various sources, the one developed for the National Library of Medicine and subsequently used in *Healthy People 2010* was the one that gained the strongest traction. This definition states that **health literacy** is "The degree to which individuals have the capacity to obtain, process, and understand basic health information and services needed to make appropriate health decisions" (Nielsen–Bohlman et al., 2004, p. 32). This definition puts the focus on the *individual* and their ability to use health information appropriately. Recent developments in the area, however, have recognized the importance of *systemic influences* on health literacy, so much so that the Healthy People initiative (see Chapter 1) now recognizes two broad areas of health literacy: personal health literacy and organizational health literacy.

The definition of **personal health literacy** is quite similar to the original definition: "the degree to which individuals have the ability to find, understand, and use information and services to inform health-related decisions and actions for themselves and others" (Healthy People 2030, n.d., para. 3). **Organizational health literacy**, though, is defined as "the degree to which organizations equitably enable individuals to find, understand, and use information and services to inform health-related decisions and actions for themselves and others" (Healthy People 2030, n.d., para. 3). The *Healthy People 2030* report highlights the ways in which these updated definitions differ from the original. First, the updated definitions emphasize that people need to be able to *use health information*, not just understand it. Second, people's health decisions should be *well informed*, not just appropriate. And third, the focus moves beyond the individual to include *organizational* and *public health perspectives*, as well as the responsibility of health organizations to play an active role in addressing and advancing health literacy. Moving forward, the literature we review will be referencing the original conceptualization of health literacy because that's what was in use at the time the work was published. However, the principles certainly apply to the updated definitions, as well.

There are four core components to health literacy (Nielsen–Bohlman et al., 2004). **Print literacy** refers to the ability to read and write. This skill is needed for anything involving printed materials, such as educational brochures and consent forms. **Oral literacy** involves the ability to listen and speak, which allows people to seek, verify, and provide information, as well as negotiate shared meaning and understanding with their healthcare providers. In other words, this skill is essential to effectively engage in patient-provider communication. **Numeracy** means having knowledge of basic mathematics and statistics, which is necessary for everything from reading nutrition labels and understanding prescription medication directions (e.g., take one teaspoon three times per day) to comparing health insurance plans (e.g., cost, co-pays, deductibles) and comprehending risks of various treatment options. Finally, having **cultural and conceptual knowledge** is necessary for understanding health and illness across cultural contexts, comprehending the meaning of health conditions, and conceptualizing the risks and benefits of treatment.

There are three additional components that should be considered as part of any comprehensive approach to health literacy. The first is media literacy. **Media literacy** originally was defined as "the ability to access, analyze, evaluate and create media in a variety of forms" (Jolls, 2008, p. 42), but the Center for Media Literacy now calls it "a 21st century approach to education" that "provides a framework to access, analyze, evaluate, create and participate using messages in a variety of forms—from print to video to the internet" (p. 42). When you consider the impact that the media can have on health (see Chapter 12; also see Chapter 11's section on direct-to-consumer advertising), it's easy to see why media literacy should be a component of health literacy: The ability to critically consume media information influences people's health decisions.

The second additional component is **eHealth literacy**, which is defined as "the ability to seek, find, understand, and appraise health information from electronic sources and apply the knowledge gained to addressing or solving a health problem" (Norman & Skinner, 2006, n.p.). As you'll learn from Chapter 5, there's a vast amount of health information available these days right at your fingertips, but not all of it is created equal. eHealth literacy is crucial to successfully navigating the online environment, knowing which information is trustworthy and which is nothing but junk. These days, eHealth literacy should also include the ability to navigate the online environment well enough to be able to use patient portals and have telehealth visits.

The third additional component is scientific literacy. Although a definitive definition of **scientific literacy** is elusive (Laugksch, 2000), it can be thought of as the ability to understand how new knowledge is created through the scientific method, from positing hypotheses to collecting and analyzing data to interpreting results and drawing valid conclusions. These days, scientific literacy is essential to avoid falling for mis- and disinformation about health. For example, the poor folks who believed that a drug made to treat parasites in animals would work to treat COVID-19, when it actually could be *lethal* to humans, clearly did not understand even the basics of the scientific method or drug development (Palmer, 2021). When the U.S. Food and Drug Administration (2021) has to issue a tweet saying, "You are not a horse. You are not a cow. Seriously, y'all. Stop it," you know we're in trouble. So, the importance of scientific literacy, as well as all the other facets, is clear. So we have all these components of health literacy, but is there a way to assess it? We're glad you asked.

Definitions and Types of Health Literacy

Health literacy was originally defined as the degree to which individuals have the capacity to obtain, process, and understand basic health information and services needed to make appropriate health decisions. The *2030 Healthy People* report, however, distinguishes between personal and organizational health literacy. This distinction recognizes that health literacy is not the responsibility of the patient alone.

Four core components of health literacy are print literacy, oral literacy, numeracy, and cultural and conceptual knowledge. Additional components include media literacy, eHealth literacy, and scientific literacy.

In health communication research, assessing health literacy levels is important, so as you might imagine, there is a multitude of measures of health literacy in the literature. They range from assessing general health knowledge to context-specific knowledge (e.g., diabetes), they assess various dimensions of health literacy (e.g., word recognition, reading comprehension, numeracy), and they range in length from a single question ("Single Item Literacy Screener"; Morris et al., 2006) to nearly 70 questions ("Test of Functional Health Literacy in Adults [TOFHLA]"; Parker et al., 1995). For many years, the TOFHLA was the preferred measure of health literacy, considered to be the most accurate assessment tool. But given difficulties in implementing it, such as the need to complete it face-to-face and its length, researchers have worked to create new scales that can be more efficiently implemented. One of the newest is called the Newest Vital Sign (NVS; Weiss et al., 2005).

It consists of six questions designed to measure reading and numeracy, and it's available in English and Spanish. It has been validated against the TOFHLA, which means it's considered to be an accurate measure of health literacy. Perhaps most important, it can be administered in under three minutes...and it comes in the form of an ice cream nutrition label. (Yum!)

The NVS questions are very much application focused (word problems—yay!). Patients are shown the nutrition label and asked to calculate how many calories they would consume if they ate the entire pint of ice cream (and come on, who doesn't do that?). They also are asked how much ice cream would contain 60 grams of carbs, how much saturated fat they would consume in their regular diet if they cut out their usual one serving of ice cream per day, and what percentage of their daily calories are in one serving of ice cream (a measly half cup takes up 10% of total daily calories). In addition, they're asked whether it would be safe to eat the ice cream if they were allergic to peanuts (the label lists peanut oil as an ingredient), and if patients answer "No," they're asked to explain why not. Patients get a point for every item they answer correctly. Scores of 0–1 indicate low health literacy; scores of 2–3 indicate limited literacy; and scores of 4–6 indicate adequate literacy. Kayce Shealy and Tiffaney Threatt (2016) conducted a systematic review of studies investigating the NVS and found that it's been used in a variety of practice settings (although mainly in primary care) and that it's been used with ethnically diverse patients who have a wide range of health conditions. Following their review, the authors conclude that the NVS has demonstrated validity as a measure of health literacy.

A very important consideration in all of this is the extent to which culture influences health literacy. This consideration includes how researchers interpret scores on measures of health literacy. On one level, considering culture involves recognizing that speaking English as a second language or not speaking English at all introduces significant challenges to understanding and acting on health information. However, on another, more sophisticated level, considering culture means recognizing that differences in health beliefs, customs, world views, and sociocultural identities will influence the way people "interpret and act on health information" (Zarcadoolas et al., 2005, p. 197), as well as how they interact with healthcare professionals. Elaine Hsieh and Eric Kramer (2021) discuss how differences in high- and low-context cultures influence perceptions of health literacy. Western medicine reflects a **low-context culture**, which means that people rely extensively on detailed, explicit information exchanged between individuals to derive meaning. In this culture, a health-literate patient would be expected to ask a lot of questions of their physician. On the other hand, people from a **high-context culture** derive meaning from implicit understandings shared among members of the community. In a high-context culture, asking direct questions of a physician, a clear figure of authority, would be well outside cultural norms—but *not* an indication of low health literacy. Hsieh and Kramer encourage everyone to remember that "The differences in patterns of information-seeking and information sharing should not be simply attributed to individuals' health literacy or lack thereof. Rather, we should reconsider the complexity and inter-relationships between the implicit cultural construction of health literacy" (p. 176). So, when it comes to measuring health literacy with an ice cream nutrition label, a low score may *not* actually reflect low health literacy for patients from diverse cultures. Instead, it "may suggest that the test-takers employ different modes of speaking, understanding, thinking, and communication than the test makers" (Hsieh & Kramer, 2021, p. 175).

You might have noticed that unlike the last three sections, this section doesn't mention communication theory. Surprisingly, there is actually a dearth of theory on the communicative processes surrounding health literacy. As Linda Aldoory (2017) notes, "There have been some beginning forays into theory development...but none of them has been replicated to

Table 4.2 U.S. National Action Plan to Improve Health Literacy

---

1. Develop and disseminate health and safety information that is accurate, accessible, and actionable
2. Promote changes in the health care system that improve health information, communication, informed decision-making, and access to health services
3. Incorporate accurate, standards-based, and developmentally appropriate health and science information and curricula in child care and education through the university level
4. Support and expand local efforts to provide adult education, English language instruction, and culturally and linguistically appropriate health information services in the community
5. Build partnerships, develop guidance, and change policies
6. Increase basic research and the development, implementation, and evaluation of practices and interventions to improve health literacy
7. Increase the dissemination and use of evidence-based health literacy practices and interventions

---

Note. From U.S. Department of Health and Human Services, Office of Disease Prevention and Health Promotion (2010).

the point of elaboration and application" (p. 215). Instead, much of the research has focused on developing valid and reliable ways to measure health literacy. Given the substantial developments in this area (as reviewed above), we anticipate that theories centered on health literacy should be forthcoming from health literacy scholars in the not-too-distant future.

When push comes to shove, what's important to remember is that health literacy is not solely the responsibility of the patient. Instead, as with everything involving communication, the responsibility rests with everyone involved, including both patients and providers, as well as the organizational structures and systems in which healthcare is delivered and the societal forces that influence health and health behavior. It's also important to recognize that although health literacy may be *necessary*, it is in no way *sufficient* to ensure that people engage in the healthy behaviors advocated by providers. Large-scale systemic change is needed to ensure that everyone has equitable access to the healthcare resources they need. A health-literate population is but one component of that. Still, it's good to know that the United States has developed a *National Action Plan to Improve Health Literacy* (U.S. Department of Health and Human Services, 2010). We present the plan's seven goals in Table 4.2. As you can see, the plan recognizes both individual and systemic influences on health literacy. We think it's a step in the right direction.

Conclusion

Hardly anybody wants to be a patient, yet nearly everyone becomes one at some point in their lives. As you've learned in this chapter, the patient experience entails uncertainty in multiple forms, involves frequently complicated decision making about not only medical treatment but also illness disclosure, requires coping in one or more forms, and benefits from proficiency in health literacy. There's a lot going on for the patient. And when you add to that the fact that patients often are in pain, afraid, and sometimes ashamed, it's not a pretty picture. That's why it's important for everyone to work together to improve the patient experience in any way we can. One person in the fight is Diana Berrent.

Diana was one of the first people to test positive with COVID-19. She worked tirelessly to seek information on testing and treatment and eventually became Participant #0001 in a clinical trial conducted by Columbia University to study how the blood and plasma of COVID-19 survivors might help with treatment for others with the virus. In the process, Diana became a fervent advocate and activist, and she established Survivor Corps, "one of the largest grassroots movements, providing education and resources for COVID-19 patients, connecting them with medical and scientific research efforts, and helping with the national response" (Survivor Corps, 2022, para 1.). Part of Survivor Corps' mission involves helping people with long COVID. If you visit one of their Facebook pages, you'll be able to read the stories of thousands of people experiencing the whims and vagaries and ravages of this disease, and in those stories, you'll witness firsthand the patient experience. Hopefully, with the help of Survivor Corps and the thousands of clinicians and scientists and others working on the frontlines of this pandemic, patients like Heidi Ferrer will soon have the treatment they need to survive.

References

Aldoory, L. (2017). The status of health literacy research in health communication and opportunities for future scholarship. *Health Communication, 32*(2), 211–218.

American Psychological Association. (2023). *Appraisal.* https://dictionary.apa.org/appraisal

Babrow, A. S., Kasch, C.R., & Ford, L. A. (1998). The many meanings of uncertainty in illness: Toward a systematic accounting. *Health Communication, 10*(1), 1–23.

Barry, M., Levin, C., MacCuaig, M., Mulley, A., & Sepucha, K. (2011). Shared decision making: Vision to reality. *Health Expectations, 14*, 1–5.

Basile, V. A., Dhillon, H. M., Spoelma, M. J., Butow, P. N., May, J., Depczynski, J., & Pendlebury, S. (2022). Medical treatment decision-making in rural cancer patients: A qualitative systematic review and meta-synthesis. *Patient Education and Counseling, 105*, 2693–2701.

Basinger, E. D. (2020). Testing a dimensional versus a typological approach to the communal coping model in the context of type 2 diabetes. *Health Communication, 35*(5), 585–596.

Benjamin, R. M. (2010). Surgeon General's perspectives: Improving health by improving health literacy. *Public Health Reports, 125*, 784–785.

Berardi, L., Glantsman, O., & Whipple, C. R. (2019). Stress and coping. In L. A. Jason, O. Glantsman, J. F. O'Brien, & K. N. Ramian (Eds.), *Introduction to community psychology* (pp. 243–261). https://open.umn.edu/opentextbooks/textbooks/738

Berg, C. A., Meegan, S. P., & Deviney, F. P. (1998). A social-contextual model of coping with everyday problems across the lifespan. *International Journal of Behavioral Development, 22*(2), 239–261.

Berger, C. R., & Calabrese, R. J. (1975). Some explorations in initial interaction and beyond: Toward a developmental theory of interpersonal communication. *Human Communication Research, 1*, 99–112.

Brashers, D. E. (2001). Communication and uncertainty management. *Journal of Communication, 51*(3), 477–497.

Brashers, D. E., & Babrow, A. S. (1996). Theorizing communication and health. *Communication Studies, 47*(3), 243–251.

Brashers, D. E., Neidig, J. L., Haas, S. M., Dobbs, L. K., Cardillo, L. W., & Russell, J. A. (2000). Communication in the management of uncertainty: The case of persons living with HIV or AIDS. *Communication Monographs, 67*(1), 63–84.

Care that Fits. (n.d.). *For care to be effective it must respond well to a patient's situation.* https://carethatfits.org/

Centers for Disease Control and Prevention. (2021). *Coping with stress.* https://www.cdc.gov/violenceprevention/about/copingwith-stresstips.html

Centers for Disease Control and Prevention. (2022, August 12). *Estimated COVID-19 burden.* https://www.cdc.gov/coronavirus/2019-ncov/cases-updates/burden.html

Clayton, M. F., Dean, M., & Mishel, M. (2018), Theories of uncertainty. In M. J. Smith & P. R. Liehr (Eds.), *Middle range theory for nursing* (4th ed., pp. 49–81). Springer.

DeRosa, A. P., Grell, Y., Razon, D., Komsany, A., Pinheiro, L. C., Martinez, J., & Phillips, E. (2022). Decision-making support among racial and ethnic minorities diagnosed with breast or prostate cancer: A systematic review of the literature. *Patient Education and Counseling, 105*, 1057–1065.

Freytag, J., & Street, R. L., Jr. (2022). Mutual persuasion as patient-centered communication. In T. L. Thompson & N. G. Harrington (Eds.), *The Routledge handbook of health communication* (3rd ed., pp. 165–178). Routledge.

Fugmann, D., Boeker, M., Holsteg, S., Steiner, N., Prins, J., & Karger, A. (2022). A systematic review: The effect of cancer on the divorce rate. *Frontiers in Psychology, 13*, Article 828656.

Garfin, D. R. (2020). Technology as a coping tool during the COVID-19 pandemic: Implications and recommendations. *Stress and Health, 36*, 555–559.

Greene, K. (2009). An integrated model of health disclosure decision-making. In T. D. Afifi & W. A. Afifi (Eds.), *Uncertainty, information management, and disclosure decisions: Theory and application* (pp. 226–253). Routledge.

Güthe, N. (2022, January 12). *My wife had long Covid and killed herself. We must help others who are suffering.* https://www.theguardian.com/commentisfree/2022/jan/12/long-covid-wife-suicide-give-others-hope

Han, P. J. K., Babrow, A., Hillen, M. A., Gulbrandsen, P., Smets, E. M., & Ofstad, E. H. (2019). Uncertainty in health care: Towards a more systematic program of research. *Patient Education and Counseling, 102*, 1756–1766.

Healthy People 2030. (n.d.). *Health literacy in Healthy People 2030.* https://health.gov/healthypeople/priority-areas/health-literacy-healthy-people-2030

Hsieh, E., & Kramer, E. M. (2021). *Rethinking culture in health communication: Social interactions as intercultural encounters.* Wiley Blackwell.

Iannarino, N. T. (2018). "My insides feel like Keith Richards' face": A narrative analysis of humor and biographical disruption in young adults' cancer blogs. *Health Communication, 33*(10), 1233–1242.

International Shared Decision Making Society. (2023). *About us.* https://www.isdmsociety.org/about-us/

Jolls, T. (2008). *Literacy for the 21st century: An overview & orientation guide to media literacy education* (2nd ed.). Center for Media Literacy.

Kutner, M., Greenberg, E., Jin, Y., & Paulsen, C. (2006). *The health literacy of America's adults: Results from the 2003 National Assessment of Adult Literacy (NCES 2006–483).* U.S. Department of Education. National Center for Education Statistics.

Laugksch, R. C. (2000). Scientific literacy: A conceptual overview. *Science Education, 84*, 71–94.

Lazarus, R. S. (1993) Coping theory and research: Past, present, and future. *Psychometric Medicine, 55*, 234–247.

Lee, C. S., Monticciolo, D. L., & Moy, L. (2020). Screening guidelines update for average-risk and high-risk women. *American Journal of Roentgenology, 214*(2), 316-323.

Lyons, R. F., Mickelson, K. D., Sullivan, M. J. L., & Coyne, J. C. (1998). Coping as a communal process. *Journal of Social and Personal Relationships, 15*(5), 579–605.

Mishel, M. H. (1988). Uncertainty in illness. *Journal of Nursing Scholarship, 20*(4), 225–232.

Mishel, M. (1990). Reconceptualization of the uncertainty in illness theory. *Journal of Nursing Scholarship, 22*(4), 256–262.

Morris, N. S., MacLean, C. D., Chew, L. D., & Littenberg, B. (2006). The Single Item Literacy Screener: Evaluation of a brief instrument to identify limited reading ability. *BMC Family Practice, 7*, Article 21.

Nielsen-Bohlman, L., Panzer, A. M., & Kindig, D. A. (Eds.). (2004). *Health literacy: A prescription to end confusion.* Institute of Medicine of the National Academies Press.

Norman, C. D., & Skinner, H. A. (2006). eHealth literacy: Essential skills for consumer health in a networked world. *Journal of Medical Internet Research, 8*(2), e9.

Ottawa Personal Decision Guide. (n.d.). *Ottawa Personal Decision Guide: For people making health or social decisions.* https://decisionaid.ohri.ca/docs/das/opdg.pdf

Palmer, A. (2021, August 31). *Amazon pushes deworming drug falsely touted as Covid treatment.* CNBC. https://www.cnbc.com/2021/08/31/amazon-pushes-deworming-drug-falsely-touted-as-covid-treatment.html

Parker, R. M., Baker, D. W., Williams, M. V., & Nurss, J. R. (1995). The test of functional health literacy in adults: A new instrument for measuring patients' literacy skills. *Journal of General Internal Medicine, 10*(10), 537–541.

Parnell, T. A. (2014). Health literacy: History, definitions, and models. In T. A. Parnell (Ed.), *Health literacy in nursing: Providing person-centered care* (pp. 3–31). Springer Publishing Company.

Perez, L., Romo, L. K., & Bell, T. (2019). Communicatively exploring uncertainty management of parents of children with Type 1 diabetes. *Health Communication, 34*(9), 949–957.

Petronio, S. (2002). *Boundaries of privacy: Dialectics of discourse.* State University of New York.

Shealy, K. M., & Threatt, T. B. (2016). Utilization of the Newest Vital Sign (NVS) in practice in the United States. *Health Communication, 31*(6), 679–687.

Simonds, S. K. (1974). Health education as social policy. *Health Education Monographs, 2*(1 supplement), 1–10.

Stacey, D., Bennett, C. L., Barry, M. J., Col, N. F., Eden, K. B., Holmes-Rovner, M., Llewellyn-Thomas, H., Lyddiatt, A., Légaré, F., & Thomson, R. (2012). Decision aids for people facing health treatment or screening decisions (Review). *Cochrane Database of Systematic Reviews 2011*, Issue 10. Article CD001431.

Stanislawski, K. (2019). The coping circumplex model: An integrative model of the structure of coping with stress. *Frontiers in Psychology, 10*, Article 694.

Survivor Corps. (2022). *Home.* https://www.survivorcorps.com/

Tufekci, Z. (2022, August 25). *If you're suffering after being sick with Covid, it's not just in your head.* https://www.nytimes.com/2022/08/25/opinion/long-covid-pandemic.html

University of Oxford. (2021, September 29). *Over a third of COVID-19 patients diagnosed with at least one long-COVID symptom.* https://www.ox.ac.uk/news/2021-09-29-over-third-covid-19-patients-diagnosed-least-one-long-covid-symptom

U.S. Department of Health and Human Services, Office of Disease Prevention and Health Promotion. (2010). *National action plan to improve health literacy.* https://health.gov/our-work/national-health-initiatives/health-literacy/national-action-plan-improve-health-literacy

U.S. Food & Drug Administration [@US_FDA]. (2021, August 21). *You are not a horse. You are not a cow. Seriously, y'all. Stop it.* [Tweet]. Twitter. https://twitter.com/us_fda/status/1429050070243192839?lang=en

Walters, R., Leslie, S. J., Polson, R., Cusack, T., & Gorely, T. (2020). Establishing the efficacy of interventions to improve health literacy and health behaviours: A systematic review. *BMC Public Health, 20*, Article 1040.

Weiss, B. M., Mays, M. Z., Martz, W., Castro, K. M., DeWalt, D. A., Pignone, M. P., & Hale, F. A. (2005). Quick assessment of literacy in primary care: The Newest Vital Sign. *Annals of Family Medicine, 3*(6), 514–522.

Zarcadoolas, C., Pleasant, A., & Greer, D. S. (2005). Understanding health literacy: An expanded model. *Health Promotion International, 20*(2), 195–203.

In-class Activities

1. Put students in small groups. Have them think about the last time they went to see a healthcare provider because they or a loved one were sick. As a group, identify at least three sources of uncertainty in each major category of uncertainty (medical, personal, and social). How was that uncertainty managed? Be specific in terms of information seeking or avoiding behaviors.

2. Divide students into small groups. Assign each group to read one of the blog entries by Dr. Elana Miller on her experience being diagnosed with and treated for cancer: https://zenpsychiatry.com/tag/elanas-personal-story/. Have them identify coping strategies used by Dr. Miller as she progressed through her cancer treatment and share them with the class. ("The Slog," dated August 27, 2014, is a particularly powerful entry.)

Discussion Questions

1. Watch the video on shared decision making from the Mayo Clinic: https://carethatfits.org/shared-decision-making/. Discuss your impressions of the shared decision-making process and outcomes as described by the physician. How does this compare to your experiences with health decision making?

2. Why is assuming that everyone wants to reduce their health and illness-related uncertainty problematic? What are some reasons that patients may want to maintain or increase uncertainty?

3. This chapter presented seven components of health literacy (print, oral, numeracy, cultural and conceptual knowledge, media, eHealth, and scientific). Do you think some components are more important than others? If you had to rank them, which would be most and least important? Why?

Searching for Information...and Hope

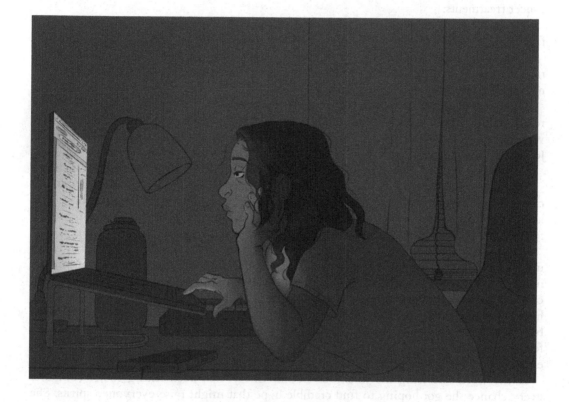

A year later, graduation was finally a few weeks away. Cheryl had already completed her coursework and was counting down the days until she was free of undergrad—albeit medical school at her first choice HBCU would start shortly after. Despite no forthcoming homework or exams, she found herself at her computer, conducting research late into the evening.

"How late are you staying up?" Liz asked, popping her head into Cheryl's room.

"I hope not much longer. But probably a bit. Are you going someplace?" Cheryl asked, noticing Liz was holding her car keys.

"I thought I'd go grab some pizza. Want some?" Liz offered.

"Sure. Thanks, Liz," Cheryl replied, forcing a smile for her friend. After living together the past four years, three of them in an off-campus apartment they decided to share after their first year in the dorm, Cheryl knew that Liz could tell that she was a bit down lately.

DOI: 10.4324/9781003214458-11

Although it had been well over a year since Helen's breast cancer diagnosis, Helen's health had been weighing heavy on Cheryl's mind lately. Initially, she'd been trying to stay out of the way of Sally and everyone attempting to help her grandmother navigate this difficult time. Maybe, deep down, she used that as an excuse to try to stay focused on finishing her schoolwork. Regardless, it was clear that she could no longer sit on the sidelines when it came to helping her grandmother make the most informed decisions regarding her treatment options. Because the chemotherapy was not working as well as hoped, Helen would need to make some difficult decisions over the next few months.

Part of Cheryl's motivation to gather more information came from her frustration with Aunt Savannah, who had called a virtual family meeting last week, getting everyone excited about what she had found online about a promising way to enhance the efficacy of breast cancer treatments.

"Okay, okay. No more waiting. What did you find?" Cheryl insisted as Samuel, the last family member to join, finally took a seat next to Sally.

A big smile came across Savannah's face. She was clearly excited to share the information she had been sitting on for a few days. "Okay," she began. "Change her deodorant to natural deodorant!"

There was complete silence on the Zoom. After a moment, Cheryl heard a small slap and realized that Monica had loudly put her hand to face. Everyone was starting to fidget as they waited for someone to say something. Uncle Michael started rubbing the bridge of his nose, Joe was looking at Sally, and even Samuel, now 15, had his head on the table.

"Savannah. Really? That was your big news?" Sally asked, finally breaking the silence.

"Wait, let me explain," Savannah insisted. "Someone posted that wearing deodorant causes breast cancer. And the reason the chemo isn't working well is because the cancer keeps coming back if the person is continuing to use deodorant. Helen just needs to switch to a natural deodorant so the chemo will work the way it's supposed to."

Cheryl was relieved that her grandmother was not on the call to hear this. It was not uncommon for her Aunt Savannah to share and recommend random things from the internet, but this was clearly the most outrageous and upsetting. Five minutes later, everyone had found their words and was making it quite clear how upset they were that Savannah had gotten their hopes up with blatant misinformation. Savannah, in turn, was so offended by their reaction that she abruptly ended the video call on the entire family. To feel for a few days that there might be hope just to be let down so quickly by misinformation took an emotional toll on Cheryl that she didn't see coming.

In the week following the infamous Zoom, Cheryl had been sitting at her computer every chance she got hoping to find credible hope that might raise everyone's spirits. She couldn't help but feel grateful for the skills she had learned in her communication classes about finding and evaluating online information. Although her Aunt Savannah was clearly the worst at information seeking, it seemed like her entire family was struggling to find health information that would actually be helpful to her grandmother—and struggling in a myriad of different ways. For instance, Cheryl had to explain to her dad that WebMD is not a credible source. And then she had to convince her mom that clinicians are not the *only* credible sources of available information. She was shocked that neither parent realized that the National Cancer Institute had amazing online information resources. She knew that seeking health information was tricky, but she was truly surprised by how differently everyone was navigating the situation. At least both her parents were receptive to Cheryl's feedback and tips.

In all fairness, she wasn't the only family member with the skills to acquire credible information. Samuel had become a regular researcher following his insistence on becoming the next Greta Thunberg. As Samuel would say, "If Greta relies on rigorous research to lead a global effort, then so can I!"

Cheryl knew that she wouldn't find everything she needed to help her grandmother in one evening. But she was ready to keep seeking health information for as long as her grandmother needed.

"Pizza!" Liz shouted from the front door of their apartment. "And because our lease ends in three weeks and we'll be going our separate ways, I've decided having dinner together from now till then isn't optional."

"I love that!" Cheryl shouted back as she closed the lid of her laptop. Maybe once she started medical school, someone in her program would have some helpful and hopeful information.

Notes

The misbelief that antiperspirants cause breast cancer is not uncommon. The American Cancer Society provides a thorough review discrediting the notion here: https://www.cancer.org/cancer/risk-prevention/chemicals/antiperspirants-and-breast-cancer-risk.html.

In addition, the National Cancer Institute provides a host of credible resources on cancer: https://www.cancer.gov/.

5   Health Information Seeking

Think about the last time you didn't feel good. Did you Google your symptoms? Call a doctor to schedule a visit? Ask a friend or relative for advice? Search online for remedies? Chances are you did at least one of these things—and maybe even all of them or more. And your goal? Seeking information to help you feel better. Information is knowledge. It's how people learn and what they use to make decisions. Seeking information is a ubiquitous part of life, and thus it deserves an entire chapter and our undivided attention.

Health information seeking research is a cornerstone of the health communication discipline. Understanding information seeking behaviors provides communication scholars with strategies for reaching individuals with credible information, for recognizing information gaps that might exist, and for identifying disparities in health information access. Within this body of research, some scholars have relied on data collected as part of an ongoing project by the National Cancer Institute (NCI; n.d.): the **Health Information National Trends Survey (HINTS)**. HINTS gathers data annually from a nationally representative sample of Americans on their health information seeking behaviors. The purpose of HINTS is to monitor changes in the rapidly evolving fields of health communication and health information technology and to develop more effective health communication strategies to reach different populations. Much of the research cited in this chapter will reference data analyzed from the HINTS project. Although the survey questions change slightly from year to year, the primary goal of describing the health information landscape remains consistent.

This chapter will explore health information seeking behaviors, including different types and sources of health information, as well as information seeking's relationship to health literacy. Following this overview, we'll present key theoretical frameworks for information seeking research. In addition, we'll examine three health-related behaviors supported by health information seeking: coping, decision making, and health management. Finally, we'll delve into the implications of online health information seeking and health reporting, areas that hold both promise and peril.

What Is Health Information Seeking?

Let's begin with exploring how we define health information. Dale Brashers and colleagues (2002) defined information as "stimuli from a person's environment that contribute to his or her knowledge or beliefs" (p. 259). **Health information**, then, is health-related stimuli contributing to people's health-related knowledge or beliefs. Many definitions of health information seeking exist throughout the communication literature. And if you're thinking that the definition is something along the lines of looking for health information, you're not far off. In a 10-year review of research on health information seeking behaviors, Margaret Zimmerman and George Shaw (2020) found that most studies defined **health information seeking** as "an active or purposeful behaviour undertaken by an individual with the

DOI: 10.4324/9781003214458-12

objective of finding information about health" (p. 176). Within the body of the literature these authors reviewed, they identified four distinct areas of research on health information seeking.

First, numerous studies explored "seeking and finding health information in order to cope with a health threatening situation" (Zimmerman & Shaw, 2020, p. 177). These studies were predominantly focused on diabetes, cancer, and chronic illness, and they described types of information sought, preferred information channels, and demographic differences in information seeking behaviors. Second, studies exploring "involvement in medical decision making" centered on determining the type and amount of information needed for individuals to feel prepared to participate in decision making (p. 178). The research in this area centered internet use and online information seeking as a means for facilitating medical decision making. Third, studies examined how health information seeking can lead to behavior change and engagement in prevention behaviors. Typically, these studies "predict that higher knowledge levels about a medical condition or practice will result in positive behaviour change" (p. 179). Finally, more recent research has focused on health information seeking when a health motivation is not present—in other words, when there's not a stimulus triggering the need to seek health information. Findings from this type of research can be helpful in identifying where information should be made available if and when it's needed. You'll find all four areas of research demonstrated throughout this chapter.

Before we move on from the definition of health information seeking, we want to draw your attention to an important phrase you might have overlooked in Zimmerman and Shaw's (2020) definition: "active or purposeful" (p. 176). Although it's not uncommon to come across health information you weren't looking for, something researchers call **passive health information seeking**, most communication research focuses on intentionally looking for health information, a behavior called **active health information seeking**. This is not to say that passive health information seeking, often called *information scanning* (Niederdeppe et al., 2007), is not important. In fact, Robert Hornik and colleagues (2013) assert that information scanning may positively influence personal health through three cognitive mechanisms. First, "scanning may increase the probability of exposure to and recall of new information" (p. 3), which may increase your health literacy. Second, "scanned exposure may reinforce descriptive or subjective norms" (p. 3), which may theoretically improve your health behavior. And third, "scanning may remind a person of the reasons for engaging in a behavior" (p. 3), which also may improve your health behavior. But unless otherwise specified, research studies reviewed in this chapter consider information seeking as active.

Health communication scholars have proposed numerous systems for organizing types of health information seeking behaviors. Many of these systems distinguish between **depth** (how long) and **breadth** (how much) of health information seeking (So et al., 2022). For example, let's pretend that we have two friends who were diagnosed with monkeypox. We'll call them Chris and Jess. Chris spends five hours reading 10 articles on treatment options, and Jess spends one hour reading two articles on treatment options. Given this information, you might assume that Chris' health information seeking behavior better prepared them to make treatment decisions than Jess'. However, depth and breadth do not account for **quality** or type of information (So et al., 2022). Going back to the example of searching for monkeypox treatment options, if all 10 of Chris' articles were on the same treatment option and written by non-medical professionals, but the two articles Jess read were on two different options and written by medical professionals, it's possible that Jess' health information seeking behavior better prepared them to make treatment decisions. The point of this scenario is that all information is not equally helpful, and you cannot assume that quantity of information is a substitute for quality of information. In fact, health information seeking behaviors are characterized by a combination of information breadth, depth, and quality. And finding a balance among the three can be difficult.

For example, Evan Kennedy and Susan Thibeault (2020) conducted a study to explore how 405 U.S. transgender individuals seek health information to navigate challenges of voice-gender incongruence (one's voice sounding inconsistent with social expectations for the pitch and timbre of gendered voices). They found that 78% of participants were concerned about the quality of information, 65% felt frustrated during their search for information, 58% reported that information seeking took a lot of effort, and 42% felt that the information was hard to understand. Regarding credibility of the source of information, 92% of participants trusted LGBTQIA+ community organizations, 88% trusted speech-language pathologists, 64% trusted clinicians, and 56% trusted websites. Such research findings provide communication researchers with a lens into how groups are currently perceiving health information, where they're searching for it, and what they feel is challenging about finding health information.

Challenges in finding, as well as understanding, health information are inextricably linked to health literacy, which, as you'll recall from the previous chapter, is an individuals' ability to obtain, process, and understand the basic health information and healthcare services needed to make good health decisions. Indeed, research shows health literacy is one of the most influential factors affecting a person's likelihood to seek health information (Chang & Huang, 2020), with greater health literacy related to greater information seeking. For example, in a survey of more than 900 Korean adults, Yong-Chan Kim and colleagues (2015) found that higher health literacy levels were associated with a wider range of accessing information sources and a higher perceived ability to find, process, and understand health information. Similar results have also been found for U.S. adults, with lower numeracy associated with increased difficulties in finding and communicating about health information (Manganello & Clayman, 2011). What about when people want to avoid information, though? How do they manage that? Joshua Barbour and colleagues can speak to that.

Barbour et al. (2012) conducted surveys with 925 students and community members to determine how prevalent **health information avoidance** was and why and how people avoided health information. They found that 52.6% of respondents reported having not wanted to hear about a health issue in the past and 34.5% said they had tried to avoid health information. The data revealed six reasons that people wanted to avoid health information: (a) *maintain hope or deniability* (e.g., postpone hearing a diagnosis), (b) *resist overexposure to information* (e.g., from the news and health campaigns), (c) *accept the limits of action* (e.g., when there was nothing they could or should do about the situation), (d) *manage flawed information* (e.g., to avoid mis- or disinformation or information that was too technical), (e) *maintain boundaries* (e.g., in relation to privacy and taboo topics), and (f) *continue with life/activities* (e.g., ignoring information about unhealthy behavior so they could continue engaging in it guilt-free). In addition, respondents reported two strategies for avoiding health information. The first was *removing or ignoring sources of health information* by controlling exposure to media and avoiding certain people, medical visits, and diagnostic tests. The second was *controlling conversations about health* by changing the subject, making jokes, interrupting, or even telling people directly that they did not want the information, as well as by withholding information that would lead to unsolicited provision of health information.

Health information seeking is an important skillset for acquiring the necessary information to make informed health decisions. In addition to depth, breadth, and quality of health information seeking, communication researchers are also interested in where people find health information. In the next section, we'll consider both online and offline channels for health information seeking.

Online and Offline Health Information Seeking

Information channels are typically classified as either *online* (e.g., social media, websites, apps) or *offline* (e.g., print, interpersonal). Given the ubiquity of the internet, the vast majority of recent communication research is focused on online health information seeking. Between 2018 and 2020, HINTS data showed that 72.1% of adults had searched online for health information for themselves, 56.9% had done so for someone else, and 72.7% most recently turned to the internet first when they needed information (NCI, n.d.). This is in stark contrast to HINTS data from 2003 showing that 59% of adults reported paying no attention to information about health online and 66% of adults reported using the internet to look for health information less than once every few months.

Research exploring online health information is broad, covering everything from the various platforms providing health information to health information seeking behaviors on a particular health topic. For example, in a study examining how the social media platform Reddit is used for health information seeking among college students, Rachael Record and colleagues (2018) found that the platform was a source of information for users on a wide range of health topics, including everything from exercise to cancer to general nutrition. They found that almost a third of Redditors used the platform for seeking health-related information. As part of their investigation, the researchers were interested in the extent to which users would try the advice they found on Reddit. They expected to find that people who used Reddit more often and users who perceived the information as credible would be the most likely to try the things they learned on Reddit. (Seems like a reasonable expectation to us.) But actually, they found neither of those things to be supported by the data. What did they find, you ask? Following the health advice was not about how often someone used Reddit generally but, instead, about how often they used it specifically to search for health information. That is, Record et al. found that the more people used the platform to search for health-related information, the more likely they were to try the things they learned on Reddit. So, it seemed that actively seeking information on the platform had a role to play in whether Redditors followed the advice they found. This was regardless of how credible they perceived the information to be. The authors postulated that the reason for this is because the platform, itself, is perceived as credible and so information posted on it would be perceived as credible by virtue of the platform.

Although offline information channels are no longer the primary channel of health information seeking for most people, they're still essential sources of information—and certainly more consistently credible than online information. HINTS data in 2019 reported that second to the internet, adults turn to providers for health information. Prior to the internet, providers were the main source of health information, serving as a form of gatekeeper between patients and health information. In fact, as recently as 2017, HINTS data showed that when adults imagined a strong need for health information, they reported that they would be most likely to reach out to a provider (NCI, n.d.).

Preferences for online and offline sources have been shown to vary by groups. For example, in a survey of more than 1,300 Asian American immigrants in New York City, Nadia Islam and colleagues (2016) found that Chinese, Korean, and Bangladeshi immigrants relied most on print media, whereas Asian Indian immigrants relied most on televised sources. In addition, Korean, Bangladeshi, and Asian Indian immigrants relied the least on radio sources, whereas Chinese immigrants relied the least on the internet. Similarly, in a comparison of American and Chinese individuals' health information seeking as reported in 2017 HINTS data, Linqi Lu and colleagues (2020) found that American adults, regardless of race or ethnicity, were more likely to seek health information online and, consistent with Islam et al.'s findings, Chinese adults were more likely to seek offline sources of health information. Knowing where communities and groups are turning for information is key to advocating for information to be available through those sources.

A final consideration for health information channels is a recognition of the disparities in health information access. These disparities can be best identified through two media frameworks (see Table 5.1). First, the **knowledge gap hypothesis** postulates that "as the infusion of mass media information into a social system increases, segments of the population with higher socioeconomic status tend to acquire this information at a faster rate than the lower status segments," which results in gaps in knowledge tending to "increase rather than decrease" (Tichenor et al., 1970, pp. 159–160). Second, recall from Chapter 1 that the **digital divide** is "the gap that exists between individuals advantaged by the internet and those individuals relatively disadvantaged by the internet" (Rogers, 2001, p. 100). Like the knowledge gap, the digital divide is perpetuated by differences in socioeconomic characteristics, such as "the disparity in access across classifications of race, gender, age, income, and education" (Colby, 2001, p. 124). Because people have to have access to information sources before they can seek health information, these two frameworks call attention to the social responsibility to recognize that health information, although at historical highs in terms of availability, is still not equally accessible, and thus not equally helpful, to all groups of people. In order to promote equitable opportunities for health information seeking, resources are needed to provide access, such as through universal broadband, and navigational support, such as through media literacy training, for underserved communities that experience these gaps at their widest.

Table 5.1 Theoretical Frameworks in Information Seeking

Theory/Model	Brief Summary	Citation
Comprehensive Model of Information Seeking (CMIS)	The act of health information seeking is a product of individual characteristics, beliefs about information seeking, and the quality of the found information.	Johnson and Meischke (1993)
Digital Divide	A gap exists between individuals advantaged by the internet and individuals relatively disadvantaged by the internet because of differences in access and utilization.	Rogers (2001)
Knowledge Gap Hypothesis	As mass media information increases, individuals with higher socioeconomic status acquire the information at a faster rate than individuals with lower socioeconomic status, furthering gaps in knowledge between the two groups.	Tichenor et al. (1970)
Risk Information Seeking and Processing Model (RISP)	There are six characteristics that influence an individual's decision to seek and process health information: individual characteristics, informational subjective norms, risk characteristics and affective response, information sufficiency, perceived information gathering capacity, and beliefs surrounding relevant channels.	Griffin et al. (1999)
Theory of Motivated Information Management (TMIM)	Individuals deciding to seek information undergo three phases during the information-seeking and management process: interpretation, evaluation, and decision.	Afifi and Morse (2009)

Note. See *Supplemental Online Theory Table* for additional theories/models.

Theoretical Perspectives on Health Information Seeking

The body of health information seeking research is arguably one of the most theoretically grounded bodies of research within the communication discipline. Indeed, numerous theoretical frameworks have been developed to explore and explain the underlying communicative processes surrounding the behavior of health information seeking. The following paragraphs will review the tenets of three of these frameworks: the comprehensive model of information seeking (CMIS; Johnson & Meischke, 1993), the risk information seeking and processing model (RISP; Griffin et al., 1999), and the theory of motivated information management (TMIM; Afifi & Morse, 2009; see also Table 5.1). For all three theories, information-seeking behaviors are understood as determined by individual difference factors and health information characteristics. There are important differences across these theories, though, which we'll highlight through presenting a recent example of how each theory has been applied in research. To conclude, we'll explore how a researcher would consider choosing between the three theories for their studies.

Comprehensive Model of Information Seeking

The **comprehensive model of information seeking** (CMIS; Johnson & Meischke, 1993) was originally proposed to highlight the processes underpinning cancer-related information seeking. CMIS argues that there are six key variables, four regarding individuals and two regarding information, that predict health information seeking actions. For individuals, the model considers *demographics* (e.g., age, race, sex), *personal experiences* (e.g., personal symptoms with the condition, knowing someone with the condition), *perceived information salience* (believing that the information about the condition is actionable), and *beliefs* (regarding the efficacy of medical treatments for the condition). For information, the model considers information carrier factors, which include *characteristics* (specifics of the message content, such as tone and style) and *utility* (the extent to which the information meets the needs of the individual). In whole, this model suggests that the act of health information seeking is a product of individual characteristics, beliefs about information seeking, and the quality of the found information. The beliefs about information are key to this model. Specifically, David Johnson and Hendrika Meischke posit that a person who does not believe having information about a problem will change the situation will never search for information related to the problem, whereas a person who does believe more information can change the situation is motivated to search for health information to make that change (Lalazaryan & Zare-Farashbandi, 2014).

Over the last three decades, the CMIS has been revisited by communication theorists to consider changes in technology and diversity of use, with much of the applied research continuing to examine the information seeking behaviors among cancer patients. For example, Stephanie Van Stee and Qinghua Yang (2018) analyzed 2014 HINTS data to examine online cancer information seeking behaviors of U.S. adults. They found that the individual health-related factors of demographics, beliefs, and interest predicted utility which, in turn, predicted online health information seeking behaviors about cancer. Similarly, they found that characteristics of information carrier predicted both utility and online health information seeking behaviors. In this study, utility was understood as a combination of trusting information about cancer from the internet, having confidence in medical safeguards protecting medical records, and having confidence that advice or information about cancer could be found if needed. In addition, and unique to the model, the researchers found that individuals who were the most worried about cancer were the most likely to have sought health information about cancer in the last year. Overall, their results demonstrate how

CMIS can help shed light on health information seeking processes within the context of online cancer-related information seeking.

Risk Information Seeking and Processing Model

The **risk information seeking and processing model** (RISP; Griffin et al., 1999) suggests that there are six characteristics that influence an individual's decision to seek and process health information. *Individual characteristics* (e.g., demographics, acceptance of risk-reduction policies, past experience with a health risk) will influence the other five characteristics of *informational subjective norms* (perceived normative influences motivating the desire for information), *risk characteristics and affective response* (sense of risk and emotional response), *information sufficiency* (confidence in the knowledge one has), *perceived information gathering capacity* (efficacy of information seeking), and *beliefs surrounding relevant channels* (e.g., trustworthiness, usefulness). Through these characteristics, the RISP model takes an audience-based focus on information seeking that considers the development and maintenance of preventive health behaviors.

The RISP model has been broadly used across the health communication literature to examine health information seeking behaviors, with research findings largely supporting the original model. For example, in a study of 1,000 South Korean adults, Doo-Hun Choi and Ghee-Young Noh (2021) applied RISP to examine how people are motivated to seek information about obesity. In their investigation, they also included measures of health consciousness (an individual's motivation to sustain good health) and autonomous motivation (the extent to which an individual endorses a behavior based on their volition and choice), anticipating that these variables would mediate the relationship between subjective norm and information sufficiency, as well as subjective norm and information seeking. Their analyses supported the propositions of RISP, including the addition of health consciousness and autonomous motivation to the model.

Theory of Motivated Information Management

The **theory of motivated information management** (TMIM; Afifi & Morse, 2009) postulates that individuals who are seeking information undergo three phases before engaging in information management. In the *interpretation phase*, individuals assess the difference between how much uncertainty they're experiencing and how much uncertainty they want to have. This difference, which produces an emotional response such as anxiety, hope, or anger, is called uncertainty discrepancy. Uncertainty discrepancy is seen as the initiating element in the decision to seek health information. In the *evaluation phase*, individuals consider two factors: (a) the positive or negative outcomes of seeking health information and (b) their health information efficacy assessment regarding *communication efficacy* (individual skills to seek information), *target efficacy* (accessibility of information being sought), and *coping efficacy* (emotional, relational, and financial ability to accept the outcome). In other words, this phase is a cost-benefit analysis for whether to seek health information. Finally, in the *decision phase*, individuals will engage in different health information management behaviors. These behaviors could include any of the following (Afifi & Robbins, 2015, p. 149):

> Direct information seeking (asking the person directly), indirect information seeking ("beating around the bush" with the person or asking a mutual friend), active avoidance (going out of their way to avoid any information on the topic) or passive avoidance (not doing much either way—not seeking information but not actively avoiding it, either).

Although most research using the TMIM focuses on the three phases for individuals seeking information, it's important to note that this model also accounts for the fact that the individuals who provide information go through the evaluation and decision phases and that their phase experiences are expected to directly affect the information seekers' decision making. For instance, if you ask a friend for their opinion on a recent diagnosis and the friend appears uninterested, you may decide to end your information seeking attempt with that friend.

In a meta-analysis of 33 studies exploring the ability of TMIM to predict information management, Kai Kuang and Steven Wilson (2021) found that research studies consistently supported the process outlined in the model. Considering TMIM's roots in the interpersonal literature, it's not surprising that the model has been predominantly used to explore health information seeking from a relational lens. For example, Katherine Rafferty and colleagues (2015) found that TMIM explained how married couples seek health information to support their partner's end-of-life preferences. Although online sources of health information seeking are less common in TMIM research than interpersonal sources, they have also supported the tenets of the model. For example, Jo-Yun Li and colleagues (2020) found that TMIM phases explained how parents navigate conflicting online health information about childhood vaccination. The TMIM's consideration of the interpersonal aspects of health information seeking has helped capture the complexity of health information seeking behavior.

Now that you have read about these three models, it's possible that you, yourself, are feeling some information overload on which model most accurately captures the processes surrounding health information seeking. We don't recommend looking at it that way. Instead, you should recognize that each model brings a unique lens for exploring the relationship between individuals, information sources, and health information seeking behaviors and so each will have different strengths depending on the goals of the research. Indeed, researchers should select theoretical frameworks on the basis of their research questions. For example, if you're interested in how COVID-19 is promoting health information seeking behaviors among young adults, then the CMIS will be most appropriate for exploring the utility of the available information. On the other hand, if you're looking to explore how individuals experience health information when considering getting a COVID-19 booster, then the RISP model is the best choice for exploring how individuals navigate information on the risks of getting boosted or not. Finally, if you're interested in how individuals who are co-parenting decide whether to vaccinate their child against COVID-19, then the TMIM is best suited for exploring that interpersonal decision-making process.

Information Management and Other Health-Related Processes

Seeking health-related information is one strategy under the larger umbrella of information management. Brashers et al. (2002) suggest that **information management** is a broad array of communicative and cognitive activities that include information seeking in addition to information avoidance, provision, appraisal, and interpretation. Together, the broader process of information management has important implications for defining moments in people's health journeys, particularly surrounding coping, decision making, and health management.

Coping

As you'll recall from the previous chapter, learning to cope with a health-related stressor is an essential skill for promoting positive health outcomes. Health communication

---

Health Information, Health Information Seeking Behaviors, and Health Information Management

Health information is health-related stimuli contributing to a person's health-related knowledge or beliefs.

Health information seeking is an intentional behavior undertaken by an individual with the objective of finding information about health.

Health information management includes a broad array of communicative and cognitive activities that entail information seeking, avoidance, provision, appraisal, and interpretation.

---

researchers typically study coping as a process, or the emotional and behavioral efforts that individuals make to navigate and work to accept challenging health situations. Efforts to cope are typically classified into one of two categories: problem-focused (addressing the external influence) and emotion-focused (addressing the negative emotions caused by the external influence; Folkman & Lazarus, 1980). Health information seeking is one type of problem-focused coping strategy. In a review of literature exploring health information seeking behaviors, Sylvie Lambert and Carmen Loiselle (2007) argue that information seeking enhances coping by helping individuals (a) understand the health threat and its associated challenges, (b) evaluate the gravity of the situation, (c) make sense of their experiences, (d) work through what is happing, (e) manage stress, (f) determine available resources, and (g) feel a sense of control over the situation.

The role of health information seeking in promoting coping is evidenced across decades of communication research. A recent example is Nia Mason and colleague's (2022) study on health information seeking as a coping strategy for caregivers of loved ones with Alzheimer's disease. In a qualitative study, the researchers analyzed 15 interviews with informal caregivers, 12 of whom were female. Most of the participants cared for a parent (67%) and identified as white (53%). In this study, coping was operationalized by stress level: The less stress caregivers reported, the more they were considered to be effectively coping with the situation. Participant responses revealed that information could increase stress if it was too difficult to understand or poorly delivered, such as through an unsupportive patient–provider interaction. On the other hand, information could also help reduce stress when it prepared caregivers for what was to come, helped them acquire new skills appropriate to the situation (e.g., completing legal paperwork), and made them feel less alone. These results show how effective health information seeking and quality health information are central tools in the coping process, allowing individuals to navigate the situations they're in and prepare for another key aspect: decision making.

Decision Making

As you'll recall from the last chapter, there are a number of strategies to promote empowered and informed medical decision making. One of the most central of them is health information seeking. Health information seeking contributes to empowered medical decision making by helping individuals identify and evaluate their options, which reduces their uncertainty about alternative choices, in order to determine the most appropriate choice for them (see Lambert & Loiselle, 2007). Both the availability and absence of health information can affect a person's ability to make decisions. Let's look at an example as to how.

In interviews with Turkish parents whose children have cancer, Ebru Kilicarslan-Toruner and Ebru Akgun-Citak (2013) found that parents almost exclusively received health information about their child's cancer from providers, predominantly oncologists and nurses. The health information centered on illness, treatment, prognosis, and childcare, which parents did feel helped inform their decision making. But there were some informational needs that parents felt were not being met. This included information on coping skills, new therapy methods, and other medication options. The authors noted one possible explanation for why some informational needs were being met and others were not: a lack of reevaluating needs throughout the care journey. Specifically, they noted that "During the long illness and therapy process, parents need to seek information about various topics. As the parents' knowledge and experiences increase, their information needs become more detailed. Each new situation required the parents to seek additional information" (p. 181). The authors concluded that for optimal support, an "evaluation of these needs must be conducted regularly throughout the care period" (p. 182). Because decision making is an ongoing activity in many health journeys, informational needs are also ongoing and ever-changing. Although information seeking is important to the decision-making process, the need for information does not end once decisions are made. Health information is also needed to facilitate health management.

Health Management

Health management centers on individual behaviors, typically focusing on whether people adhere to recommended health behaviors or attempt to change poor health behaviors. Adherence encompasses a person's ability to follow medical recommendations or treatment plans as outlined by their clinician. For instance, taking medication as prescribed, completing physical therapy at home, or monitoring blood sugar or blood pressure all count as adherence behaviors. Behavior change encompasses efforts by individuals to adjust one or more aspects of their life in order to live healthier. For instance, stopping smoking, eating more vegetables, and exercising regularly all count as behavior change. Both adherence and behavior change are important aspects of successfully managing health. Information seeking has been shown to be a major factor influencing the extent to which individuals engage in such health management behaviors. Of course, information in and of itself does not guarantee that individuals will engage in healthy behaviors. If only, right? Instead, acquiring credible and accurate information is key to motivating individuals to successfully manage their health (see Lambert & Loiselle, 2007). (Obviously, behavior change involves much more than gathering information, but our point is that it's a start.)

Of interest to health communication researchers is the ways in which health information seeking assists individuals with managing their health. A leading explanation for why health information seeking is essential to health management is that it reduces uncertainty, which allows individuals to feel more capable of engaging in whatever behaviors they need to adopt. Research has shown this to be especially true for health information seeking with clinicians. For example, in a study of more than 200 U.S. adults with heart conditions, actively seeking information during an office visit was associated with greater confidence in managing heart health, which, in turn, was associated with having a lower body mass index—a key measure of heart health (Checton et al., 2017). Health management is also easily integrated into online systems for organizing, finding, and acting on health information.

Indeed, searching for health information online is so universal that online communities for health information management and exchange have become standard options for patients—and rich sources of data for health communication researchers interested in information exchange processes. Research shows that online health communities provide essential spaces for the exchange of health information to assist patients with health management. For example, in Erin Willis and Marla Royne's (2017) analysis of almost 2,000 online exchanges from four arthritis-centered communities, they concluded that online health communities act as informal health management programs, allowing patients to hold each other accountable and promoting positive health behavior changes. These communities are seen as informal because they appear in online spaces not specifically dedicated to health management, such as on Facebook or Reddit. But there are also spaces entirely dedicated to facilitating the exchange of health information. One such space is *Patients Like Me* (PatientsLikeMe.com), a large, health-centered social networking site where patients can connect over a common disease. With more than 850,000 members, the site is designed to facilitate the exchange of information about illnesses, treatments, and health outcomes between patients with the same health condition. And consistent with findings from studies of informal communities, findings from a survey of users of *Patients Like Me* revealed strong support for the site's use motivating both patients and caregivers to take more control over health management (Wicks et al., 2010).

Implications of Health Information Seeking and Management

Coping: Health information seeking promotes the ability to process and manage the implications of a health condition.

Decision Making: Health information seeking facilitates the ability to make informed choices.

Health Management: Health information seeking promotes and supports ongoing adherence and positive health behaviors.

Health Reporting

Media organizations such as newspapers and broadcasting corporations are typically perceived by the public as credible sources of information (with the caveat that in our currently partisan nation, different groups of people perceive different outlets as more or less credible). Given this perceived credibility, these organizations and their editors and reporters bear a social responsibility for how they decide to share health information. Even if you don't work for one of these organizations or you're not planning to become a journalist yourself, as a media consumer you also bear a social responsibility for any health information you choose to promote in your own social networks. This responsibility begins with building literacy skills for finding and selecting health information and evaluating its quality. But even with such skills, there is a lot to consider regarding how health information is disseminated online. The following paragraphs will highlight what journalists consider when creating health information content, review the role of citizen engagement in journalistic practices, and demonstrate the risks of media mis- and disinformation to public health.

Journalistic Considerations for Creating Health Content

How a news story is developed plays a role in what information it communicates. Vish Viswanath and colleagues (2008) note that media outlets tend to follow a four-step process in the creation of news: (1) determine whether a story is interesting, exciting, or unique enough to be told, (2) select sources of accurate and reliable information and translate that information for lay audiences, (3) gather supplemental information to make the story appealing, such as personal testimonies and analogies, and (4) widely disseminate the story. These guidelines apply to all reporting, of course, not just to health reporting. However, health topics tend to be more sensitive than other topics, so special care should be taken at each of these steps. For instance, due to the potential impact on life or death decision making, health stories might require additional time to create, skills to translate medical jargon, and verification by medical experts. In addition, there are no universal standards that delineate what information should be highlighted in health-related news stories (although there are guidelines available for particularly sensitive topics such as mental illness and suicide; see Chapter 9). Fortunately, there are some organizations working to promote ethical standards in health reporting, such as the **Association of Health Care Journalists (AHCJ)**.

The AHCJ (n.d.) is a nonprofit organization dedicated to advancing public understanding of healthcare issues and improving the quality, accuracy, and visibility of healthcare reporting, writing, and editing. The organization lists seven goals that guide their mission for healthcare journalism (para. 2):

1. To support the highest standards of reporting, writing, editing, and broadcasting in health care journalism for the general public and trade publications
2. To develop a strong and vibrant community of journalists concerned with all forms of health care journalism
3. To raise the stature of health care journalism in newsrooms, the industry, and the public, as a whole
4. To promote understanding between journalists and sources of news about how each can best serve the public
5. To advocate for the free flow of information to the public
6. To advocate for the improvement of professional development opportunities for journalists who cover any aspect of health and health care
7. To advocate for and work toward diversity, equity, and inclusion in media outlets and within AHCJ

Although not officially recognized as universal standards among journalistic organizations, the AHCJ goals are among the closest you'll find, and they're an important tool for journalists who want to improve and hone their health reporting skills. But other organizations have additional ideas for how to enhance the quality of health reporting.

The **Alan Alda Center for Communicating Science** (n.d.) operates under the premise that the solution to improving the quality of health reporting is by prioritizing the relationships between the scientific and journalistic communities. Center staff train scientists how to effectively share the results of their research with the press. Through the center, they seek to reduce the burden of health reporting on journalists by preparing researchers to disseminate their findings themselves. Outside of the Alan Alda Center, academic journals are taking a similar approach by encouraging researchers who are submitting their studies for publication consideration to also submit a tweet about their study along with their manuscript. If the manuscript is accepted for publication, the journal can then use the tweet to disseminate news of the study to the public. Both approaches can help journalists recognize credible sources, navigate scientific jargon, and provide quality health information for audiences. Although efforts to promote health reporting among journalists are important to ensure accessible and credible health information, not all health reporting is done by trained journalists. Sometimes, journalistic practices are taken into the hands of citizens.

Citizen Journalism

The ability for any person to create and upload content that can immediately reach mass audiences marked a sea change in media reporting. Today, it's not uncommon for news to be broken online—particularly on social media—by an average user. Those users are called citizen journalists. **Citizen journalism** is "the act of a citizen, or group of citizens, playing an active role in the process of collecting, reporting, analyzing and disseminating news and information" (Bowman & Willis, 2003, p. 9). What information individuals choose to post online is typically protected under the First Amendment as freedom of speech—regardless of its accuracy or credibility. Citizen journalists are not held to the same standards of investigative integrity as trained, professional journalists. In theory and practice, though, citizen journalism has the potential to give platforms to historically unheard voices, such as marginalized groups, and provide opportunities for new perspectives to engage in online discourse.

In recounting his witnessing of the transition from traditional journalistic reporting to the inclusion of citizen journalists in today's reporting, Dan Gillmor (2004), journalist, author, professor of practice, and co-founder of the News Co/Lab at Arizona State University's Walter Cronkite School of Journalism and Mass Communication, shares the following (p. 60):

> Journalism is transforming from a twentieth-century mass-media structure to something profoundly more grassroots and democratic. This transformation is a story, first, of evolutionary change. Humans have always told each other stories, and each new era of progress has led to an expansion of storytelling. It is, however, also a story of a modern revolution because technology has given us a communications toolkit that allows anyone to become a journalist at little cost and (in theory) with global reach. Nothing like this has ever been possible before.

Gillmor (2004) adds that citizen journalism provides an affordable channel to an often voiceless group and holds the potential to "help spark a renaissance of the notion, now threatened, of a truly informed citizenry" (p. 63). Although he was not alone in his optimism that citizen journalism would enhance democratic practices and create a more level playing field when it came to information dissemination (e.g., Allan & Thorsen, 2009), citizen journalism also created new challenges, particularly in health reporting, that have not been so positive. One of these challenges has implications for people seeking health information: the accuracy of the information reported. When information is not accurate, things can go sideways fast. One of the most striking examples of this is the anti-vaccine movement.

Vaccine hesitancy and refusal is not a new phenomenon. Scientists have been navigating anti-vaccination perspectives (or anti-vaxxers) since the first vaccine was developed. What is new, however, is the ability of anti-vaxxer messages to reach mass audiences so easily (Hussain et al., 2018). Many experts point to the 2008 Oprah interview with actress and model Jenny McCarthy as the fuel that ignited the festering embers of anti-vax perspectives, sparking a full-fledged online movement (Gottlieb, 2016). In the interview, McCarthy, who has no medical expertise or training, chose to use her platform to engage in irresponsible citizen journalism and argue that vaccines contain toxins that cause autism. She cited a controversial study that was being refuted by numerous scientists, including most of the original authors (we'll provide more detail about this study in the next section). In less than two years, the study would be officially retracted by the journal. Although there was no credible evidence to support McCarthy's claim, the damage was done. Following media backlash against McCarthy's demonstrably false claim, a minority of online users with anti-vax perspectives flocked to her defense. This collection of defenders served as citizen journalists to echo the false claims. Despite the vast, vast, vast (we cannot emphasize this enough) majority of the scientific community arguing that vaccines do not cause autism, the opinion of one celebrity helped derail decades of public health protections through her promotion of disinformation.

Media Misinformation and Disinformation

In today's media environment, inaccurate, misleading, and incomplete health information is a common challenge. Journalists, medical professionals, and public health professionals have raised serious concerns regarding the effects of misinformation on public perceptions and health behaviors. Recently, contentious political rhetoric has made way for a new classification of misinformation: disinformation. Whereas **misinformation** is understood to be inaccurate due to a lack of credible sources or misinterpretation of science, **disinformation** is the weaponization of misinformation for personal, and often political, gain (Guess & Lyons, 2020). When someone posts information they believe to be true, but it's actually false, they're promoting misinformation. However, if someone is given the facts to correct the misinformation and continues to perpetuate the falsehoods, or if they want only to spread lies from the outset, that is disinformation.

Misinformation and Disinformation

Misinformation: False information that is unknowingly promoted.
Disinformation: False information that is knowingly promoted.

Due to the nature of online spaces serving as echo chambers for particular perspectives on topics, it can sometimes seem like more people are engaging in mis- and disinformation than not. But a study by the **Center for Countering Digital Hate** (2021), a nonprofit organization that seeks to disrupt the architecture of online hate and misinformation, shows that's not the case. In examining online promotions of anti-vax conspiracy theories, they found that only 12 users are responsible for 65% of all disinformation surrounding vaccines on social media. Labeling these problem children the "disinformation dozen," the center calls for social media companies to close their accounts as a way to reduce the threat of mis- and disinformation about vaccines. Although the disinformation dozen are a clear and present danger to public health, they did not start the online epidemic of mis- and disinformation, they're just riding the wave.

Indeed, many researchers point to the rise of the misinformation era following the 1998 publication of an article in the British medical journal *The Lancet* reporting a link between the measles, mumps, and rubella (MMR) vaccine and autism in children. By the time physicians and national and international health organizations were able to refute the study's false claims, it was too late: Media coverage of the report spurred the creation of an organized anti-vax movement that, reignited partially thanks to Jenny McCarthy's interview, is still prevalent today (Hussain et al., 2018). The initial reporting of research findings was misinformation (among many other ethical violations that will be explored in more detail in Chapter 11) that was quickly identified as such by the medical community. The perpetuation of these claims was disinformation because there is no credible evidence to support them. Given the magnitude of such disinformation efforts, it can feel impossible to combat, particularly online. But researchers and activists are not ready to stand down just yet.

Wen-Ying Sylvia Chou and colleagues (2020) call for five areas of research that should be continued to combat the mis- and disinformation on social media. First, they suggest additional efforts to gather data from lesser-studied platforms, such as WeChat, Tumblr, and Pinterest. This information can provide further understanding of mis- and disinformation efforts outside of mainstream platforms. Second, they call on social scientists to draw on their theoretical understanding of human emotion, cognition, and identity to effectively inform needed interventions. Third, little is known about the consequences of exposing online misinformation as false. The authors call for additional investigations of strategies for successfully correcting mis- and disinformation and holding posters who knowingly and willfully spread lies accountable. Fourth, they call for an increased focus on vulnerable populations in order to help those most in need of accurate health information be able to access and utilize it. Finally, they suggest that evidence-based standards for situational responses be developed that consider optimal timing (when), appropriate manner (how), and suitable forum (where) for responding to misinformation. Although these suggestions cannot happen overnight, they can begin a movement that over years could gain the traction needed to counter the devastating impacts of mis- and disinformation. You might be wondering what to do in the meantime, especially if you're feeling a little hopeless about countering mis- and disinformation. If so, maybe the story of Maranda Dynda will inspire you.

In an episode of National Public Radio's (NPR) podcast *Hidden Brain*, host Shankar Vedantam (2019) explored the psychology of false beliefs by highlighting the story of Maranda Dynda. When Maranda was 18 years old and about to give birth, she hired a midwife for the delivery. Although the midwife was experienced and friendly, she convinced Maranda that vaccines gave her son autism. Worried about vaccines giving her soon-to-be-born child autism, Maranda joined an online group of moms against vaccination to learn more. She recalls what happened next:

> To me, it seemed so clear. It seemed like I had just found this secret information that only some people come across. And I thought, why would I not use this information? Why would I not use this to my benefit, to my child's benefit? So it did not take me very long at all before I was solidly saying I will not vaccinate my child when she is born.

Over the next two years, Maranda actively worked against the recommendation of medical professionals to not vaccinate her daughter. But the longer she stayed in the online groups, the more skeptical she became of their credibility. She recalled seeing posts about "People denying that AIDS exists, people saying that the reason there's gay people is vaccines - on and on and on with really crazy conspiracy theories" (n.p.) Vendantam (2019) states, "Then it hit her. If she didn't believe those ideas, why was she trusting them on vaccines?" (n.p.).

After considering the risks she was taking with her daughter's health by not vaccinating her and after researching information from credible sources that the online groups discouraged, such as the Centers for Disease Control and Prevention and medical journals, Maranda changed her mind and vaccinated her daughter. She gives the following advice to new moms: "Don't try to confirm your own fears online. It is so, so easy to Google, what if this happens, and find something that's probably not true that confirms your fear, that confirms your anxieties. Don't do that." We would like to extend that advice beyond new moms and suggest that everyone can benefit from Maranda's cautionary tale. This means to sharpen your information seeking and media literacy skills, trust credible sources of information, and don't, for your own sake and the sake of those around you, go down conspiracy theory rabbit holes.

Conclusion

Today, health information is widely accessible to most individuals. However, the skills needed to find and process the information vary across communities and groups. Health information seeking is a central behavior for promoting and maintaining overall health. Health communication researchers have made important contributions to the scientific understanding of how health information seeking can promote important health behaviors, including coping, decision making, and health management. In addition, theoretical contributions shed light on the underlying processes that individuals go through when navigating vast spaces of health information. Although it can feel overwhelming to navigate the sea of health information, particularly online, reporting and research efforts continue to advocate for standards that promote access to credible, understandable health information. Regardless of who you are or where you are in life, one day you are bound to find yourself seeking some form of health information. This universal experience will continue to drive important research questions among health communication scholars.

References

Afifi, W. A., & Morse, C. R. (2009). Expanding the role of emotion in the theory of motivated information management. In T. D. Afifi & W. A. Afifi (Eds.), *Uncertainty, information management, and disclosure decisions: Theories and applications* (pp. 87–105). Routledge.

Afifi, W. A., & Robbins, S. (2015). Theory of motivated information management: Struggles with uncertainty and its outcomes. In D. O. Braithwaite & P. Schrodt (Eds.), *Engaging theories in interpersonal communication: Multiple perspectives* (2nd ed., pp. 143–156). Sage.

Alan Alda Center for Communicating Science. (n.d.). *Home.* https://aldacenter.org/index.php

Allan, S., & Thorsen, E. (2009). *Citizen journalism: Global perspectives* (Vol. 1). Peter Lang.

Association of Health Care Journalists. (n.d.). *Mission & goals.* https://healthjournalism.org/about-missionGoals.php

Barbour, J. B., Rintamaki, L. S., Ramsey, J. A., & Brashers, D. E. (2012). Avoiding health information. *Journal of Health Communication, 17*(2), 212–229.

Bowman, S., & Willis, C. (2003). We media: How audiences are shaping the future of news and information. *The Media Center at the American Press Institute.* http://www.flickertracks.com/blog/images/we_media.pdf

Brashers, D. E., Goldsmith, D. J., & Hsieh, E. (2002). Information seeking and avoiding in health contexts. *Human Communication Research, 28*(2), 258–271.

Center for Countering Digital Hate. (2021, March 24). *The disinformation dozen: Why platforms must act on twelve leading online anti-vaxxers.* https://252f2edd-1c8b-49f5-9bb2-cb57bb47e4ba.filesusr.com/ugd/f4d9b9_b7cedc0553604720b7137f8663366ee5.pdf

Chang, C.-C., & Huang, M.-H. (2020). Antecedents predicting health information seeking: A systematic review and meta-analysis. *International Journal of Information Management, 54*, 102115.

Checton, M. G., Greene, K., Carpenter, A., & Catona, D. (2017). Perceptions of health information seeking and partner advocacy in the context of a cardiology office visit: Connections with health outcomes. *Health Communication, 32*(5), 587–595.

Choi, D.-H., & Noh, G.-Y. (2021). Information seeking behavior about obesity among South Koreans: Applying the risk information seeking and processing model. *Journal of Applied Communication Research, 49*(2), 228–245.

Chou, W.-Y. S., Gaysynsky, A., & Cappella, J. N. (2020). Where we go from here: Health misinformation on social media. *American Journal of Public Health, 110*(S3), S273–S275.

Colby, D. (2001). Conceptualizing the" digital divide": Closing the" gap" by creating a postmodern network that distributes the productive power of speech. *Communication Law & Policy*, *6*(1), 123–173.

Folkman, S., & Lazarus, R. S. (1980). An analysis of coping in a middle-aged community sample. *Journal of Health and Social Behavior*, *21*(3), 219–239.

Gillmor, D. (2004). We the media: The rise of citizen journalists. *National Civic Review*, *93*(3), 58–63.

Gottlieb, S. D. (2016). Vaccine resistances reconsidered: Vaccine skeptics and the Jenny McCarthy effect. *Biosocieties*, *11*(2), 152–174.

Griffin, R. J., Dunwoody, S., & Neuwirth, K. (1999). Proposed model of the relationship of risk information seeking and processing to the development of preventive behaviors. *Environmental Research*, *80*(2 Pt 2), S230–S245.

Guess, A. M., & Lyons, B. A. (2020). Misinformation, disinformation, and online propaganda. In N. Persily & J. A. Tucker (Eds.), *Social media and democracy: The state of the field, prospects for reform* (pp. 10–33). Cambridge University Press.

Hornik, R., Parvanta, S., Mello, S., Freres, D., Kelly, B., & Schwartz, J. S. (2013). Effects of scanning (routine health information exposure) on cancer screening and prevention behaviors in the general population. *Journal of Health Communication*, *18*(12), 1422–1435.

Hussain, A., Ali, S., & Ahmed, M. (2018, July 3). The anti-vaccination movement: A regression in modern medicine. *Cureus*, *10*(7), e2919.

Islam, N. S., Patel, S., Wyatt, L. C., Sim, S.-C., Mukherjee-Ratnam, R., Chun, K., Desai, B., Tandon, S. D., Trinh-Shevrin, C., Pollack, H., & Kwon, S. C. (2016). Sources of health information among select Asian American immigrant groups in New York City. *Health Communication*, *31*(2), 207–216.

Johnson, J. D., & Meischke, H. (1993). A comprehensive model of cancer-related information seeking applied to magazines. *Human Communication Research*, *19*(3), 343–367.

Kennedy, E., & Thibeault, S. L. (2020). Voice–gender incongruence and voice health information–seeking behaviors in the transgender community. *American Journal of Speech-Language Pathology*, *29*(3), 1563–1573.

Kilicarslan-Toruner, E., & Akgun-Citak, E. (2013). Information-seeking behaviours and decision-making process of parents of children with cancer. *European Journal of Oncology Nursing*, *17*(2), 176–183.

Kim, Y.-C., Lim, J. Y., & Park, K. (2015). Effects of health literacy and social capital on health information behavior. *Journal of Health Communication*, *20*(9), 1084–1094.

Kuang, K., & Wilson, S. R. (2021). Theory of motivated information management: A meta-analytic review. *Communication Theory*, *31*(3), 463–490.

Lalazaryan, A., & Zare-Farashbandi, F. (2014). A review of models and theories of health information seeking behavior. *International Journal of Health System and Disaster Management*, *2*(4), 193–203.

Lambert, S. D., & Loiselle, C. G. (2007). Health information—Seeking behavior. *Qualitative Health Research*, *17*(8), 1006–1019.

Li, J.-Y., Wen, J., Kim, J., & McKeever, R. (2020). Applying the theory of motivated information management to the context of conflicting online health information: Implications for childhood vaccination communication with parents. *International Journal of Strategic Communication*, *14*(5), 330–347.

Lu, L., Liu, J., & Yuan, Y. C. (2020). Health information seeking behaviors and source preferences between Chinese and U.S. populations. *Journal of Health Communication*, *25*(6), 490–500.

Manganello, J., & Clayman, M. (2011). The association of understanding of medical statistics with health information seeking and health provider interaction in a national sample of young adults. *Journal of Health Communication*, *16*, 163–176.

Mason, N. F., Francis, D. B., & Pecchioni, L. L. (2022). Health information seeking as a coping strategy to reduce Alzheimer's caregivers' stress. *Health Communication*, *37*(2), 131–140.

National Cancer Institute (NCI). (n.d.). *Health Information National Trends Survey: All HINTS Questions.* https://hints.cancer.gov/view-questions-topics/all-hints-questions.aspx

Niederdeppe, J., Hornik, R. C., Kelly, B. J., Frosch, D. L., Romantan, A., Stevens, R. S., Barg, F. K., Weiner, J. L., & Schwartz, J. S. (2007). Examining the dimensions of cancer-related information seeking and scanning behavior. *Health Communication*, *22*(2), 153–167.

Rafferty, K. A., Cramer, E., Priddis, D., & Allen, M. (2015). Talking about end-of-life preferences in marriage: Applying the theory of motivated information management. *Health Communication*, *30*(4), 409–418.

Record, R. A., Silberman, W. R., Santiago, J. E., & Ham, T. (2018). I sought it, I Reddit: Examining health information engagement behaviors among Reddit users. *Journal of Health Communication, 23*(5), 470–476.

Rogers, E. M. (2001). The digital divide. *Convergence, 7*(4), 96–111.

So, J., Ahn, J., & Guan, M. (2022). Beyond depth and breadth: Taking "types" of health information sought into consideration with cluster analysis. *Journal of Health Communication, 27*(1), 27–36.

Tichenor, P. J., Donohue, G. A., & Olien, C. N. (1970). Mass media flow and differential growth in knowledge. *Public Opinion Quarterly, 34*(2), 159–170.

Van Stee, S. K., & Yang, Q. (2018). Online cancer information seeking: Applying and extending the comprehensive model of information seeking. *Health Communication, 33*(12), 1583–1592.

Vedantam, S. (Host). (2019, July 22). Facts aren't enough: The psychology of false beliefs [Audio podcast episode]. In *Hidden Brain*. National Public Radio. https://www.npr.org/transcripts/743195213

Viswanath, K., Blake, K. D., Meissner, H. I., Gottlieb Sointz, N., Mull, C., Freeman, C. S., Hesses, B., & Croyle, R. T. (2008). Occupational practices and the making of health news: A national survey of U.S. health and medical science journalists. *Journal of Health Communication, 13*(8), 759–777.

Wicks, P., Massagli, M., Frost, J., Brownstein, C., Okun, S., Vaughan, T., Bradley, R., & Heywood, J. (2010). Sharing health data for better outcomes on PatientsLikeMe. *Journal of Medical Internet Research, 12*(2), e1549.

Willis, E., & Royne, M. B. (2017). Online health communities and chronic disease self-management. *Health Communication, 32*(3), 269–278.

Zimmerman, M. S., & Shaw, G. (2020). Health information seeking behaviour: A concept analysis. *Health Information and Libraries Journal, 37*, 173–191.

In-class Activities

1. Put students in small groups and assign each group a health topic (e.g., exercise, eating a balanced diet, consuming alcohol in moderation or not at all, getting vaccinated, preventative cancer screening). Have the group provide an example of how a researcher would approach the topic through the lens of CMIS, RISP, and TMIM. Bonus points for including specific details on the characteristics within each framework.
2. Below are scenarios of mis- and disinformation. In pairs, have students work through the implications of the mis- and disinformation and come up with a counter message for each scenario.
   a. Wearing bras can cause breast cancer by obstructing lymph flow.
   b. HIV/AIDs is airborne and can be spread through close contact.
   c. Smoke emitted from vape devices is just water vapor.
   d. Smoking cigarettes doesn't cause lung cancer.
   e. The flu vaccine is ineffective against the flu virus.

Discussion Questions

1. When you're sick, where do you turn for health information? How have these sources helped or hindered your ability to cope, make decisions, and manage your healing needs? Would you say they've improved your health literacy?
2. In your own words, how would you describe the distinction among the depth, breadth, and quality of health information seeking?
3. Recall Viswanath et al.'s (2008) four-step process that media outlets follow for creating news. How can these steps be specifically applied to the coverage of health topics?

Unit III
Caring for Patients

Sally Reflects on Helen's Healthcare Providers

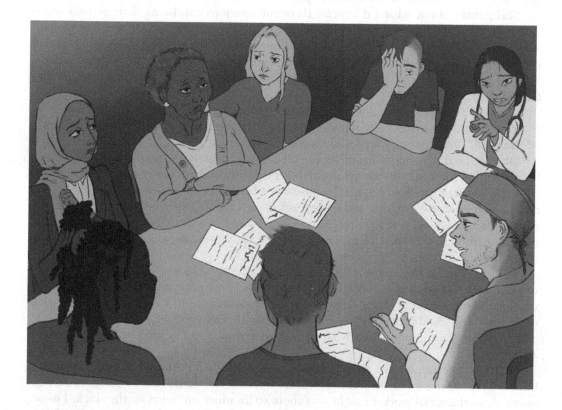

Another year had passed, and Cheryl was about to finish her second semester of medical school. To her delight, her grades were consistently at the top of her class, and she was finally feeling confident in her ability to become a doctor. That feeling of confidence, however, was currently taking a backseat to feelings of anxiety as Cheryl and Sally discussed Helen's health.

"We're just so proud of you, sweetie," Sally said supportively. "And I promise, we won't hide anything from you. As soon as we know, you'll know."

"Thanks" Cheryl replied. "And thanks for continuing to be Grams' 'doctor buddy.' If I've learned anything in class so far, it's that when the stress piles up, patients can shut down and not process information during medical visits. Having someone there can be so important."

"Of course, I'm glad to be there with her," Sally replied sincerely. "And between your Grams and my mother, I completely understand why that happens to patients. I swear, in one short meeting I could fill multiple notebooks with all the information the doctors are

DOI: 10.4324/9781003214458-14

sharing." Sally shook her head slightly. "I mean, just the names of all the doctors and their specialties could fill a single notebook *alone*."

Cheryl chuckled a little before replying, "Before starting medical school, I had no idea how common healthcare teams were. And how much they can vary from patient to patient. Does Grams tend to have the same people each visit or are they changing from visit to visit?"

"Um, let me think," Sally paused for a moment, attempting to recall all of the providers she'd met over Helen's last few appointments. "Her oncologist has definitely been consistent. He's just the best. And the same surgeon has been in the last two or three meetings. Oh, and the social worker's always there. But the residents and nurses always seem to change, and there's a nutritionist who comes and goes."

"Yeah, that's about what I'd expect. Resident rotations can be as short as two weeks depending on the program, and nurses will vary depending on shift," Cheryl explained. "Unless an emergency meeting is called and her oncologist and surgeon are unavailable, though, those two should be consistent throughout her care."

"You know another person who has been consistent on our visits?" Sally asked with a teasing tone.

"Uh, no," Cheryl replied, not entirely sure what to expect.

"Your friend Nathian," Sally stated. "He's the patient care advocate at your grandmother's hospital. We've actually seen him on every visit."

"Oh, yes, he did mention that he'd been seeing you all lately," Cheryl shared. She should have seen this coming. Sally always insisted that there was a spark between her and Nathian. And maybe there was at some point, but between Nathian being enrolled in a health communication graduate program and Cheryl off at med school, their relationship had dwindled to the occasional text message. Even Cheryl and Liz weren't talking as often as they used to. Although they went to medical schools in the same state, neither of their schedules really allowed for trips away.

"I didn't even know there was such a thing as a patient advocate," Sally continued, unaware that Cheryl's thoughts had drifted slightly. "And how perfect for him to have that job while he works on his graduate degree. And it's so wonderful to have a friendly face greet us on each visit. And Helen just loves talking to him about you."

"Oh, great. I can only image what she's been saying. But I'm glad he's there," Cheryl added.

"Me, too, sweetie. It's just all so exhausting," Sally sighed. "And what I didn't realize is how exhausting it is for some of the healthcare workers, too. In the last meeting, I heard the nurse say to the social worker that he was about to hit nineteen hours on the clock. I mean, that's a lot. And it's not like we were having a casual conversation about the weather. These are life or death conversations. Everyone was clearly doing their best to be fully present for Helen, which I appreciate, but a person can only give so much."

"Speaking of overworked and exhausted providers, have you talked to Monica this week?" Cheryl asked.

"No, what's happening?" Sally asked, a little worried.

"She's just exhausted," Cheryl shared. "She loves being a nurse, but the ER position seems to really be wearing on her. I'm worried she's burning out."

"Have you mentioned this to your uncle? Or encouraged Monica to talk to him about it?"

"I did suggest she talk to Uncle Michael. I'm hoping he'll have some good advice for her," Cheryl replied.

"He's been in healthcare for over twenty years. I'm sure he'll have some great suggestions for her," Sally shared, hoping she was right.

"Fingers crossed," Cheryl replied.

And with that, Cheryl and Sally said their goodbyes. Despite Cheryl's busy schedule, she always made time to check in with her mom. And it didn't matter where she was or what she was doing, Sally always answered when Cheryl called. That's just the kind of person Sally was— always answering the call from family.

Note

A patient advocate is one of many possible careers for a health communication major. They serve as liaisons between patients and health providers, and they help patients and families navigate the healthcare system. The Alliance of Professional Health Advocates (https://aphadvocates.org/) serves as a resource for members to help them establish and navigate their patient advocacy goals.

6 Healthcare Provider Roles and Perspectives

If two families were playing a game of Family Feud and host Steve Harvey said, "Name someone who provides healthcare," we'd bet good money that the top answer would be doctor. As Mr. Harvey went from family member to family member, they would probably guess nurse and dentist, and someone might even say pharmacist. At that point, though, the family member next in line might start sweating a bit and scratching their head. But they needn't do that because there are numerous types of health professionals who provide patient care. For example, there are also physician assistants, nurse practitioners, dental hygienists, pharmacy technicians, paramedics, physical therapists, clinical psychologists, and many, many more.

Up to this point in the book, we've been focusing almost exclusively on the perspective of patients and their communication experiences in the healthcare system. This chapter is going to take a slight turn and consider what it's like to be a healthcare provider. Because these professionals are on the frontline of patient care, gaining insight into their experiences and perspectives will give you a more comprehensive understanding of the patient care environment.

We're going to begin with a review of the literature on healthcare teams. We'll provide a definition and characterization of teams and present two examples of healthcare teams in action. After that, we'll discuss how healthcare provider communication is integral to patient safety yet can result in medical errors. As a part of that discussion, we'll delve into the context of patient handoffs, and we'll present research on interventions to improve communication among members of healthcare teams. Next, we'll consider the experiences of providers in the healthcare system, including how providers can suffer from burnout and encounter discrimination. As you read through this chapter, it's important to remember that healthcare providers are people, too. Although patients trust them with their lives and they're esteemed members of our society, they face all the challenges that go with being human.

Healthcare Teams

Several decades ago, healthcare was typically provided by a doctor who worked in a solo practice, lived in the community they served, and even made house calls. Advances in medicine and the complexity of medical treatment, though, have turned healthcare into more of a "team sport" (Mitchell et al., 2012). A **healthcare team** is defined as "an identifiable group of two or more people working interdependently toward shared, mutual goals that could not be accomplished effectively, if at all, by a single person" (Weaver et al., 2017, p. 52). A key point with teams is that team members work interdependently, which is another way to say they engage in teamwork. **Teamwork** is defined as

> the behaviors (e.g., communicating and sharing information, checking for mutual understanding), attitudes (e.g., belief in the collective ability of the team and need for

DOI: 10.4324/9781003214458-15

teamwork), and cognitions (e.g., shared mental models) teams use to communicate, coordinate, and collaborate their efforts to achieve shared, collective goals.

(Weaver et al., 2017, p. 52)

As anyone who has played sports will tell you, teamwork is essential to any group activity, particularly when health is on the line.

Who Are Healthcare Providers?

Healthcare providers are physicians, nurses, dentists, pharmacists, physician assistants, nurse practitioners, dental hygienists, paramedics, physical therapists, clinical psychologists, and any other person working to provide direct patient care.

There are also numerous other people working in healthcare who provide patient support outside of direct care, such as health educators, lab technicians, social workers, chaplains, housekeeping staff, administrators, and volunteers.

Teams can be defined along several dimensions (Weaver et al., 2017). For example, teams may be characterized by the patient population they serve, such as surgical teams treating patients receiving surgery or hospice teams treating patients in the last months of their lives. Teams also may be defined by the type of disease they treat, such as a cardiovascular team that treats heart disease or an oncology team that treats cancer, or the setting in which they practice, such as intensive care units. There are also **rapid response teams**, which are groups of healthcare providers brought together quickly to respond to crisis situations, such as the COVID-19 pandemic (Schilling et al., 2022).

A frequent assumption about teams is that their composition is relatively stable and team members typically perform the same roles over time. This is true in many cases, such as in aviation, the military, and sports. For example, in football, although new players may be brought on each year and players sometimes will be traded, team composition throughout a season tends to remain the same, and players tend to stay in their lanes (because you wouldn't want your kicker taking over as quarterback). Pamela Andreatta, however, wondered whether the same stability was true of healthcare teams. This is an important question because if healthcare teams do have more variability than other types of teams, the theoretical models currently in use for those teams would not apply as well to healthcare settings.

Andreatta (2010) designed an observational study to assess the stability of the personnel comprising healthcare teams and the roles they perform. She recruited 25 interdisciplinary teams to participate. The theoretical framework she used to guide her research was **team member schema similarity** (see Table 6.1). This framework suggests that teams function better when "team members have similar knowledge structures for perceiving, interpreting, and organizing team-related phenomena" (p. 346). Similar knowledge structures, or schemas, develop over time through member interaction, socialization, and training and include perceptions of members' "competence, cooperativeness, reliability, communicativeness, and interpersonal skills" (p. 346). Organizations can promote the development of similar schemas among team members by providing decision support systems, facilitating team communication, and establishing a supportive organizational culture and quality performance reward system (Rentsch & Hart, 1994). When team members share similar schemas, team performance will be enhanced, which should lead to improved patient outcomes, stronger team members bonds, and team member personal growth and well-being.

Table 6.1 Theoretical Frameworks in Provider Communication

Theory/Model	Brief Summary	Citation
Communication Competence Model	Competent communication has two dimensions: appropriateness and effectiveness. A communicator's knowledge, skill, and motivation lead them to be able to produce messages that are perceived as appropriate and effective, thus competent.	Spitzberg and Cupach (1984)
Systems Model of Clinician Burnout and Professional Well-being	External environmental factors, healthcare organization factors, and frontline care delivery factors influence clinician burnout and professional well-being as mediated by individual differences among clinicians. Burnout and well-being have consequences for patients, clinicians, healthcare organizations, and society.	National Academy of Medicine (2019)
Team Member Schema Similarity	Each member of a healthcare team has a schema for perceiving, understanding, and organizing knowledge about their team. Schema similarity is influenced by team member individual differences and team-related schema communication that occurs during team member interaction, socialization, and training. If there is an optimal level of high-quality schema similarity among team member schemas, team performance will be enhanced and lead to improved patient outcomes, stronger team members bonds, and team member personal growth and well-being.	Rentsch and Hall (1994)

Note. See *Supplemental Online Theory Table* for additional theories/models.

Andreatta (2010) used nonparticipant observation methodology to observe the activity of each of the 25 teams on two separate occasions for multiple hours on each occasion. Her observations led to the identification of four types of healthcare teams: stable role/stable personnel (SrSp), variable role/stable personnel (VrSp), stable role/variable personnel (SrVp), and variable role/variable personnel (VrVp). Figure 6.1 provides examples of the four types of teams. Andreatta found that only six teams were SrSp, the configuration assumed by traditional models of team development and performance (stable roles and stable personnel). The most common configuration, characterizing 12 of her 25 teams, was SrVp (stable roles but variable personnel). She concluded, therefore, that "team models and associated competencies from other domains may not wholly transfer to health care or adequately inform training specific to the challenges of interdisciplinary teamwork in health care" (p. 350). This raises the stakes for healthcare teams, then, making those teams with variability in roles and personnel have to work harder to develop cross-disciplinary competencies and interpersonal relationships. As they do, they should keep in mind the values and principles of highly effective teams that were identified by Pamela Mitchell and her colleagues in a project that came out of a meeting on innovation and best practices for team-based healthcare (National Academy of Medicine, 2022).

Mitchell et al. (2012) identified five **personal values of highly effective team members**. First, highly effective team members are *honest*, which promotes transparency, continual improvement, and mutual trust. Second, they are *disciplined*, which allows them to know they can depend on themselves and one another to carry out responsibilities and follow protocols. Third, they need to be *creative* so they can solve unanticipated problems effectively and use the problems as learning opportunities. Fourth, they need to be *humble*, which means that they perceive all members' contributions as valuable and believe that no

TEAM ROLE			
		Stable	**Variable**
TEAM PERSONNEL	**Stable**	**SrSp** **Example**: A pediatric medicine team that provided well- and sick-child care. Members were physicians, nurses, and administrative staff. Team members never changed and always performed the same roles.	**VrSp** **Example**: A physical medicine and rehabilitation therapy team that provided in-home care for adults with physical disabilities. Members were physical and occupational therapists, therapy aids, and administrative staff. Team members never changed but sometimes performed roles outside the scope of their normal duties depending on patient needs.
	Variable	**SrVp** **Example**: A surgical team that performed surgeries on adult patients. Members included surgeons, residents, nurses, anesthesiologists, and technicians. Team members frequently changed but always performed the same roles.	**VrVp** **Example**: An emergency flight team that provided urgent care on site or air transport to medical facilities. Members included physicians, nurses, pilots, and technicians. Team members sometimes changed, and roles varied depending on the situation and patient needs; however, there was always a pilot and a nurse.

Figure 6.1 Four Types of Healthcare Teams as Defined by Personnel and Role Stability or Variability.
Source: Andreatta (2010).

one is superior to anyone else; it also means that they acknowledge everyone is human and capable of mistakes. And fifth, they need to be *curious* in looking for ways to continuously improve the quality of team performance. To demonstrate these values in an example that should be familiar to you, consider the infamous group project you sometimes get assigned in classes. When group members engage in honest communication, create a timeline of responsibilities to which members adhere, consider creative responses to assignment prompts, value all member contributions, and take the time to double check the final product, they are much more likely to earn an "A" on the assignment. (Hint, hint.)

Mitchell et al. (2012) also identified five **principles of team-based healthcare** that are necessary for optimal performance: *shared goals, clear roles, mutual trust, effective communication,* and *measurable processes and outcomes.* First, highly effective healthcare teams develop goals that are shared not only among the healthcare professionals on the team but also by the patient and their family. The teams involve the patient in goal setting, and they continually monitor progress toward achieving the goals. Second, the members have clear expectations and an understanding of each other's roles and responsibilities. This is especially important when personnel or roles vary within teams (Andreatta, 2010). It's also important when integrating patients and family members as part of the team because they don't share the same knowledge base and language as healthcare providers. Thus, they may have unclear expectations, and understanding roles and responsibilities may be difficult for them. The principle of clear roles also includes understanding when certain tasks are better accomplished individually versus collaboratively, knowing who is responsible for team administrative tasks, and identifying who takes on team leadership roles in which contexts.

Third, highly effective healthcare teams establish and maintain mutual trust so they can depend on and learn from one another, respect each other, and acknowledge every member's contributions. They also have processes in place to deal with breaches of trust, should they occur. Fourth, they demonstrate exemplary interpersonal and professional communication skills. Members are active listeners, they seek and share information on an ongoing basis, they check to verify their understanding of information, and they demonstrate person-centered communication, which means they show respect for emotional and relational aspects of interactions. Team members have clear channels of communication in place (e.g., electronic medical records, email, web portals, smartphones) and use them across all care settings. Finally, highly effective healthcare teams agree upon and establish reliable and valid means of evaluating both the processes and outcomes of team activities. This applies to both patient care goals and team functioning goals. Feedback should be timely and ongoing, and it should be used for continuous quality improvement.

Mitchell et al. (2012) also identified **organizational factors** that support and promote each of these principles. We won't go into all of them here, but we will cover the ones for effective communication. First, to establish and maintain effective healthcare team communication, organizations must provide necessary resources. These resources include time for teams to meet, space to meet in person, and technology and support for virtual meetings. Second, they must make sure that team members have training in communication skills because, as any student of communication knows, competent communication is not a natural-born ability. Finally, for optimal communication, organizations need to adopt and effectively implement applicable technology, including electronic medical records, patient portals, and email systems, to support and encourage communication among team members, as well as patients and their families.

In their report, Mitchell et al. (2012) describe several highly functioning healthcare teams in place at institutions across the United States. We'll briefly highlight two of them. The first is the Department of Veterans Affairs (VA) Patient Aligned Care Teams (PACT). PACT teams operate nationwide through the VA health system (U.S. Department of Veterans Affairs, 2022). They are based on the concept of a patient-centered medical home, a model of patient care that emphasizes comprehensive, patient-centered, and coordinated care that is easily accessible and promotes quality and safety (Agency for Healthcare Research and Quality [AHRQ], 2021). PACTs are composed of a veteran (who is the patient), a primary care provider, a nurse care manager, a clinical associate, and an administrative clerk. Members undergo formal training in team functioning. The goal is to establish a partnership between the veteran and members of the team to provide coordinated, personalized, whole-person care that emphasizes disease prevention and health promotion. All team members have clearly defined roles and responsibilities, and all work toward establishing trusted, personal relationships.

The second example is the Mt. Sinai Palliative Care team (Icahn School of Medicine at Mount Sinai, 2023). Operating through five of Mt. Sinai's eight hospitals in New York, members of the palliative care team number more than 80 and include nurses, doctors, social workers, a chaplain, and others to provide comprehensive inpatient, outpatient, or home-based palliative care that is available around the clock. Teams provide coordinated care that includes symptom management, discussion about the patient's condition and treatment options, and physical, psychosocial, spiritual, emotional, and social services support. The goal is to center patients and their families to relieve suffering and attain the highest possible quality of life for the patient when curative treatment is no longer an option. In interviews with members of this team, Mitchell et al. (2012) discovered that they had established a selective hiring process to ensure that anyone brought onto the team shared the team's values so that trust and mutual continuous learning would be maintained and nurtured.

If we haven't said so explicitly yet, there is good evidence that interdisciplinary healthcare teams can lead to several positive outcomes, including improved patient safety and quality of care, increased efficiency and reduced cost, improved patient health outcomes, a safer workplace, increased provider satisfaction, and reduced staff turnover (Rosen et al., 2018). However, working in teams is complicated and challenging, particularly when dealing with hierarchical relationships (e.g., physician–nurse, specialist–general practitioner) and implicit biases and stereotyping (Sukhera et al., 2021). Poor communication resulting from these complications and challenges can lead to a host of negative outcomes, including threats to patient safety. It is to the connection between healthcare provider communication and patient safety that we turn our attention next.

Healthcare Provider Communication and Patient Safety

In 2000, the Institute of Medicine (IOM) issued its landmark report, *To Err is Human* (Kohn et al., 2000), documenting the impact of adverse events on patient morbidity and mortality. An **adverse event** is a medical error that results in "an undesirable clinical outcome—an outcome not caused by underlying disease—that prolonged the patient stay, caused permanent patient harm, required life-saving intervention, or contributed to death" (U.S. Department of Health and Human Services, 2022, n.p.). Such events include failing to make a timely diagnosis, procedural complications, and medical errors. Martin Makary and Michael Daniel (2016) estimated that preventable adverse events account for between 250,000 and 400,000 deaths annually in U.S. hospitals, making medical errors the third leading cause of death in the nation. The number one cause for these errors? Communication problems.

In a report identifying the eight most common root causes of medical errors, AHRQ (2003) put communication problems at the top of the list. The report noted that such problems could cause all sorts of errors (e.g., incorrect medication, incorrect dosage, operating on the wrong surgical site or wrong patient) and that the problems could happen in all sorts of circumstances (n.p.):

> Communication failures (verbal or written) can take many forms, including miscommunication within an office practice as well as miscommunication between different components of the health care system or health care providers working different shifts. These problems can occur between health care providers such as primary care physicians and emergency room personnel, attending physicians and ancillary services, and nursing homes and patient services in hospitals. Communication problems can result in poorly documented or lost information on laboratory results, diagnostic testing, or medication information, and can occur at any point along the communication chain. Communication problems can also occur within a health care team in one location, between providers at different locations, between health care teams and other non-clinician providers (such as labs or imaging centers), and between health care providers and patients.

In other words, there is a multitude of opportunities for communication problems in healthcare. One of the most significant is the patient handoff.

Healthcare Team Communication and Patient Safety

A healthcare team is an identifiable group of two or more people working interdependently toward shared, mutual goals that could not be accomplished effectively, if at all, by a single person.

Members of highly effective teams are honest, disciplined, creative, humble, and curious. Teams should have shared goals, clear roles, mutual trust, effective communication, and measurable processes and outcomes. Healthcare organizations need to provide adequate resources and support to promote team effectiveness.

Poor communication among healthcare providers can lead to medical errors and patient harm.

Patient Handoffs

A **patient handoff** is defined as the transfer of patient care from one healthcare provider to another (The Joint Commission, 2017). Handoffs happen between all different types of healthcare providers, such as nurse to nurse, therapist to physician, and paramedic to emergency department staff. They happen between units within hospitals (e.g., emergency department to surgery) and between different care facilities (e.g., hospital to nursing home). Handoff communication may be verbal (either in person or recorded) or written. These days, technology can also be used to facilitate patient handoffs. Examples include cloud-based applications designed specifically for handoffs (Albanese et al., 2022) and electronic health records (EHR) that organize all patient information into one portal (Panda, 2020).

With the latest data showing nearly 33 million total admissions to U.S. hospitals each year (American Hospital Association, 2022), the opportunity for miscommunication during handoffs leading to adverse events is unsettling. Adverse events can result from patient handoffs in which the information exchanged about the patient is incomplete, inaccurate, unclear, not timely, or misunderstood. Michael Rosen and colleagues (2018) described patient handoffs as "high-risk interactions in which critical information about the patient's status and plan of care can be miscommunicated, leading to delays in treatment or inappropriate therapies" and said they were "leading opportunities for communication failures directly causing patient harm" (p. 435). **The Joint Commission (TJC),** an organization that provides accreditation to healthcare organizations across the nation, deemed communication during the handoff so essential to patient safety that it made standardization of patient handoffs a part of their standards for accreditation, stating that the handoff process needed to include the opportunity for discussion between the healthcare providers giving and taking responsibility for the patient (TJC, 2017).

In addition, TJC listed five expectations for the discussion: (a) it should be interactive, (b) it should include up-to-date information about the patient, (c) there should be a process for verifying the information received, (d) the provider receiving the handoff information should be able to review any relevant historical patient data, and (e) interruptions during the handoff should be minimized to keep the discussion focused (Arora & Johnson, 2006). TJC also suggested that providers use a standardized checklist or another tool to help organize and ensure consistency and clarity of the information transferred from one provider to another.

There are several patient handoff checklists available. One of the most common is called **SBAR,** for **Situation-Background-Assessment-Recommendation**. Interestingly, SBAR has its roots in the military and aviation industry (Narayan, 2013). It was initially developed by the U.S. Navy for use in nuclear submarines (where it's sorta important to get things right), and then it was adopted and modified for the aviation industry (you know, the preflight checklist we've all had to wait on before our flight could take off). Eventually, Kaiser Permanente developed the tool for use in healthcare. (A quick aside: The SBAR can be used in healthcare contexts beyond the patient handoff, such as a nurse calling a physician to report a concern about a patient, but we're focusing our discussion here on using SBAR for patient handoffs.)

The specifics of each handoff will vary with each patient, of course, but broadly, the SBAR protocol involves the following four steps. First, the provider handing off the patient, let's call them Nurse Judy, tells the provider receiving the patient, let's call them Nurse Tyler, a concise statement of the *situation*. For example, Judy would state the patient's name and condition. Next, Judy would provide pertinent *background information* on the patient, such as the most recent vital signs, any new lab results, and any changes in patient status. Then, Judy would provide an *assessment* of the situation, noting any particular concerns.

Finally, Judy would make any *recommendations* that they think Tyler should follow during the upcoming shift. Along the way, Tyler should be able to clarify or verify any of the information Judy provides. Checklists such as SBAR are useful to promote consistency and clarity of information. Evaluations of their effectiveness, though, suggest there may be room for improvement. For example, a systematic review of the use of SBAR in handoffs showed only five of 11 studies found statistically significant improvements in patient outcomes (Müller et al., 2018). One reason for this may be that SBAR and other checklists lack a foundation in communication theory. Would a theoretical framework help to provide greater guidance in applying the SBAR to patient handoffs? This is what Anne Streeter and her colleagues wanted to find out.

Streeter et al. (2015) applied principles of communication competence (Spitzberg & Cupach, 1984; see Table 6.1) and Don Cegala's PACE model (see Chapter 3) to see how nurses differentiated the "best" from the "worst" patient handoffs. Their goal was to identify specific communication behaviors that would characterize competent, or high-quality, handoffs. They hypothesized that high-quality handoffs would have higher ratings of information exchange behaviors (giving, seeking, and verifying information) and higher ratings of socioemotional behaviors (being warm and friendly, being open and honest, showing compassion, showing they care, making the other nurse feel comfortable, using understandable language, and contributing to a trusting relationship) than poor quality handoffs. They recruited 286 nurses to complete an anonymous online questionnaire assessing handoff quality. The focus on nurses was important because they provide or coordinate more than 80% of patient care (Keenan et al., 2008), so finding a way to improve the quality of handoff communication between nurses could make a substantial contribution to healthcare quality and safety.

The study asked participants to reflect on a specified role during a shift change (incoming nurse vs. outgoing nurse) and handoff quality (best vs. worst). Specifically, the questionnaire instructions read as follows:

> Think back to a time when you were the (incoming/outgoing) nurse and participated in the (best/worst) handoff of a patient's care at the nursing change of shift. Describe below what made this handoff the (best/worst) one that you can remember as the (incoming/outgoing) nurse.
>
> (Streeter et al., 2015, p. 300)

After providing an open-ended description of the handoff, nurses completed a scale that assessed their perceptions of their own and the other nurse's information seeking, giving, and verifying behaviors and socioemotional communication.

Results of Streeter et al.'s (2015) study showed that mean scores on all information exchange and socioemotional variables were higher in the best-quality handoffs than the worst-quality handoffs. This indicates that specific communication behaviors associated with seeking, giving, and verifying information, as well as with being socioemotionally supportive, can lead to higher quality handoffs as perceived by nurses. Interestingly, perceptions of which nurse was responsible for these behaviors varied in three key ways. Specifically, all nurses regardless of their role generally thought the incoming nurse should be the one asking questions, should verify information provided by the outgoing nurse, and should set a positive socioemotional climate (quite possibly because the outgoing nurse would be exhausted).

Streeter and Harrington (2017) subsequently analyzed the qualitative data gathered in response to the open-ended question asking for a description of the best/worst handoff. They found that the qualitative data supported the quantitative results but provided more detail. For example, incoming nurses described the types of patient information they wanted the outgoing nurse to give (e.g., status/results of lab and radiology tests, personal/social information about the patient or family that might influence care), and they described the order in which they preferred to receive patient information (a "head-to-toe" body systems approach). Incoming nurses emphasized the importance of being able to seek information so they could "hit the ground running." For socioemotional communication, incoming nurses appreciated when outgoing nurses would introduce them to patients and families, saying something to instill confidence in quality of care, such as "I know I'm leaving you in good hands" (Streeter & Harrington, 2017, p. 5). Outgoing nurses appreciated being thanked by the incoming nurse, complimented for quality care, and not judged if they couldn't complete a task during their shift. The open-ended data also revealed four other characteristics that differentiated best from worst-quality handoffs: *location* (bedside was best), *environment* (quiet and calm with minimal distractions), *type* (face-to-face to facilitate discussion), and *time* (having enough of it). Interestingly, one nurse added insight into why the patient's bedside was the preferred location for a handoff (Streeter & Harrington, 2017, p. 5):

> The patient is involved and has the opportunity to listen to our report, get involved, correct us if we are wrong about any history or information or anything else. This gives them the opportunity to ask questions and really be an active part in our care for them.

Streeter and Harrington (2017) used the results of their qualitative analysis to create tables that included specific "handoff tips" for change of shift and tips for building trust and rapport. They also created a PACE Nurse Handoff Tool, which organized results into Present, Ask, Check/clarify, and Express concerns categories. They published their work in a nursing journal to reach the nursing audience, making this an example of translational research.

Use of Technology in Healthcare Provider Communication

We mentioned that technology can assist with patient handoffs, but we haven't considered the broad impact of technology on interprofessional healthcare provider communication and whether it helps or hurts. The answer is yes. As always, it's not the technology itself that necessarily makes a difference. It's how the technology is introduced and integrated into the workflow. Introducing technology seamlessly is basically impossible, but on the continuum of good to bad integration, our read of the literature is that it leans toward the bad. For example, Ilinca Popovici and colleagues (2015) designed a study to assess how technology-based communication tools influenced communication between providers and to identify any major technology-related barriers. The goal of their study was "to provide the necessary domain knowledge for designers to anticipate the impact that their communication tools will have on the workflow of the healthcare team" (p. 184). The researchers did 123 hours of observational research at three large teaching hospitals in Toronto. They also conducted in-depth interviews with three clinicians at each hospital to contextualize their data. They conducted a thematic analysis of their observational and interview data and identified six issues of concern related to technology. We summarize those findings in Table 6.2.

Popovici et al. (2015) also identified two issues not directly related to technology but that could potentially be improved by it. One was the "Ineffectiveness of the paper chart for storing and accessing patient information" (p. 186). The problems with the paper chart were illegible handwriting (a notorious problem) and troubles with organizing the charts and finding needed information in them, especially updates or changes. The risks to patients were orders that were duplicated, incomplete, incorrect, or even missing, as well as

Table 6.2 Communication Issues Identified in the Use of Technology during Patient Handoffs and the Risk to Patients

Communication Issue	Risk to Patients
High Reliance on Interruptive Communication The prevalence of face-to-face, interruptive communication devices such as pagers, shared phone lines, and overhead paging contributed to a chaotic, distracting work environment, with interruptions leading to errors because working memory was disrupted.	Errors in patient care.
Severe Workflow Inefficiencies and Delays Due to Numeric Pagers The workflow for numeric pagers involved the caller waiting for a call back near the nursing station phones, but the receiver of the page lacked awareness of the urgency of the issue. Delayed and unanswered pages were the norm, and user feedback was very poor.	Delays in patient care.
Multitude of Specialized, Unintegrated Tools Physicians often carried multiple devices (e.g., multiple pagers, hospital-provided smartphone, personal phone), which made prioritizing and answering medical requests difficult. Work duplication was often an issue because clinicians were required to chart similar patient-related information in up to four different systems. Accessing the multiple information sources was also difficult and time consuming.	Delays in patient care and inaccessible patient information.
Lack of Awareness of Completion Status of Patient Tests and Consultations Clinicians were often unaware of the completion status of tests or consultations, which introduced delays in patient care.	Delays in patient care.
Unintuitive User Interfaces for Software Tools The EHR systems in use at each site had usability issues in terms of entering orders and viewing test results. The interfaces of other software programs (e.g., electronic whiteboards, smart web paging) were over-crowded with symbols. Clinicians were repeatedly observed to struggle when interacting with these systems.	Errors with order entry and delays in retrieving information (e.g., test results, medication list).
Delays and Errors Stemming from Mixed Use of EHR and Paper Ordering The transition phase from a paper system to an EHR system carried a high risk of delays and errors in patient care.	Duplicated or incomplete orders and delays in patient care.

Note. Adapted from Popovici et al. (2015).

delays in patient care while sorting out the paper chart information. With proper design and implementation, EHRs could alleviate this issue. The second issue was "Lack of timely and accurate contact information for clinicians" (p. 186). Basically, providers had a hard time figuring out which other providers were working when, who was on call, and how to contact anybody. Surprisingly, "All hospitals lacked an accessible and comprehensive hospital-wide contact information list or on-call schedule. Clinicians involved in the care of one patient often meet when both parties attempt to use the paper chart simultaneously" (p. 186). An accessible, user-friendly, technological interface containing all this information could go a long way to solving this issue. Until that time, though, maybe hanging on to the paper charts isn't such a bad idea. As this study shows, there is room for improvement in how communication technology is used in hospitals. But what about improving healthcare team communication in general? It's to those interventions that we turn next.

Interventions to Improve Healthcare Team Communication

Given the essential role of competent communication in promoting the quality and safety of patient care, you won't be surprised to learn that many interventions have been developed to improve communication in healthcare teams. Interestingly, there is considerable variety in the approach to these trainings. Sallie Weaver and colleagues (2017) described several broad team training strategies, including *assertiveness training*, which covers principles such as conflict management, mutual trust, psychological safety, and leadership, and *error management training*, which teaches trainees how to recognize and manage errors in a controlled training environment. Another training strategy they identified was cross-training. *Cross-training* focuses on teaching healthcare team members "the roles that comprise the team and the tasks, duties, and responsibilities fulfilled by fellow team members" (p. 61). This kind of training is also known as **interprofessional education (IPE)**. Such education emphasizes developing mutual understanding and respect for each member's disciplinary expertise and contributions. Mutual understanding and respect, in turn, are meant to promote collaboration and coordination among team members. Mitchell et al. (2012) have noted that "Health education groups in the United States and abroad have called for improved interprofessional education in the preclinical and clinical settings" (p. 22).

Although IPE can be offered to practicing healthcare professionals, many universities offer IPE opportunities for their health professions students to better prepare them to enter the workforce. There is even a national organization devoted to it, called the **Interprofessional Education Collaborative (IPEC)**. The IPEC was established in 2009 and now comprises 21 national health professions associations. Its mission is "to ensure that new and current health professionals are proficient in the competencies essential for patient-centered, community- and population-oriented, interprofessional, collaborative practice" (IPEC, 2022, para. 6). With such a focus on IPE, you might wonder whether there is any evidence for its effectiveness. The literature in this area is still young, but a number of systematic reviews have found evidence that IPE can improve student attitudes toward interdisciplinary teamwork, as well as interprofessional collaborative knowledge, skills, and/or behaviors (e.g., Marcussen et al., 2019; Riskiyana et al., 2018).

One widely used intervention for healthcare team training is called **TeamSTEPPS**. This program was released in 2006 by the AHRQ and the U.S. Department of Defense, and it has been implemented by healthcare organizations and health professionals across the United States (King et al., 2008). TeamSTEPPS is an evidence-based program that focuses on communication and teamwork skills to improve patient safety (AHRQ, 2019). It was recently updated to its 2.0 version. Updates included adding a measurement module to provide users with validated measures to evaluate the impact of the program and enhancing the communication module. TeamSTEPPS 2.0 has an "essentials" version (two hours of training) that is designed for staff who do not provide direct patient care (e.g., administrators) and a "fundamentals" version (four to six hours of training) that is designed for those who do (e.g., nurses, physicians, dentists). The fundamentals course consists of seven modules: introduction, team structure, communication, leading teams, situation monitoring, mutual support, and summary. There also are supplemental modules to aid in program implementation, which is exceedingly important to promote implementation fidelity (i.e., teaching the program the way it was meant to be taught).

You might be wondering whether TeamSTEPPS has positive outcomes. So did Alissa Chen and colleagues (2019). These researchers conducted a comprehensive review of the literature to be able to describe approaches to the implementation and evaluation of Team-STEPPS and its outcomes in IPE. They identified 22 programs across the nation and one in Singapore that had implemented TeamSTEPPS in some way, shape, or form and then reported on it. The researchers found that a wide variety of health professions students participated in the programs, including medical, nursing, pharmacy, dental, and public health students and medical and pharmacy residents, among several others. Programs involved anywhere from 2 to 10 types of health professions, the most common combination being medical and nursing students. The most common instructional strategy was small or large group didactic sessions, but programs also used simulations and online instruction. Only five of the programs explicitly described which parts of the TeamSTEPPS program they implemented, and only one of those fully implemented the formal program (i.e., had 100% fidelity). Thirteen programs used validated measures to evaluate the impact of the curriculum, although only four of them used the measures provided by TeamSTEPPS. Chen et al. concluded that "the results of all the programs are generally positive" (p. 802). Given the challenges inherent in implementing curricula in busy academic and practice settings, we consider that an encouraging outcome.

The Experience of Being a Healthcare Provider

We've covered a lot so far about healthcare teams, patient safety, and IPE, including communication training. When things go smoothly in healthcare, providers can feel a great sense of professional satisfaction and derive great meaning from their work. When things don't go smoothly, though, and workplace stress builds, it can lead to burnout. In addition, like any other workplace, healthcare is not immune to problems of discrimination. That means added stress for women, people of color, and other marginalized groups. It's those darker sides of the healthcare provider experience that we address in this section.

Burnout

You know that feeling when you've been working so hard and been under so much stress, all you want to do is quit and run away? That's burnout. In the 11th revision of its International Classification of Diseases, the World Health Organization (2019) defines **burnout** as "a syndrome conceptualized as resulting from chronic workplace stress that has not been successfully managed" (para 4). Burnout has three components. First, there is *emotional exhaustion*, when a person's energy has been depleted by overwhelming and incessant demands. Second, there are feelings of *negativism, cynicism, and depersonalization*, where people feel detached from their jobs. Finally, there's a sense of *reduced personal accomplishment*, where a person lacks self-efficacy and a sense of achievement.

Although burnout can happen in any profession, it is a particularly significant problem among healthcare providers. Since 2011, Tait Shanafelt and colleagues (2022) have been conducting triennial surveys among physicians and adults working in a variety of other professions in the United States. They consistently find that physicians are at increased risk of burnout and have lower satisfaction with work-life balance than other adults in the U.S. workforce. Their latest survey revealed that 38.2% of physicians reported experiencing at least one symptom of burnout. Likewise, a report by the National Academy of Medicine (2019), which was written by its Committee on Systems Approaches to Improve Patient Care by Supporting Clinician Well-Being, indicates that "between 35 and 54 percent of U.S. nurses and physicians have substantial symptoms of burnout; similarly, the prevalence of burnout ranges between 45 and 60 percent for medical students and residents" (p. 1).

The causes of burnout are multiple and systemic. To demonstrate, let's consider physicians. Burnout for them likely starts in residency, when they are still in training yet engaged in substantial patient care for long stretches of time. Ingrid Philibert and Cynthia Taradejna (2011) noted that the long hours residents are expected to work were rooted in "traditional models of physician education as brief periods of intense training, during which responsibility for patients rested with residents 24 hours a day, 7 days a week" (p. 6). When a study in the early 1970s showed that residents coming off call made more errors reading an electrocardiogram than residents who had not been on call (Friedman et al., 1971), concern about the impact of sleep deprivation on patient safety began to mount. But it wasn't until the mid-1980s that things began to change. An advisory committee recommended that residents work no more than 80 hours/week (which, you realize, is twice that of a regular work week), work no more than 24 hours consecutively, and always be supervised by a senior physician. Adoption of these recommendations was spotty, but then the Accreditation Council for Graduate Medical Education (ACGME) stepped in. In 2003, the organization mandated a maximum of 80 hour/week, no more than 30 hours of consecutive duty, being on call no more than every third night, and getting one day off per week. In 2011, it added further requirements: first-year residents (sometimes called interns) should work no more than 16 hours in a row, and senior residents should work no more than 24 hours in a row; all residents should get at least 8 hours off between scheduled shifts; and all residents should get at least 14 hours off after 24 hours of being on call at work (Philibert & Amis, 2011).

Although these requirements may help somewhat to mitigate physician fatigue, there are other systemic factors that increase the likelihood of burnout, such as heavy workload, time pressures, lack of autonomy, technology challenges, inadequate resources, and healthcare worker shortage (National Academy of Medicine, 2019). As you might imagine, there are several negative outcomes of burnout. Risk to patient safety is one of the greatest, along with broader costs to organizations and society. At the provider level, though, there are also serious personal consequences. Burned-out providers are more likely to experience career regret and quit their jobs. They are more likely to experience depression and substance misuse. And they are more likely to commit suicide. For example, approximately 400 physicians commit suicide each year (Kishore et al., 2016). Among male physicians, the rate of suicide is 1.41 times higher than adult males in the general population, and among female physicians, the rate is 2.27 times higher than adult females in the general population (Schernhammer & Colditz, 2004). To show you the devastating impact of burnout and physician suicide, we'll share the story of one physician who took her life in the throes of the COVID-19 pandemic, Dr. Lorna Breen. *The New York Times* (Knoll et al., 2020) reported her story.

Dr. Breen had been an overachiever her whole life and always knew she wanted to be a doctor. She did residencies in both emergency medicine and internal medicine, and she became supervisor of the emergency department at New York-Presbyterian Allen Hospital. She enjoyed running, snowboarding, and salsa dancing, and she played the cello. She also was in a dual-degree master's program at Cornell University, even while she was a practicing physician. Just before the pandemic hit, Dr. Breen and her sister, Jennifer Feist, went on a planned vacation. By the time she returned to work on March 14, 2020, a state of emergency had been declared in New York, and her emergency department was overwhelmed with COVID-19 patients. Four days later, she came down with the virus, and it hit her hard. She came back to work on April 1 to discover complete chaos. On April 9, Dr. Breen called her sister and said, "I don't know what to do. I can't get out of the chair." Her sister took her to the University of Virginia Medical Center, where Dr. Breen checked herself into the psychiatric ward. She spent about 11 days there before being discharged and going to stay with her mother. Although she showed some signs of improvement, she never returned to her old self. On April 26, she committed suicide. She did not leave a note.

Devastated, her sister Jennifer and Jennifer's husband, Corey, established the Dr. Lorna Breen Heroes' Foundation (drlornabreen.org), an organization dedicated to reducing burnout among healthcare professionals and protecting their well-being and job satisfaction. Part of their efforts included working with Senator Tim Kaine (D-VA), other members of Congress, and healthcare industry leaders to develop the **Dr. Lorna Breen**

Health Care Provider Protection Act. On March 18, 2022, President Biden signed the Act into law. It provides funding for training and education grants for healthcare providers and students, establishes an awareness campaign to reduce stigma and encourage help seeking, and works to identify and disseminate best practices to reduce and prevent burnout and suicide. That is certainly a step in the right direction. But is there anything else being done? Yes.

Alex Anderson and colleagues (2022) report on a study that the Institute for Healthcare Improvement conducted with help from the Health Research and Educational Trust and the Centers for Disease Control and Prevention. The goal was to identify what changes needed to be made to prevent healthcare provider suicide. The report identified three areas for change. First, stigma associated with burnout, suicide, and help seeking needs to be reduced and psychological safety needs to be prioritized. Second, there needs to be increased access to mental health services for healthcare providers. Finally, job-related challenges that lead to burnout, such as mandatory overtime and administrative burden, need to be reduced. But how should healthcare organizations go about making such changes?

The National Academy of Medicine (2019) report we mentioned earlier is meant to be a resource for healthcare organizations nationwide in their efforts to reduce burnout and promote provider well-being. The committee members who produced the report developed a **systems model of clinician burnout and professional well-being** that drew on theories and concepts from multiple social science and engineering disciplines to identify multilevel factors contributing to burnout that should be taken into account when designing interventions to improve well-being (see Table 6.1). Factors at the external environmental level are the healthcare industry, societal values, and laws, regulations, and standards. At the healthcare organization level, factors include leadership and management, governance, and organizational rewards and benefits. At the center are the frontline care team members (providers, staff, learners, patients, and families) who are affected by local conditions within the healthcare organization, technologies (including EHRs), the physical environment, and the various tasks that comprise healthcare. These multilevel factors influence clinician burnout and professional well-being (as mediated by individual difference characteristics such as clinician age, experience, role, and personality characteristics), which in turn have consequences for patients, clinicians, healthcare organizations, and society.

The report offers guidelines for designing "well-being systems" within care facilities (National Academy of Medicine, 2019). First, organizations need to adopt a systems approach to align the structures and functions of the organization with its values, and it needs strong leadership to reduce burnout, increase professional wellness, and support patient care. Second, there needs to be a work system redesign that provides adequate resources to facilitate clinicians' work and promotes a sense of meaning and purpose, as well as teamwork, collaboration, communication, and professionalism. Finally, there needs to be a comprehensive and concerted implementation strategy for the redesigned well-being system that addresses infrastructure, reward systems, organizational culture, and human-centered design processes. To accomplish all of this, the committee set forth six goals: (a) create positive work environments, (b) create positive learning environments, (c) reduce administrative burden, (d) enable technology solutions, (e) provide support to clinicians and learners, and (f) invest in research on professional well-being. For each goal, the report provides detailed action steps to facilitate progress. Does all of this sound "pie in the sky"? Perhaps. As ER doctor Thomas Fisher observed of the U.S. healthcare system, "It took generations to build this, it's gonna take generations to dismantle it, and there's going to be a lot of setbacks along the way" (Weissman, 2022). But reports like this one from the National Academy of Medicine and efforts like those from the ACGME are steps in the right direction.

What Is Burnout?

Burnout is a syndrome resulting from chronic workplace stress that has not been successfully managed.

Burnout consists of emotional exhaustion; feelings of negativism, cynicism, and depersonalization; and a sense of reduced personal accomplishment.

Burnout can be reduced through systemic efforts to reduce stigma, increase access to mental health services, and deal with job-related challenges, as well as making changes to the workplace environment to promote professional well-being.

Discrimination

As you learned in Chapter 2, discrimination continues to be a significant problem in the United States, and the healthcare system is no different. In this section, we'll focus on discrimination against people of color (Filut et al., 2020) and women (e.g., Newman et al., 2020), although other groups of healthcare providers face discrimination, as well (e.g., providers with disabilities; Lindsay et al., 2022). We'll start with brief statistics and then describe experiences and effects of discrimination. We'll wrap up the section with suggestions for reducing discrimination in healthcare.

The Association of American Medical Colleges (AAMC) represents the 125 accredited allopathic (i.e., conventional) medical schools in the United States. The organization maintains a host of statistics on medical students and physicians in the workforce, including figures on sex and race (AAMC, 2023). For example, in the 1980–1981 academic year, approximately 70% of applicants to medical school were male and 30% were female. In the 2018–2019 academic year, it was 49% male and 51% female. Longitudinal data isn't available on medical school applications by race/ethnicity. However, the 2018–2019 data shows the following percentages: 46.8% white, 21.3% Asian, 9.2% multiple race/ethnicity, 8.4% Black or African American, 6.2% Hispanic or Latino, 0.2% American Indian or Alaskan Native, and 0.1% Native Hawaiian or Pacific Islander; 4.1% were other or unknown, and 3.7% were non-U.S. citizen or nonpermanent resident. Figures for sex and race/ethnicity shift, however, when you look at students who become practicing physicians. In 2018, 64% of practicing physicians were male and 36% were female. In terms of race/ethnicity of practicing physicians, 2018 data showed the following: 56.2% white, 17.1% Asian, 1.0% multiple race/ethnicity, 5.0% Black or African American, 5.8% Hispanic, 0.3% American Indian or Alaskan Native, and 0.1% Native Hawaiian or Pacific Islander; 14.5% were other or unknown. So, there is a drop-off among women and African Americans from the time they enter medical school to the time they enter the workforce. Discrimination, either overt or systemic, is sure to play some role in that.

What does discrimination look like for women and African American doctors? In their review of the literature on sex discrimination, Connie Newman and colleagues (2020) identified substantial differences in the experience of discrimination between men and women physicians. One study showed that whereas 9% of men reported gender bias that hurt their professional advancement, 60% of women did so. Another study showed that whereas 10% of men perceived gender bias directed at them personally, 66% of women did so. The authors summarized the negative effects of sex bias toward women doctors. First, their careers are negatively affected. They are underrepresented in leadership positions, are less likely to be promoted in academic positions (and are promoted more slowly), receive fewer professional awards, lead fewer grand rounds, present fewer national lectures, and are more likely to leave the profession. Second, there are negative financial impacts, with women doctors earning lower salaries and receiving less grant funding (which is essential for tenured academic positions). Third, they face harassment, burnout, and imposter syndrome (doubting their skills and accomplishments and worrying about being called a fraud). The situation for physicians of color is no better.

In a systematic review of the literature on discrimination against physicians of color, Amarette Filut and colleagues (2020) found widespread evidence of discrimination, especially toward Black physicians. Specifically, discrimination was experienced by 59–71% of Black physicians, 20–27% of Hispanic/Latino physicians, 31–50% of Asian physicians, and 6–29% of white physicians. The types of discrimination were vast. There were many examples of overt statements of prejudice, but there were also examples of "inadequate institutional support, exclusion from social networks, devaluation of research on minority health or health disparities, and a lack of institutional commitment to advancing diversity" (p. 4). In addition, "Physicians of color described facing greater scrutiny, being held to higher standards, having their competence questioned, needing to justify their credentials, and being mistaken for maintenance, housekeeping, or food service workers in the workplace" (p. 4). The impact of this discrimination led to negative outcomes such as lack of career advancement, lower career satisfaction, changing specialties, leaving medicine entirely, and reporting being in poorer health.

You might recall the discussion of intersectionality from Chapter 2. As a reminder, intersectionality describes the experience of having multiple social identities (e.g., Black, female, disabled) and how those intersecting identities affect the experience of privilege and oppression in society. In medicine, the intersection of sex and race is particularly fraught. To show you how, we'll share quotes from two women physicians of color:

- Being a Black woman and a physician has often felt like an existence of opposing identities. As a physician, I am entrusted with protecting the bodies, health, and well-being of my patients and am told all lives matter. Yet as a Black woman I carry the legacy of enslavement, experimentation, eugenics, and disenfranchisement. I have attempted to lead with my professional identity as a means of subverting the oppositional nature of my dual identities, yet have often failed, as I have found the first and often only thing I am judged by is the color of my skin. On countless occasions people have assumed that I am anything other than a physician. –Kameelah Lanette Gateau (2021, p. 327)
- As a Hispanic woman, a number of reasons explain why I am meticulous about how I present myself. Often, I am the only minority and female rounding on a team. During one such time, a patient called my tall, male peer Clark Kent. Another patient called me Margarita. At first, I dismissed it with a chuckle to save face, but a hidden inuendo lurks beneath these monikers, and it must be understood. Clark Kent is a quintessential savior who leads an insurmountable alliance. Margarita is an alcoholic beverage. –Natalie A. Moreno (2021, p. e32)

Highly trained professionals providing life-saving healthcare to patients should not find themselves in these positions, and so there must be systemic change to prevent such discrimination. What should that change look like?

Newman et al. (2020) offer nine recommendations to reduce sex discrimination. Eugenia South and colleagues (2020) detail several action steps that could be implemented to establish an equitable culture of antiracism in healthcare organizations. We present the recommendations in Table 6.3 and the actions steps in Table 6.4. Such change will not be easy, but it's necessary if our society is to ever achieve a healthcare system in which everyone can thrive. As South et al. observe, if interpersonal, institutional, and structural racism could

Table 6.3 Strategies for Improving Gender Inequities in Healthcare

1. Introduce implicit bias training for physicians and healthcare staff
2. Develop a compensation plan based on position only
3. Establish safe and clear processes for reporting incidents of bias in the workplace
4. Have transparent hiring procedures and promotion requirements
5. Develop career advancement plans for women and men physicians
6. Provide family leave for women regardless of their career stage
7. Nominate women physicians for leadership positions and other career advancement opportunities
8. Provide funding and support for women physicians to be able to participate in leadership and other career advancement opportunities
9. Be transparent about organizational commitment to equity and inclusion

Note. Based on Newman et al. (2020).

Table 6.4 Action Steps to Establish a Culture of Antiracism in Healthcare

1. Establish a network of supported leaders to oversee health system antiracism efforts
2. Empower existing health system teams to leverage strengths to address racism
3. Implement antiracism-focused training and education
4. Reevaluate institutional policies and practices with a lens of antiracism
5. Deploy accountable systems for racism reporting, feedback, and intervention
6. Reconfigure health systems as key actors in addressing structural barriers
7. Reorganize power structures and accountability in support of antiracism
8. Support scientific research focused on addressing and eliminating racism

Note. Based on South et al. (2020).

ever be overcome, "Many Black health care providers and patients could experience a sense of belonging and being treated fairly for the first time" (p. 5039). Imagine.

Conclusion

When doctors, nurses, and other health professionals care for patients, they accept a lot of responsibility. Despite potential challenges and pressures, these people dedicate themselves to serving patients. We hope this chapter has given you some insight into the experiences and perspectives of healthcare providers and the teams they work in. With so many people involved in patient care, exemplary communication is essential to avoid errors, yet it is a major challenge in the healthcare environment. Although a lot of research has sought to improve communication among members of healthcare teams, there is still room for more research. This research is especially needed to address the increasing rate of burnout and to reduce discrimination experienced by healthcare providers. Doing so will go a long way to helping healthcare providers thrive in their chosen professions. And when healthcare providers thrive, the entire healthcare system benefits.

References

Agency for Healthcare Research and Quality. (2003). *AHRQ's patient safety initiative: Building foundations, reducing risk.* https://archive.ahrq.gov/research/findings/final-reports/pscongrpt/psini2.html
Agency for Healthcare Research and Quality. (2019). *About TeamSTEPPS.* https://www.ahrq.gov/teamstepps/about-teamstepps/index.html
Agency for Healthcare Research and Quality. (2021). *Defining the PCMH.* https://www.ahrq.gov/ncepcr/research/care-coordination/pcmh/define.html

Albanese, E., Cameron T., Gervacio, J., & Van de Castle, B. (2022). Standardization of oncology nursing shift handoff utilizing a cloud-based application. *Oncology Nursing Forum, 49*(2), E99–E100.

American Hospital Association. (2022). *Fast facts on U.S. hospitals, 2022.* https://www.aha.org/statistics/fast-facts-us-hospitals

Anderson, A., Davidson, J., & Gold, K. (2022). Preventing healthcare workforce suicide. *Healthcare Executive, 38*(3), 54–57.

Andreatta, P. B. (2010). A typology for health care teams. *Health Care Management Review, 35*(4), 345–354.

Arora, V., & Johnson, J. (2006). A model for building a standardized hand-off protocol. *Journal on Quality and Patient Safety, 32*(11), 646–654.

Association of American Medical Colleges. (2023). *Data & reports.* https://www.aamc.org/

Chen, A. S., Yau, B., Revere, L., & Swails, J. (2019). Implementation, evaluation, and outcome of TeamSTEPPS in interprofessional education: A scoping review. *Journal of Interprofessional Care, 33*(6), 795–804.

Filut, A., Alverez, M., & Carnes, M. (2020). Discrimination toward physicians of color: A systematic review. *Journal of the National Medical Association, 112*(2), 117–140.

Friedman, R. C., Bigger, J. T., & Kornfeld, D. S. (1971). The intern and sleep loss. *New England Journal of Medicine, 285*(4), 201–203.

Gateau, K. L. (2021). White Coats for Black Lives. *Journal of Graduate Medical Education, 13*(3), 327–328.

Icahn School of Medicine at Mount Sinai. (2023). *Palliative care.* https://www.mountsinai.org/care/palliative-care

Interprofessional Education Collaborative. (2022). *About us.* https://www.ipecollaborative.org/about-us

Keenan, G. M., Tschannen, D., & Wesley, M. L. (2008). Standardized nursing terminologies can transform practice. *JONA, 38*(3), 1031–1106.

King, H. B., Battles, J., Baker, D. P., Alonso, A., Salas, E., Webster, J., Toomey, L., & Salisbury, M. (2008). TeamSTEPPS™: Team strategies and tools to enhance performance and patient safety. In *Advances in patient safety: New directions and alternative approaches* (Vol. 3: Performance and Tools). Agency for Healthcare Research and Quality.

Kishore, S., Dandurand, D. E., Mathew, A., & Rothenberger, D. (2016). *Breaking the culture of silence on physician suicide.* National Academy of Medicine.

Knoll, C., Watkins, A., & Rothfeld, M. (2020, July 11). "I couldn't do anything": The virus and an E.R. doctor's suicide. *The New York Times.* https://www.nytimes.com/2020/07/11/nyregion/lorna-breen-suicide-coronavirus.html

Kohn, L. T., Corrigan, J. M., & Donaldson, M. S. (Eds.). (2000). *To err is human: Building a safer health system* (Vol. 627). National Academies Press.

Lindsay, S., Fuentes, K., Ragunathan, S., Lamaj, L., & Dyson, J. (2022). Ableism within health care professions: A systematic review of the experiences and impact of discrimination against health care providers with disabilities. *Disability and Rehabilitation.* Advance online publication. doi: 10.1080/09638288.2022.2107086

Makary, M. A., & Daniel, M. (2016). Medical error—The third leading cause of death in the US. *BMJ, 353*, i2139.

Marcussen, M., Norgaard, B., & Arnfred, S. (2019). The effects of interprofessional education in mental health practice: Findings from a systematic review. *Academic Psychiatry, 43*(2), 200–208.

Mitchell, P., Wynia, M., Golden, R., McNellis, B., Okun, S., Webb, C. E., Rohrbach, V., & Von Kohorn, I. (2012). *Core principles & values of effective team-based health care.* Institute of Medicine.

Moreno, N. A. (2021). Of capes and white coats: Championing diversity and inclusion in medicine. *Annals of Surgery, 273*(2), e32–e33.

Müller, M., Jürgens, J., Redaèlli, M., Klingberg, K., Hautz, W. E., & Stock, S. (2018). Impact of the communication and patient hand-off tool SBAR on patient safety: A systematic review. *BMJ Open, 8*, e022202.

Narayan, M. C. (2013). Using SBAR communications in efforts to prevent patient rehospitalizations. *Home Healthcare Nurse, 31*(9), 504–515.

National Academy of Medicine. (2019). *Taking action against clinician burnout: A systems approach to professional well-being.* The National Academies Press.

National Academy of Medicine. (2022). *Event: Best practices innovation collaborative.* https://nam.edu/event/best-practices-innovation-collaborative-3/

Newman, C., Templeton, K., & Chin, E. L. (2020). Inequity and women physicians: Time to change millennia of societal beliefs. *The Permanente Journal, 24*, 1–6.

Panda, S. (2020). Nursing shift handoff process: Using an electronic health record tool to improve quality. *Clinical Journal of Oncology Nursing, 24*(5), 583–585.

Philibert, I., & Amis, S. (Eds.). (2011). *The ACGME 2011 duty hour standard enhancing quality of care, supervision, and resident professional development.* Accreditation Council for Graduate Medical Education.

Philibert, I., & Taradejna, C. (2011). A brief history of duty hours and resident education. In I. Philibert & S. Amis (Eds.), *The ACGME 2011 duty hour standard enhancing quality of care, supervision, and resident professional development* (pp. 5–11). Accreditation Council for Graduate Medical Education.

Popovici, I., Morita, P. P., Doran, D., Lapinsky, S., Morra, D., Shier, A., Wu, R., & Cafazzo, J. A. (2015). Technological aspects of hospital communication challenges: An observational study. *International Journal for Quality in Health Care, 27*(3), 183–188.

Rentsch, J., & Hall, R. (1994). Members of great teams think alike: A model of team effectiveness and schema similarity among team members. In M. Beyerlein & D. Johnson (Eds.), *Advances in interdisciplinary studies of work teams* (Vol. 1, pp. 223–262). JAI Press.

Riskiyana, R., Claramita, M., & Rahayu, G. R. (2018). Objectively measured interprofessional education outcome and factors that enhance program effectiveness: A systematic review. *Nurse Education Today, 66*, 73–78.

Rosen, M. A., DiazGranados, D., Dietz, A. S., Benishek, L. E., Thompson, D., Pronovost, P. J., & Weaver, S. J. (2018). Teamwork in healthcare: Key discoveries enabling safer, high-quality care. *American Psychologist, 73*(4), 433–450.

Schernhammer, E. S., & Colditz, G. A. (2004). Suicide rates among physicians: A quantitative and gender assessment (meta-analysis). *American Journal of Psychiatry, 161*(12), 2295–2302.

Schilling, S., Armaou, M., Morrison, Z., Carding, P., Bricknell, M., & Connelly, V. (2022). Understanding teamwork in rapidly deployed interprofessional teams in intensive and acute care: A systematic review of reviews. *PLoS ONE, 17*(8), e0272942.

Shanafelt, T. D., West, C. P., Sinsky, C., Trockel, M., Tutty, M., Wang, H., Carlasare, L. E., & Dyrbye, L. N. (2022). Changes in burnout and satisfaction with work-life integration in physicians and the general US working population between 2011 and 2020. *Mayo Clinic Proceedings, 97*(3), 491–506.

South, E. C., Butler, P. D., & Merchant, R. M. (2020). Toward an equitable society: Building a culture of antiracism in health care. *The Journal of Clinical Investigation, 130*(10), 5039–5041.

Spitzberg, B. H., & Cupach, W. R. (1984). *Interpersonal communication competence.* Sage.

Streeter, A. R., & Harrington, N. G. (2017). Nurse handoff communication. *Seminars in Oncology Nursing, 33*(5), 536–543.

Streeter, A. R., Harrington, N. G., & Lane, D. R. (2015). Communication behaviors associated with the competent nursing handoff. *Journal of Applied Communication Research, 43*(3), 294–314.

Sukhera, J., Bertram, K., Hendrikx, S., Chisolm, M. S., Perzhinsky, J., Kennedy, E., Lingard, L., & Goldszmidt, M. (2021). Exploring implicit influences on interprofessional collaboration: A scoping review. *Journal of Interprofessional Care, 36*(5), 716–724.

The Joint Commission. (2017, September 12). Inadequate hand-off communication. *Sentinel Event Alert 58.* Author.

U.S. Department of Health and Human Services. (2022). *Adverse events.* https://oig.hhs.gov/reports-and-publications/featured-topics/adverse-events/

U.S. Department of Veterans Affairs. (2022). *Patient care services: Patient Aligned Team Care (PACT.)* https://www.patientcare.va.gov/primarycare/PACT.asp

Weaver, S. J., Benishek, L. E., Leeds, I., & Wick, E. C. (2017). The relationship between teamwork and patient safety. In J. A. Sanchez, P. Barach, J. K. Johnson, & J. P. Jacobs (Eds.), *Surgical patient care: Improving safety, quality and value* (pp. 51–66). Springer.

Weissmann, D. (Host). (2022, July 7). On ER doc's journey through the pandemic—and the healthcare system. [Audio podcast episode]. In *An Arm & A Leg.* https://armandalegshow.com/episode/one-er-docs-journey/

World Health Organization. (2019, May 28). *Burn-out an "occupational phenomenon": International Classification of Diseases.* https://www.who.int/news/item/28-05-2019-burn-out-an-occupational-phenomenon-international-classification-of-diseases

In-class Activities

1. Separate the class into small groups. Assign each group one of the three types of communication trainings (assertiveness, error management training, and cross-training). Task groups with the following:

   > You've been hired to develop a communication skills training program to promote communication among members of a healthcare team. Select a type of healthcare team and propose a communication intervention program for your group's assigned training. Be prepared to share the details of your intervention, including what the focus will be, who will go through the training, and how you expect the training to improve healthcare team communication.

2. Have the students read the story of Dr. Lorna Breen: https://www.nytimes.com/2020/07/11/nyregion/lorna-breen-suicide-coronavirus.html. Then in small groups, have them identify the personal and systemic factors that led to her experiencing severe burnout.

Discussion Questions

1. Think about the last time you had a doctor's appointment or had to go to the hospital. How many different healthcare providers did you see? Did they seem to be working as a team? What did they do and say that made you answer the way you did?
2. Review the four types of healthcare teams identified by Andreatta (2010). Using Figure 6.1 as a reference, what are other examples of each of the four types of healthcare teams?
3. Why are Mitchell et al.'s (2012) five personal values of highly effective team members (i.e., honest, disciplined, creative, humble, and curious) particularly important for healthcare teams? Provide examples as to how the values could contribute to team effectiveness.

The Montgomery Family Needs Support

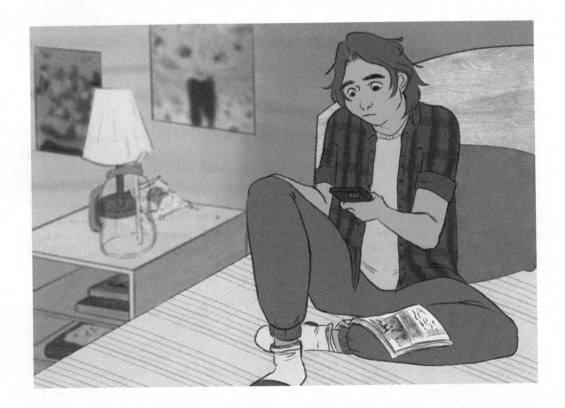

Throughout Helen's challenging breast cancer journey, no one could (or would) deny that Sally had fully stepped into the role of caregiver. Joe's recent promotion to superintendent of a large K-12 school district meant a lot of early-morning and late-night meetings—in addition to his regular eight-to-five work hours. Similarly, Michael had just accepted a job managing a 24-hour pharmacy. Although he typically worked the standard eight-to-five shift, he was often covering shifts for his team. Luckily for the family, not only was Sally more than willing to serve as an informal caregiver to Helen but her career as an independent artist provided her the flexibility she needed to be available to Helen. Of course, that meant Sally had to cut back significantly on her painting.

Sally may have been the primary caregiver, but Helen never found herself short of support from her family. Michael had taken lead on managing all of the paperwork associated with her treatment, which was nearly overwhelming. Joe was ensuring that all of the day-to-day activities stayed on track, such as paying the bills, keeping the house full of groceries, and

DOI: 10.4324/9781003214458-16

even making sure the car was always clean. One form of support that Helen hadn't expected to appreciate so much was Monica's and Cheryl's insistence on moderating all questions from friends and family far and wide. Cheryl had set up a CaringBridge page where she and Monica could post updates on Helen and answer questions, all without anyone having to bother Helen. This way, Helen could decide when and with whom she discussed her cancer. Even Savannah was helping, insisting on being the person to take Helen to get her hair done each week. Despite all of the help that everyone was trying to provide, Sally was still carrying a lot, including now being worried about Monica.

Following Michael's advice, Monica was about to quit her job. Working as an ER nurse during the COVID-19 pandemic had taken its final toll. Although Monica was insistent that quitting was the right decision, Sally worried about the lack of a clear plan for Monica's next steps. For the time being, Monica was contemplating using this time to be Helen's home care nurse. Although Sally was grateful, she was worried about the financial and emotional toll this might take on Monica.

And on top of Monica adding worry to Sally's plate, there was Samuel. His teenage mood swings had not ceased as the family had hoped. Although he'd seemed to be a little more comfortable at school lately, it was clear that he was still struggling to make friends. Sally thought not having anyone his age to talk to might be why he was on edge so often. But Cheryl knew the real reason. Last week, in a swirl of emotions, Samuel called her, and it all came out.

"So, did you hear the news about Elliot Page?" Samuel asked Cheryl. The actor was a favorite of both of theirs.

"Yes, I heard," Cheryl replied. "There was even a Time magazine feature on it."

"What did you think?" Samuel asked.

"I thought it was really brave, Samuel," Cheryl replied. She paused for a second before saying something she had been trying to say for the last year. "It must have been really hard for him to come out. He'd probably been thinking about how to tell people for a long time. You know? Trying to find the right moment?"

There was a short pause on the phone before Samuel responded, "I have no doubt."

"You know," Cheryl continued, as sincerely as possible, "I bet he started with a single person before working his way up to telling the entire world. Because telling one person is often a great place to start."

There was another short pause before Samuel asked, "How long have you known?"

"Samuel, you're my brother—my sibling. Sorry. I love you and I see you. Since we were kids I've known that you weren't like most other boys. And I figured that was why school had been so hard these last few years. I just want you to be happy," Cheryl said, feeling tears start to well.

"I just can't believe you knew," he said. There was a long pause before he choked, "You don't hate me, do you?"

"Of course, I don't hate you!" Cheryl said with conviction, starting to cry now herself. "Don't ever think that. I love you. The family loves you. You are who you are," Cheryl added, desperately hoping this was a remotely "right" thing to say. "What do you need?"

Samuel took another few moments to catch his breath. After thinking for a second he said, "I need to tell mom."

"That seems like a good idea," Cheryl said. "She'll probably be surprised, but she loves you, and nothing's going to change that. She's going to be glad you told her."

"Okay," Samuel said, still trying to stop crying.

"So, should I start using they/them pronouns?" Cheryl asked.

"Um, no. Thanks for asking, but I'm not ready. I need to tell mom first, and dad, I think. I don't know. And I don't know exactly how I want to label who I am or how I identify," Samuel admitted.

"I understand," Cheryl replied. "You just let me know what you need. And call anytime. Okay? Promise?"

"Promise," Samuel replied, feeling seen for the first time in his life.

To Cheryl's surprise, she would keep Samuel's secret for longer than expected. With all that was going on with Helen's health, Samuel kept finding reasons not to tell Sally. Although Cheryl had no doubt that Sally would be supportive, telling her seemed to be a step that Samuel just wasn't ready to take.

Notes

CaringBridge is a free online program for sharing health updates with family and friends. You can learn more about it here: https://caringbridge.org

If you want to read more about Elliot Page and his reflection on coming out, here is the *Time Magazine* story: https://time.com/5947032/elliot-page-2/

There are many resources available to support the LGBTQ+ community. If you are looking for such a resource, we recommend the following:

- https://gaycenter.org/
- https://www.thetrevorproject.org/
- https://www.cdc.gov/lgbthealth/index.htm

Knowing what to say when someone comes out to you can be difficult. Below are resources to assist with the conversation.

- From the University of North Carolina at Chapel Hill's LGBT Center, here is a guide for when a friend comes out to you (note that many of these tips apply to more than just friends): https://lgbtq.unc.edu/resources/how-to-support-lgbtq-people-on-campus/if-someone-comes-out-to-you/
- Rebecca Thompson from the Huffington Post (UK) provides reaction ideas to keep in mind when someone comes out to you: https://www.huffingtonpost.co.uk/entry/how-to-react-someone-comes-out_uk_5a688e34e4b072371ece73c0

If you're thinking about coming out but haven't quite figured out how to navigate the conversations, here are some resources intended to help.

- The University of California, Berkley Division of Equity & Inclusion provides a thoughtful review of what it means to come out and some ideas for how to navigate the conversations: https://cejce.berkeley.edu/geneq/resources/lgbtq-resources/coming-out
- NPR's *Life Kit* created a 23-minute episode to support both sides of the coming out conversation: https://www.npr.org/2020/06/01/867059156/navigating-the-coming-out-conversation-from-both-sides

7   Social Support and Informal Caregiving

You just got dumped by a longtime love. In response, your best friend tells you that you really are a terrific person and your ex is a jerk. Your instructor tells you about all the mental health resources your college offers free of charge to students. And your mom comes and cooks dinner for you every night for a week. Despite feeling awful, you listen to your friend, you call the number for a counselor, and you don't starve. You have just been the beneficiary of lots of social support. And like millions of other people on the planet who also receive social support, you're better off because of it. Indeed, understanding the positive relationship between social support and improved health outcomes, including a decreased rate of mortality, has kept researchers occupied for decades (MacGeorge & Zhou, 2022; Reblin & Uchino, 2008). And it's a relationship we'll be taking a close look at in this chapter.

We'll begin by presenting the foundations of social support, which include conceptual and operational definitions and theoretical models of how social support operates. We'll also cover research on how to effectively give advice and how to be an ally to members of marginalized groups that need support. Next, we'll turn our attention to online social support, an area that has attracted considerable attention from researchers. Then, we'll transition to informal caregivers—those friends and family members who provide support to people who are ill—and address the impact of providing care on their health and well-being. Finally, we'll consider interventions that have been developed to provide support for caregivers. As a human on this planet, you undoubtedly will both need and provide support in some way, shape, or form throughout your life. We hope, therefore, that you'll find this chapter helpful, if not now, in your future.

Foundations of Social Support

If you ask a bunch of people what social support is, their informal definitions probably will converge around the idea that social support is the things that people do and say to help one another in times of need. The American Psychological Association (2023) would mostly agree, but they'd elaborate slightly, stating that **social support** is "the provision of assistance or comfort to others, typically to help them cope with biological, psychological, and social stressors" (para. 1). These are fine definitions for a start, but as with all things academic, the concept is a little more complicated than that. To have a firm grasp of social support, you'll need to understand various distinctions in conceptual and operational definitions, as well as the different types of support that people provide. Let's start with how different disciplines approach the subject.

Erina MacGeorge and colleagues (2011) provide an instructive review of different disciplinary approaches to social support. A *sociological approach* emphasizes social support as **social integration**, which is the nature of a person's social network and how well integrated they are into it. For example, are you in a committed romantic relationship, do you

DOI: 10.4324/9781003214458-17

have a large family, and are you a member of a community organization? To the extent that you have such ties, you theoretically have access to greater social support resources. In other words, the more social connections you have, the more support you have. Measuring social support from a sociological perspective is relatively objective given that relationships and memberships can be reliably counted.

A *psychological approach*, on the other hand, emphasizes three aspects of social support: enacted support, received support, and perceived availability of support. These three aspects vary in how they are measured. **Enacted support** is actual supportive behaviors performed by others. Because valid measures of enacted support technically require observational research (e.g., a researcher observes your friend driving you to a doctor's appointment) or reports from support providers (e.g., a researcher talks to your friend or someone else who observed the friend driving you to your appointment), psychologists made a shift to studying received support. **Received support** is defined as support that a person says they have received. It has the benefit of being measured by self-report (e.g., you simply report that your friend drove you to the doctor's office). Both enacted and received support measures are retrospective, of course, and some psychologists were more interested in prediction. So, they turned to **perceived availability of support**, which is defined (via self-report) as how much support a person *believes* they have available to them if they would ever need it.

The discipline of *communication* takes a third approach, one that MacGeorge et al. (2011) distinguish along several lines. First, our discipline recognizes that communication itself is central to social support. This means that no matter which approach you take, verbal and nonverbal communication are required to function within a social network and to enact, receive, or perceive support. Second, the communication of social support is understood to have a direct effect on improving well-being, like the direct path between communication and health outcomes in Street et al.'s (2009) model of how communication heals (see Chapter 3, Figure 3.1). It also can have an indirect effect, of course (e.g., communication strengthens social integration, which improves well-being), but our discipline emphasizes the direct effect, whereas others do not. Third, there is a focus on the support provider's intention to help a person in need, along with attempting to understand how and why they perceive that the person needs help and how the recipient is or isn't helped. This focus emphasizes the *transactional* (back and forth) nature of communication. Fourth, instead of focusing only on psychological or physiological outcomes related to health and well-being, the communication discipline also emphasizes relationship outcomes, such as relational satisfaction. Finally, communication takes a normative approach to the study of social support, which means we consider the quality of supportive messages and their contextual appropriateness, we don't just assume that more support is better.

MacGeorge et al. (2011) define **supportive messages** as "verbal and nonverbal behavior produced with the intention of providing assistance to others perceived as needing that aid" (p. 317). Supportiveness in messages is operationalized as **person-centeredness**, which is "an awareness of and adaptation to the subjective, affective, and relational aspects of communicative contexts" (Burleson, 1987, p. 305). Supportive messages are typically categorized as being low, moderate, or high in person-centeredness. A good example of this comes from Colter Ray and Alaina Veluscek (2018), who conducted a study to see how breast cancer patients or survivors would respond to messages that varied in person-centeredness. They recruited 224 women to participate, asking them to think of "someone they would expect to receive emotional support from following the announcement of their breast cancer diagnosis on social media" (p. 650). These women then read either a low, moderate, or high person-centered message or the following statement: "Nothing was said. Although you expected the person to provide a supportive message, the person never reaches out to you to provide emotional support in regard to your diagnosis" (p. 650). (Ouch!) Table 7.1 provides definitions of the levels of person-centeredness and the test

Table 7.1 Low, Moderate, and High Person-Centered Breast Cancer Diagnosis Support Messages

Person-Centeredness	Definition	Example
Low	Challenges or ignores the legitimacy of the person's feelings. Tells the recipient how they ought to act or places blame on the recipient.	"I think this shows you have to start living a healthier lifestyle. You have to take care of yourself and not rely on luck when it comes to your health."
Moderate	Acknowledges the person's feelings but does not help the person elaborate their feelings or understand their experience in a broader sense.	"I'm really sorry to hear the news of your diagnosis. However, I'm sure you'll be okay."
High	Explicitly acknowledges the person's feelings. Helps elaborate these feelings to gain understanding and perspective on the broader context of the situation.	"I am really sorry. You must be devastated by the news. You're probably feeling uncertain and anxious and all sorts of other emotions, and that's completely understandable. I hope you know that myself and others are feeling for you and are here to support you. Let me know if there is anything you need or if you just need to talk through your thoughts and feelings."

Note. From Ray and Veluscek (2018).

messages. Study results showed that the higher the person-centeredness of a message, the more positively the women rated it. High person-centered messages also were associated with greater emotional improvement and fewer relationship consequences. Interestingly, women receiving the low person-centered message said they would have been better off receiving no message at all. The take-home message here is that supportive messages should be person-centered. But what kind of support are we talking about exactly?

Across the social science disciplines, researchers have identified several kinds of social support. Although you'll find different typologies that provide somewhat different terms and distinctions, we find that the one from Karen Glanz and colleagues (2008) offers the best balance of being comprehensive while being concise. **Emotional support** is expressing empathy and caring. An example would be a son telling his father, who has just been diagnosed with cancer, that he loves him and is there for him. **Instrumental support** is providing tangible forms of assistance. Perhaps the son drives his father to medical appointments. **Informational support** is providing knowledge relevant to the situation. The son may visit websites to learn more about cancer and provide that information to his father. Finally, **appraisal support** is a specific kind of information that can be used for self-evaluation to better navigate the situation. For example, the son could remind his father that he's gotten through other health problems in the past and remind him how much support he has from his extended family. All these types of support can be offered in more or less person-centered ways, depending on how messages are crafted.

Interestingly, social support sometimes can come in the form of **invisible support**, meaning the receiver is unaware that support was given or doesn't interpret the supportive behavior as help. An example of this would be the abovementioned son fielding family questions without his dad's awareness or telling the father how someone he knew managed nausea when they had chemotherapy (instead of simply telling the father how to manage nausea). In some cases, invisible support can actually have better outcomes than visible support.

Definition, Disciplinary Approaches, and Types of Social Support

The American Psychological Association defines social support as the provision of assistance or comfort to others, typically to help them cope with biological, psychological, and social stressors.

Sociology emphasizes social support as social integration. Psychology emphasizes social support as enacted, received, and perceived availability of support. Communication emphasizes social support as the quality of support messages.

Types of social support include emotional, instrumental, informational, and appraisal support.

Support can be visible or invisible.

Katherine Zee and Niall Bolger (2019) considered the literature on visible versus invisible support to figure out why this might be. They developed three propositions. *Proposition 1* states that how enacted support is delivered will determine whether it's visible or not. Visible support is more direct and is interpreted by the receiver as "help," whereas invisible support is more indirect and is not interpreted as help. This distinction is important because some people can be reluctant to receive help, believing that doing so implies they are unable to take care of themselves. Providing invisible support avoids such implications.

Indeed, *Proposition 2* says that invisible support will be more beneficial when it protects receivers' self-efficacy or sense of competence. Another way to say this is that invisible support protects a receiver's face (Burleson, 2003). The concept of **face** stems from Penelope Brown and Stephen Levinson's (1987) politeness theory (see Table 7.2), which states that people have positive and negative face wants. This basically means that people want to be

Table 7.2 Theoretical Frameworks for Social Support

Theory/Model	Brief Summary	Citation
Appraisal Theory	Stress results not from external events but from a person's appraisal of events as stressful or not. Appraisals include a person's perceived available social support.	Lazarus and Folkman (1984)
Buffering Effects Model of Social Support	Social support improves well-being by providing positive experiences, predictability and stability in daily life, and feelings of self-worth.	Cohen and Wills (1985)
Direct Effects Model of Social Support	Social support improves well-being by interrupting a person's appraisal of an event as stressful or helping them to reappraise a stressful event in a way that reduces negative affect and behavioral responses.	Cohen and Wills (1985)
Integrated Model of Advice Giving	To be most effective, advice should be given following emotional support and problem analysis.	Feng (2009)
Optimal Matching Model of Social Support	Social support will be most beneficial when it meets the needs of the receiver.	Cutrona and Russell (1990)
Politeness Theory	People have two types of face wants: positive face and negative face. Positive face is the desire to be liked and perceived in a positive light. Negative face is the desire to not have autonomy impeded. Face wants can be supported or threatened by other people's words and actions.	Brown and Levinson (1987)

Note. See *Supplemental Online Theory Table* for additional theories/models.

perceived in a good light (positive face) and not have their autonomy impeded (negative face). Visible social support can suggest that a person is not competent to handle their own problems (threatening positive face) and that they should change their behavior to fall in line with whatever support the provider is suggesting (threatening negative face). Invisible support would *not* pose these threats.

Finally, *Proposition 3* states that whether a person needs invisible or visible support depends on their motivational orientation, or their needs and expectations at the time. For example, if someone is clearly emotionally distressed at, say, learning about an unwanted pregnancy, providing visible support is called for. Likewise, if a person directly asks for support, then saying you intend to help and following through is appropriate. Alternately, if a person is concerned that a diagnosis threatens to cast them in a "sick role" and lead people to pity them, or if they are newly diagnosed and have not yet had time to process the implications of the diagnosis, invisible support would be more appropriate.

In summary, social science disciplines have conceptualized and operationalized social support differently. Across these distinctions, social support can be examined based on the social connections people have; how people enact, receive, or perceive support; and the types and quality of support messages. Theoretical models build on these foundations.

Theoretical Models of Social Support

Early theorizing on social support presented two models of how social support operated (Cohen & Wills, 1985). The first is the **direct effects model** (also called the main effects model). This model says that social support will have a positive effect on people regardless of circumstances. It emphasizes the social integration conceptualization of social support advanced by the sociological perspective. The second is the **buffering effects model**. This model says that social support has a positive effect on people by reducing the impact of, or buffering, the effects of stressors. In other words, a stressor needs to be present before social support can help. This model emphasizes the enacted or received conceptualization of social support advanced by the psychological perspective and highlights how social support helps people cope. It also includes the conceptualization of social support as perceived availability of support. Cohen and Wills (1985) concluded that there is evidence for both models depending on how you conceptualize and operationalize social support. That was then. What about now?

MacGeorge and Zhou (2022) write that subsequent research on social support has led to more "nuanced theorizing about multiple causal mechanisms through which social support operates" and that the mechanisms can be

> behavioral (i.e., social support influences the recipient's adoption, maintenance, or termination of health–relevant behaviors), psychological (i.e., social support affects factors such as stressor appraisal, emotional distress, and mental illness), or biological (i.e., social support affects cardiovascular, neuroendocrine, metabolic, and immune function, either directly or indirectly).
>
> (p. 136)

In the *behavioral* sense, you can think about coping. **Adaptive coping** behavior may include adopting healthier eating, sleeping, or exercising patterns or being more adherent to treatment recommendations. So, for example, after a medical diagnosis, your friends may involve you in a cooking or exercise class, or your mom may call with daily reminders to take your medicine. This contrasts with **maladaptive coping**, which people may engage in without appropriate social support. Maladaptive strategies could include socially isolating yourself and possibly turning to alcohol or other drugs.

In the *psychological* sense, you can think of social support as influencing a person's cognitive appraisal of their situation. **Appraisal theory** (Lazarus & Folkman, 1984; see Table 7.2) suggests that it's not the situation itself that influences outcomes but a person's appraisal of it as positive or negative. Appraisals may be more positive if a person perceives they have more social support available to them, and positive appraisals can lead to reduced emotional distress, anxiety, and depression. In the *biological* sense, researchers consider how various measures of social support are related to important biological markers of health. Bert Uchino and colleagues (2020) detail how social support is related to lower cardiovascular reactivity, lower blood pressure, lower catecholamine levels, lower levels of inflammatory cytokines, and multiple measures of oxytocin response. Clearly, theorizing on social support has identified many pathways through which it can lead to positive health outcomes. It's important to remember, though, that not all social support has positive outcomes.

Indeed, Carolyn Cutrona and Daniel Russell (1990) proposed an **optimal matching model of social support** to emphasize that "all support, all the time" may not be desirable in the least. Specifically, the model predicts that social support will be most beneficial when it meets the needs of the receiver. Too little support, and the receiver is bereft. Too much support, and the receiver may become overwhelmed, potentially lose self-confidence and hope, and possibly become angry or depressed. A study by Chris Segrin and colleagues (2011) demonstrates the optimal matching hypothesis in action. The researchers surveyed 71 prostate cancer patients three times over four months, analyzing the relationship between stage of cancer diagnosis (newly diagnosed vs. advanced), social support from family and friends, and depression. They found that social support differentially predicted changes in depression in the men depending on the stage of their disease. For men with more advanced prostate cancer, social support was associated with improvements in depression. The support these men received helped them to deal with their advanced illness, serving as a buffer between illness and depression. For men with an early-stage prostate cancer diagnosis, though, social support was associated with worsening of depression. Prostate cancer doesn't necessarily have symptoms in its early stages, so men who are newly diagnosed may not even consider themselves to be ill. Therefore, they wouldn't feel the need for support from others, and if they received it, the support would suggest that family and friends viewed the men differently (i.e., threatened their positive and/or negative face) and serve as an unwanted reminder of the prostate cancer. Clearly, it's important for family and friends to be sensitive to what support people need and when. The same can be said of a particular kind of support: advice giving.

Advice Giving

Advice can be a valuable form of social support, but how it is given will affect how it is received, or so says Bo Feng (2009) in her work on developing an **integrated model of advice giving** (see Table 7.2). Feng noted that although research had established that the quality of advice is assessed according to who gives it, how they give it, and what they say when giving it, research had not established what the *timing* of advice should be in terms of when to say what. According to the model, when you see someone who appears to need advice, you should *not* just jump in and start holding forth. Why? Well, you may have misjudged the situation, and giving "unwanted, irrelevant, or redundant advice is counterproductive" (Feng, 2009, p. 118). Instead, you first should provide *emotional* support by responding to the person's sadness, anxiety, fear, or anger. Second, still not assuming that the person needs advice, you should ask about their perspective of the *problem* and analyze the situation. Only then are you in a sound position to be able to offer *advice*. When you do, the advice should support the receiver's positive and negative face, and it should also emphasize response efficacy (the advice will work) and feasibility (it's possible to take the advice).

Feng (2009) conducted a large-scale experiment to test her model, recruiting 752 college students to participate. She developed three scenarios, none of which were directly related to health but were still quite relevant to social support: failing an exam, fighting with parents, and being underpaid. To test her model, she developed advice messages whose parts she could rearrange or leave out. For example, one message might consist of just advice (A). Another might start with advice (A), move on to assess the problem (P), and end with emotional support (E). In all, there were 11 message variations (EPA, EAP, PAE, PEA, AEP, APE, EA, AE, PA, AP, and A) for each of the three scenarios. Feng hypothesized that messages that offered emotional support before they offered advice would be rated as higher quality than messages in which emotional support followed advice (EA > AE) or was not offered at all (EA > A). She also hypothesized that messages that analyzed the problem before they offered advice would be rated as higher quality than messages in which problem analysis followed advice (PA > AP) or was not offered at all (PA > A). Finally, she hypothesized that the EPA order would be rated as higher quality than the PEA order. In terms of results, with one minor exception (PA = A), that's exactly what she found. Even though this study was conducted outside the context of health, its findings are still applicable to such scenarios. If someone is distressed about a health problem, consider being emotionally supportive first. Then, if they're receptive, ask about their perspective and analyze the problem. Only then should you consider offering advice. Another form of support to consider offering, if you're in a position to do so, is to be an ally.

Allyship

An **ally** is "a person who is a member of the 'dominant' or 'majority' group who works to end oppression in his or her personal and professional life through support of, and as an advocate with and for, the oppressed population" (Washington & Evans, 1991, p. 195). **Allyship** is "a lifelong process of building relationships based on trust, consistency, and accountability with marginalized individuals and/or groups of people" (The Anti-Oppression Network, n.d.). Stephanie Nixon (2019) uses a coin metaphor to illustrate this. The coin is the system of oppression (e.g., sexism, racism, ableism). On the top of the coin are people with privilege (e.g., able-bodied, cisgender), and on the bottom of the coin are people who are oppressed (e.g., disabled, transgender). Privileged people have advantages others do not because of who they happen to be, not because they earned the privileges (i.e., they were born on top of the coin). Oppressed people have disadvantages others do not because of who they happen to be, not because they deserve them (i.e., they were born at the bottom of the coin). The goal of allyship is for "people who find themselves on the top of a coin...to understand that there is a coin, that it has two sides, and that they occupy the position of unearned advantage (i.e., privilege) on the top" (p. 5). This will poise them to use their privilege and power to become allies. To see an example of allyship in action, we turn to Kenji Yoshino and his research on covering in the workplace.

Allyship

An ally is a member of the "dominant" or "majority" group who works to end oppression in their personal and professional lives through supporting and advocating with and for members of oppressed populations. Allyship involves building relationships based on trust, consistency, and accountability with marginalized individuals and/or groups of people. Allyship is a lifelong process.

Table 7.3 Four Strategies for Covering

Axis	Definition and Example
Appearance	How individuals alter their self-presentation—including grooming, attire, and mannerisms—to blend into the mainstream. For example, a Black woman might straighten her hair to de-emphasize the natural hair of her race.
Affiliation	How individuals avoid behaviors widely associated with their identity, often to negate stereotypes about that identity. For example, a woman might avoid talking about being a mother because she does not want her colleagues to think she is less committed to her work.
Advocacy	How much individuals "stick up for" their group. For example, a veteran might refrain from challenging a joke about the military, lest she be seen as overly strident.
Association	How individuals avoid contact with other group members. For example, a gay man might refrain from bringing his same-sex partner to a work function so as not to be seen as "too gay."

Note. Based on Yoshino and Smith (2013).

The term **covering** comes from sociologist Erving Goffman (1963). It's a strategy in which people with stigmatized identities (i.e., people on the bottom of the coin) work to downplay those identities as much as possible to attempt to conform more with the mainstream or dominant group. The extent to which people engage in covering can reveal which side of the coin they're on. Yoshino (2006) elaborated the concept of covering by identifying four axes along which people can cover: appearance, affiliation, advocacy, and association (see Table 7.3).

Yoshino and Smith (2013) report the results of a study to identify the extent of covering in the workplace. They surveyed 3,129 people across organizations representing a variety of industries. There was a range of age, gender, race/ethnicity, sexual orientation, and organizational seniority. The survey asked how often respondents covered at work, how important covering was to their career advancement, and how harmful covering was to their sense of self, among other questions. On average, 61% of respondents said they covered on at least one of the axes. By group, covering ranged from a low of 45% among straight, white men to a high of 83% for LGBT individuals. In other words, findings demonstrated that *everybody* covered to some extent, so this should matter to all of us. As you can imagine, covering who you are caused stress and harm (Yoshino & Smith, 2013, p. 11):

> The impact of certain kinds of covering behavior will be immediately evident, such as the physical pain suffered by the person who forgoes a cane to cover his disability, the juggling act conducted by the woman who must not only care for her children but also pretend she is not doing so, or the personal humiliation suffered by the gay person who feels he should not bring his spouse to an event where significant others are invited.

Indeed, results of the survey showed the extent to which covering results in harm. Depending on the axis, 60%–73% of respondents said that covering was somewhat to extremely harmful to their sense of self. So, what can an ally do to help individuals navigate the burden of covering?

In a talk given at the 9th Annual Inclusion Summit, Yoshino (2021) offers three strategies to redress covering demands in the workplace, one of which is allyship. He argues that it's important to engage in allyship because social science research overwhelmingly shows that confronting offenses such as microaggressions is more effective coming from an ally than what he calls the "affected person" (i.e., the person affected by the covering demands). This is because the affected person is stuck between the proverbial rock and hard place: They either speak up and risk appearing too sensitive, or they silently bear the offense and feel like they didn't stand up for themselves. Allies are not in that position.

But before you think the ally should just rush in to call out an offender, Yoshino (2021) actually recommends that the ally ask themselves whether the affected person actually wants help and whether the kind of help they'd offer as an ally might cause even more burden (e.g., potentially embarrass the person). Then, the ally should approach the affected person after whatever offense may have occurred (such as a microaggression), say that they noticed what happened, cared about it, and would like to be an ally. Then they can ask whether there is anything they can do to be helpful. If yes, then the ally and affected person can strategize about how to respond in the future. If no, then at least the affected person knows they have an ally they could call upon in the future if needed. Yoshino's work focuses on covering demands in the workplace. But there are several healthcare contexts that call for allyship. One such context is healthcare for transgender persons.

There is compelling evidence that transgender persons do not receive adequate medical care because of systemic issues such as lack of provider training and negative attitudes toward LGBTQ+ patients (Obedin-Maliver, 2015). In addition, the stigmatization experienced by the transgender community can lead to increased covering behaviors. Therefore, it's essential to have allies in the healthcare community. Ash Alpert and colleagues (2021) conducted a study to explore barriers to healthcare for transgender persons with cancer. Focus groups with patients and physicians revealed several disturbing themes related to stigmatization and paternalism stemming from gendered expectations regarding cancer care. For example, physicians simply expected that biological women would prefer to avoid radical mastectomies or hysterectomies and that biological men would prefer to avoid oriectomies, but such surgeries actually align with transitioning needs for trans men and trans women, so these were assumptions patients needed to either actively resist or succumb to. Allyship in healthcare, then, consists of raising awareness of the trans identities of patients and never making gender-conforming assumptions. Allyship also consists of using preferred names and pronouns (in conversations and on forms) and resisting family member stigmatization. Demonstrating the value of healthcare allyship, one cancer patient shared their experience (Alpert et al., 2021, p. 2556):

> My family had to deal with me initiating my medical transition right before I got diagnosed with cancer and came to associate the two, so my doctors were really excellent in helping me have information for my parents and help keep them at bay and talking me through what kind of care I needed.

As Alpert et al. (2021) conclude, "Patient-centered care takes into account the values, needs, and desires of patients and prioritizes shared decision-making" (p. 2557). That includes recognizing and respecting the values, needs, and desires of transgender patients in a system that currently defaults to cisgender assumptions.

Although allyship, advice giving, and other forms of social support (as we've discussed them so far) sound like they're being offered in person, that doesn't have to be the case. Indeed, these days there's plenty of opportunity to provide social support through online channels. It's to those channels that we turn next.

Online Social Support

The online environment has a plethora of social support resources available, and these resources have become central to seeking and receiving support. MacGeorge and Zhou

(2022) summarize the characteristics of online social support that make it popular. First, assuming that people have internet access, it's easy to access social support. You don't have to travel anywhere, you can be online any time of the day or night, and a lot of online support has no monetary cost. Second, you gain access to a potentially vast group of people who can give you greater perspective on your problem. Although people in your face-to-face social networks might want to help, they may not always be able to fully understand exactly what you're going through, whereas someone online might. Finally, you can maintain your anonymity and present yourself in a more curated manner than you could in face-to-face interactions. But is social support online as good as in-person?

Elizabeth Nick and colleagues (2018) developed a scale to measure online social support and found evidence that it can provide the same kind of support as in-person. They recruited three samples (one undergraduate and two community based) for a total of 1,090 participants in their multi-part study. They found that people can seek and receive emotional support, informational support, instrumental support, and social companionship online and that such support has similar (though somewhat weaker) effects as in-person support in terms of bolstering people's self-esteem and reducing depression. They also found that for online social support, participants turned to social media (e.g., Facebook), text (e.g., email), and forum (e.g., Reddit) platforms more than other types of platforms (such as dating and gaming). This latter finding is echoed in many other studies, as demonstrated in a systematic review by John Gilmour and colleagues.

Gilmour et al. (2020) reviewed 27 studies that investigated social support obtained through Facebook to assess its impact on health outcomes. Overall, they concluded that the literature shows that "Facebook-based social support is generally beneficial to physical and mental health outcomes" (p. 345). However, they noted that there were several factors that moderated an overall positive effect. For example, although self-disclosure tended to lead to greater social support, too much self-disclosure, especially of intimate information, had a negative effect. Social comparison also had a negative effect. They suggested that "greater education around the positive use (of) Facebook and how to effectively use SNSs for supportive social interactions is required" (p. 344) so that people seeking social support via Facebook do so appropriately. They also suggested that it may be better to use Facebook with social support goals in mind because another study found that general Facebook use was related to poorer mental health outcomes (see Frost & Rickwood, 2017).

More subtleties of how online social support operates were revealed in a study by Siyue Li and colleagues (2022). The researchers were interested in determining whether online social support influenced perceived risk from the COVID-19 virus and perceived efficacy to prevent the spread of the virus, as well as determining the effect of risk and efficacy on preventive behaviors. They made a distinction between passive and active online involvement, noting that *passive involvement* meant simply viewing online content without interacting with others, whereas *active involvement* meant some kind of interaction between two or more people. Active involvement was further differentiated as either *public* (e.g., posting on a wall) or *private* (e.g., direct messaging). The researchers looked specifically at informational and emotional support as the most common forms of social support online (Rains et al., 2015).

Li et al. (2022) surveyed 555 U.S. adults in April 2020, about a month after COVID-19 had been declared a pandemic. All in all, it appeared that online emotional support obtained through private interactions could have an impact on perceived efficacy, which then could influence preventive behaviors. However, even though informational support was related to increased perceptions of risk, those risk perceptions did not influence preventive behaviors. The relative effectiveness of emotional online support over informational online support in changing health behavior seems clear, at least in this particular pandemic context.

Informal Caregiving

We've talked a lot about healthcare providers in previous chapters—the doctors, nurses, and allied health professionals who work in clinics, hospitals, and other healthcare settings. But when you think of it, a lot of healthcare is provided by people outside of the formal healthcare system. Whether we're talking about short-term, acute care, like a friend bringing you chicken soup and ibuprofen for a week when you have mono, or long-term, chronic care, like a daughter providing assistance over the course of several years for a mother with Alzheimer's disease or cancer, a lot of people are providing a lot of informal care. An **informal caregiver** is defined as "an unpaid individual (e.g., a spouse, partner, family member, friend, or neighbor) involved in assisting others with activities of daily living and/or medical tasks" (Family Caregiver Alliance, 2016, para. 1).

Although caregiving commitments vary, the research on informal caregivers has focused on those providing long-term care to a family member or friend with a serious, chronic disease or physically disabling condition. In the United States, approximately 40% of the population has provided such care (Titus et al., 2020). Research in this area tends to emphasize instrumental support, such as shopping and preparing meals; feeding, bathing, grooming, dressing, and toileting; doing housework or laundry; and transporting patients to appointments (both medical and other). This instrumental support also includes keeping track of medical records, filling out insurance forms, paying bills, and acting as a patient advocate, as well as providing actual medical care such as giving medications, changing bandages, and checking blood pressure or glucose levels (Family Caregiver Alliance, 2016). Of course, along with such instrumental support, caregivers will provide informational, appraisal, and emotional support, as well.

On average, caregivers spend about 24 hours/week providing care, although 25% of caregivers spend more than 40 hours/week doing so (Family Caregiver Alliance, 2016). Most informal caregivers are not paid for their work. Instead, 80% of them end up spending their own money to cover caregiving costs (Titus et al., 2020). The value of the unpaid care informal caregivers provide is enormous, estimated at approximately $470 billion annually (Reinhard et al., 2019).

Women and people of color are disproportionately overburdened as caregivers (Family Caregiver Alliance, 2016). Approximately 75% of caregivers are women. Women caregivers spend more time providing care than their male counterparts (21.9 vs. 17.4 hours/week), and women are more likely to help with things like bathing and toileting, whereas men are more likely to help with managing finances and care planning. Although most adult caregivers in the United States are white, the prevalence of caregiving breaks down as follows: 21% of Hispanics, 20.3% of African Americans, 19.7% of Asians, and 16.9% of whites.

Informal Caregivers

An informal caregiver is an unpaid individual who assists others with activities of daily living and/or medical tasks. About 40% of the U.S. population has provided informal care at some point in time. On average, caregivers spend about 24 hours/week providing care. The value of informal care is estimated to be approximately $470 billion annually. Women and people of color are disproportionately overburdened as caregivers.

Burdens and Benefits of Caregiving

Caregiver burden is defined as "the extent to which caregivers perceived their emotional or physical health, social life, and financial status as suffering as a result of caring for their relative" (Zarit et al., 1986, p. 261). The literature on caregiving has identified numerous such burdens to caregivers resulting from their roles and responsibilities. A report from the National Alliance for Caregiving (NAC) and the American Association of Retired Persons (AARP; 2020) based on a nationally representative sample of 1,392 caregivers provides a snapshot of these burdens and how they may have increased over time. For example, whereas 48% of caregivers rated their health as good or excellent in 2015, only 41% did so in 2020; this compares to a 2018 national estimate of 62% of people rating their health as good or excellent. Conversely, 17% of caregivers rated their health as fair or poor in 2015, but 21% did so in 2020; this compares to a 2018 national estimate of 12% of people rating their health as fair or poor. In addition, 23% of caregivers say caregiving has made taking care of their own health more difficult and made their health worse. These caregivers were the ones more likely to provide more hours of care per week, to provide more instrumental support, and to live with a care recipient who had multiple health conditions.

Although there are a lot of stressors involved in caregiving, there are benefits associated with caregiving, as well. For example, the NAC/AARP (2020) survey found that half of caregivers agreed or strongly agreed that their role gave them a sense of purpose. This feeling was enhanced when the caregiver felt they had a choice in their role. There is also evidence that caregivers experience feelings of gratitude and accomplishment from their role, as well as developing skills such as assertiveness and advocacy (Anderson & White, 2018). Beyond these benefits, a review of five population-based mortality studies found that "Caregivers, as a general group, have significantly reduced mortality rates compared to their respective noncaregiving reference groups" (Roth et al., 2015, p. 312). David Roth and colleagues (2018) wanted to investigate what they called this "seemingly paradoxical finding," given all the literature demonstrating caregiver burden.

Drawing on the stress-buffering model of social support, the researchers investigated whether caregiving, as a prosocial helping behavior, would buffer the negative impact of the stressors experienced from caregiving. Using data from a larger study, they compared 3,580 family caregivers to 3,580 noncaregivers matched on multiple variables (i.e., they were comparing "apples to apples"). They found that whereas caregivers experienced greater depression and higher stress than noncaregivers, depression and stress levels predicted mortality for noncaregivers but *not* for caregivers. This was evidence that caregiving acted as a stress buffer. The authors concluded that "Family caregiving appears to be similar to other prosocial helping behaviors in that it provides stress-buffering adaptations that ameliorate the impact of stress on major health outcomes such as mortality" (Roth et al., 2018, p. 619).

To take more of a communication focus, let's now consider the impact of caregiving on the caregiver-receiver relationship. Catherine Riffin and colleagues (2018) conducted in-depth dyadic interviews with caregiver–patient pairs to investigate their experiences, attitudes, and perspectives around providing and receiving care associated with medical tasks. They recruited 20 adults aged 65 years or older who had at least two chronic conditions and their caregivers to participate. In the interview, patients were asked to list their chronic conditions, describe the activities undertaken to manage the conditions, and describe their reaction to the assistance their caregiver provided. The caregiver then was asked to respond to what the patient had said, elaborating and providing examples and describing how they felt about their caregiving assistance. The authors transcribed and coded their data, identified overarching themes, and then established a typology of two types of caregiving: *supportive dyadic relationships* and *conflicted dyadic relationships*. These relationships differed along five themes.

First, whereas supportive relationships saw agreement on how much assistance the caregiver would provide, conflicted relationships did not. For example, there was either agreement or disagreement about how much the caregiver would participate in doctor's visits. Second, in supportive relationships, caregivers and patients saw each other as being competent in performing disease management tasks, but in conflicted relationships, they did not. Tasks included things like reading medication directions, taking medications, and communicating with healthcare providers. Third, whereas caregivers and patients in supportive relationships expressed mutual understanding, those in conflicted relationships felt underappreciated by one another. Fourth, in supportive relationships, there was collaborative decision-making in regard to health management, whereas in conflicted relationships, there was disagreement. Finally, although those in supportive relationships preferred to rely on family caregiving, when that was not possible, caregivers and patients would problem-solve to identify alternative solutions that were acceptable to both of them (e.g., hire hourly help). In contrast, those in conflicted relationships went straight to formal caregiving solutions regardless of patient preference. The authors emphasized the strength of their dyadic approach by saying it allowed them to observe caregiver–patient language use in interactions, which shed light on the relationship. For example, a patient in a conflicted relationship said that "he was fighting a gang" (his family), and his caregiving wife replied that "she felt like the mother of a toddler" (Riffin et al., 2018, p. 1996).

Clearly, there's stress involved in caregiving for both the caregiver and patient, and as we've seen, relationships can be either supportive or conflicted in that respect. One factor that could influence the extent to which the relationship is supportive or conflicted is the caregiver's motivations and willingness to provide care. Mikolaj Zarzycki and colleagues (2022) used a cultural lens in conducting a meta-ethnographic review to explore this question. They searched the literature for studies that involved adult informal caregivers and that "reported qualitative data on motivations and/or willingness to provide care that pertained to culture-specific norms of informal care provision" (p. 1576). Their search revealed 37 eligible studies that involved 833 participants whose ethnicities included Asian, Caucasian, non-Caucasian American, Black African, and Arab.

The authors identified six motivations for providing care. *Cultural self-identity* as a caregiver was developed through socialization via role modeling and embracing the cultural values, norms, and beliefs that supported and promoted caregiving. The authors noted that this theme served as an overarching explanatory concept. *Cultural duty and obligation* were closely related to gendered expectations, which cast women in the role of primary caregivers. *Cultural values* involved respect for parents and the elderly, family loyalty and solidarity, and religious and philosophical ideas. *Love and emotional attachments* related to how sociocultural norms and expectations led to showing love through caregiving behavior or how experiencing feelings of love led to caregiving behavior. *Repayment and reciprocity* stemmed from cultural expectations regarding mutual obligations. Finally, *competing demands and roles* were influenced by expectations about having a paying job. This factor negatively influenced motivation and willingness to provide care. The authors drew the following conclusions (Zarzycki et al., 2022, p. 1583):

Our findings demonstrate that people's motivations for caring are underpinned by specific cultural values, religious and philosophical beliefs, and cultural norms of informal care provision and as such they hold potential implications for culturally sensitive assessment, support planning and for service development. Caregiving, for some, can be a taken for granted activity whilst for others it is a source of pride and a behaviour congruent with important cultural values. It can also be resented as limiting an individuals' ability to take up educational, employment and social opportunities, or as initiating role/identity conflicts.

Given these cultural tensions, as well as potential relationship tensions and the tensions between caregiving burdens and benefits, it's important to consider what resources and interventions are available to support caregivers in their roles.

Interventions to Support Caregivers

In an article on the impact of COVID-19 on caregivers, Steven Cohen and colleagues (2021) point out that there are several federal, state, and local policies and programs aimed at providing support and assistance for caregivers. At the federal level, they cite the **Recognize, Assist, Include, Support, and Engage (RAISE) Family Caregivers Act**, which was passed by the 115th Congress (2017–2018). (Ever note how Congress can't pass anything without making an acronym out of it?) The RAISE Act requires the Secretary of Health and Human Services "to develop, maintain, and update an integrated strategy to recognize and support family caregivers" (p. 1034). That's all well and good, but given the extent of caregiving and caregiver needs, more assistance seems warranted. In this last section of our chapter, we look at interventions designed specifically to support caregivers, including one that takes advantage of technology.

We'll start with a focus on interventions targeted at caregivers of dementia patients. The interventions we've selected to highlight take a unique approach in that they're based on creative arts participation. The premise is that such programs provide life-enriching experiences that promote well-being and, because they take place in public settings, help participants feel more connected to their broader communities. In addition, such programs can also have positive impacts on dementia patients and the caregiver–patient relationship.

The first intervention is a music-focused intervention called *B Sharp Arts Engagement*®. It provides caregivers and dementia patients with season tickets to their local symphony and arranges for them to attend social receptions with other intervention recipients before performances and during intermissions. In a randomized controlled trial over a three-year period, Meara Faw and colleagues (2021) demonstrated through a thematic analysis that participation in the program helped caregivers to build relationships with other participants and within the broader community, experience increased personal dignity and have moments when they felt things were back to normal, and experience positive emotions while engaged in the program.

The second intervention involves an art gallery program in which caregivers and dementia patients participate in eight weekly sessions during which they spend one hour viewing and discussing art in a gallery and then spend an additional hour creating art based on what they had seen in the gallery. Paul Camic and colleagues (2014) demonstrated through a qualitative thematic analysis that participation in this arts program led caregivers to feel more socially included and to have improved quality of life. A systematic review found that social engagement and leisure activities were two of the three self-care needs reported by informal caregivers of dementia patients (sleep was the third; Waligora et al., 2019), so these creative arts interventions clearly are meeting caregiver needs.

To wrap up this section, let's take a quick look at an innovative technology-based intervention that uses social robots to help caregivers manage the stress and demands of caregiving. **Social robots** are machines that are programmed to communicate autonomously or semi-autonomously with humans (think of a less life-like Baymax from Disney's© *Big Here 6*). Guy Laban and colleagues (2022) developed an intervention in which "Pepper," a social robot, would interact with caregivers via Zoom in a way that encouraged caregivers to self-disclose. The researchers based this strategy on studies showing that self-disclosure has a positive impact on health, both mental and physical, and that emotional disclosure in particular can be therapeutic. The researchers recruited 34 British adult caregivers to participate in the experiment, which involved two 5–10 minute sessions per week over five weeks.

Each session began with Pepper offering a short greeting (e.g., "Hi! How are you?") and then asking a general, predefined question to build rapport (e.g., "How was your day?"). Then, Pepper stated that it was going to ask a question about one of 10 topics (work situation, leisure and passions, finances, relationships, social life, mental health, physical health, personality, goals and ambitions, and routine daily activities). Participants had been instructed to respond as they saw fit and to be honest to the extent that they felt comfortable. With the aid of an experimenter, Pepper would respond throughout the conversation with statements that were neutral (e.g., "I see"), positive (e.g., "That's amazing"), or negative (e.g., "These are not easy times"). The researchers measured the duration (in seconds) and length (in words) of participants' self-disclosures during the conversations. Results showed that over the five-week period, participant duration and length of disclosure with Pepper increased significantly, which the researchers interpreted as "meaningful evidence for user experience, acceptance, and trust of social robots in care settings" (Laban et al., 2022, p. 5). These results are preliminary, of course, and they do not consider the breadth and depth of participants' self-disclosures. However, they suggest that there is promise in using social robots to engage caregivers in an easy-to-use support intervention.

Conclusion

Social support is a central and essential part of the human experience. It comes in all shapes and sizes, and it can be measured in multiple ways. Through behavioral, psychological, and biological mediators, it affects our mental, physical, and emotional health. Although it often has positive effects, it also can backfire, especially if communicated poorly. And although giving support as an informal caregiver can cause significant stress, caregiving also brings rewards.

We mentioned at the start of this chapter that as a human on this planet, you will both need and provide social support throughout your life. To make the most of it, we suggest you appraise it as an opportunity, not a burden. In the words of Seneca, Roman Stoic philosopher and statesman, "Nature bids us to do well by all…Wherever there is a human being, we have an opportunity for kindness." And in the words of James M. Barrie, Scottish novelist and playwright best known for creating Peter Pan, "Always be a little kinder than necessary." We think those are fine words to live by.

References

Alpert, A. B., Gampa, V., Lytle, M. C., Manzano, C., Ruddick, R., Poteat, T., Quinn, G. P., & Kamen, C. S. (2021). I'm not putting on that floral gown: Enforcement and resistance of gender expectations for transgender people with cancer. *Patient Education and Counseling, 104*, 2552–2558.

American Psychological Association. (2023). *Social support.* APA Dictionary of Psychology. https://dictionary.apa.org/social-support

Anderson, E. W., & White, K. M. (2018). "It has changed my life": An exploration of caregiver experiences in serious illness. *American Journal of Hospice and Palliative Medicine, 35*(2), 266–274.

Brown, P., & Levinson, S. C. (1987). *Politeness: Some universals in language usage.* Cambridge University Press.

Burleson, B. R. (1987). Cognitive complexity. In J. C. McCroskey & J. A. Daly (Eds.), *Personality and interpersonal communication* (pp. 305–349). Sage.

Burleson, B. R. (2003). Emotional support skills. In J. O. Greene & B. R. Burleson (Eds.), *Handbook of communication and social interaction skills* (pp. 551–594). Erlbaum.

Camic, P. M., Tischler, V., & Pearman, C. (2014). Viewing and making art together: An eight-week gallery-based intervention for people with dementia and their caregivers. *Aging & Mental Health, 18*(2), 161–168.

Cohen, S., & Wills, T. A. (1985). Stress, social support, and the buffering hypothesis. *Psychological Bulletin, 98*(2), 310–357.

Cohen, S. A., Nash, C. C., & Greaney, M. L. (2021). Informal caregiving during the covid-19 pandemic in the US: Background, challenges, and opportunities. *American Journal of Health Promotion, 35*(7), 1032–1036.

Cutrona, C. E., & Russell, D. W. (1990). Types of social support and specific stress: Toward a theory of optimal matching. In B. R. Sarason, I. G. Sarason, & G. R. Pierce (Eds.), *Social support: An interactional view* (pp. 319–366). Wiley.

Family Caregiver Alliance. (2016). *Caregiver statistics: Demographics.* https://www.caregiver.org/resource/caregiver-statistics-demographics/

Faw, M. H., Luxton, I., Cross, J. E., & Davalos, D. (2021). Surviving and thriving: Qualitative results from a multi-year, multidimensional intervention to promote well-being among caregivers of adults with dementia. *International Journal of Environmental Research and Public Health, 18*, Article 4755.

Feng, B. (2009). Testing an integrated model of advice giving in supportive interactions. *Human Communication Research, 35*, 115–129.

Frost, R. L., & Rickwood, D. J. (2017). A systematic review of the mental health outcomes associated with Facebook use. *Computers in Human Behavior, 76*, 576–600.

Gilmour, J., Machin, T., Brownlow, C., & Jeffries, C. (2020). Facebook-based social support and health: A systematic review. *Psychology of Popular Media, 9*(3), 328–346.

Glanz, K., Rimer, B. K., & Viswanath, K. (2008). *Health behavior and health education: Theory, research, and practice* (4th ed.). Jossey-Bass.

Goffman, E. (1963). *Notes on the management of spoiled identity.* Prentice Hall.

Laban, G., Kappas, A., Morrison, V., & Cross, E. S. (2022, April–May). Informal caregivers disclose increasingly more to a social robot over time. *CHI '22 Extended Abstracts*, New Orleans, LA.

Lazarus, R. S., & Folkman, S. (1984). *Stress, appraisal, and coping.* Springer.

Li, S., Liao, W., Kim, C., Feng, B., & Pan, W. (2022). Understanding the association between online social support obtainment and coping during a public crisis. *Journal of Health Communication, 27*(5), 343–352.

MacGeorge, E. L., Feng, B., & Burleson, B. R. (2011). Supportive communication. In M. L. Knapp & J. A. Daly (Eds.), *Handbook of interpersonal communication* (4th ed., pp. 317–354). Sage.

MacGeorge, E. L., & Zhou, Y. (2022). Supportive communication and health. In T. L. Thompson & N. G. Harrington (Eds.), *The Routledge handbook of health communication* (3rd ed., pp. 136–148). Routledge.

National Family Alliance and AARP. (2020). *Caregiving in the U.S.* https://www.caregiving.org/wp-content/uploads/2021/01/full-report-caregiving-in-the-united-states-01-21.pdf

Nick, E. A., Cole, D. A., Cho, S-J., Smith, D. K., Carter, T. G., & Zelkowitz, R. (2018). The Online Social Support Scale: Measure development and validation. *Psychological Assessment, 30*(9), 1127–1143.

Nixon, S. A. (2019). The coin model of privilege and critical allyship: Implications for health. *BMC Public Health, 19*, Article 1637.

Obedin-Maliver, J. (2015). Time for OBGYNs to care for people of all genders. *Journal of Women's Health, 24*(2), 109–111.

Rains, S. A., Peterson, E. B., & Wright, K. B. (2015). Communicating social support in computer-mediated contexts: A meta-analytic review of content analyses examining support messages shared online among individuals coping with illness. *Communication Monographs, 82*(4), 403–430.

Ray, C. D., & Veluscek, A. M. (2018). Nonsupport versus varying levels of person-centered emotional support: A study of women with breast cancer. *Journal of Cancer Education, 33*(3), 649–652.

Reblin, M., & Uchino, B. (2008). Social and emotional support and its implication for health. *Current Opinions in Psychiatry, 21*(2), 201–205.

Reinhard, S., Feinberg, L., Houser, A., Choula, R., & Evans, M. (2019). Valuing the invaluable: 2019 update. *Insight on the Issues, AARP Public Policy Institute*, 1–32.

Riffin, C., Van Ness, P. H., Iannone, L., & Fried, T. (2018). Patient and caregiver perspectives on managing multiple health conditions. *Journal of the American Geriatric Society, 66,* 1992–1997.

Roth, D. L., Brown, S. L., Rhodes, J. D., & Haley, W. E. (2018). Reduced mortality rates among caregivers: Does family caregiving provide a stress-buffering effect? *Psychology and Aging, 33*(4), 619–629.

Roth, D. L., Fredman, L., & Haley, W. E. (2015). Informal caregiving and its impact on health: A reappraisal from population-based studies. *The Gerontologist, 55*(2), 309–319.

Segrin, C., Badger, T. A., & Figueredo, A. J. (2011). Stage of disease progression moderates the association between social support and depression in prostate cancer survivors. *Journal of Psychosocial Oncology, 29,* 552–560.

Street, R. L., Jr., Makoul, G., Arora, N. K., & Epstein, R. M. (2009). How does communication heal? Pathways linking clinician-patient communication to health outcomes. *Patient Education and Counseling, 74*(3), 295–301.

The Anti-Oppression Network. (n.d.). *Allyship.* https://theantioppressionnetwork.com/allyship/

Titus, J., Malato, D., Benz, J., Kantor, L., Bonnell, W., Okal, T., Smith, C., Tompson, T., Swanson, E., & Fingerhut, H. (2020). Long term caregiving: The true costs of caring for aging adults. *The Associated Press-NORC Center for Public Affairs Research,* 1–20. https://www.longtermcarepoll.org/long-term-caregiving-the-true-costs-of-caring-for-aging-adults/

Uchino, B. N., Cronan, S., Scott, E., Landvatter, J., & Papadakis, M. (2020). Social support and stress, depression, and cardiovascular disease. In P. D. Chantler & K. T. Larkin (Eds.), *Cardiovascular implications of stress and depression* (pp. 211–223). Elsevier.

Washington, J., & Evans, N. J. (1991). Becoming an ally. In N. J. Evans & V. Wall (Eds.), *Beyond tolerance: Gays, lesbians and bisexuals on campus* (pp. 195–204). American College Personnel Association.

Waligora, K. J., Bahouth, M. N., & Han, H-R. (2019). The self-care needs and behaviors of dementia informal caregivers: A systematic review. *The Gerontologist, 59*(5), e565–e583.

Yoshino, K. (2006). *Covering: The hidden assault on our civil rights.* Random House.

Yoshino, K. (2021). *Uncovering talent: A new model of equity, diversity, inclusion and belonging.* Annual Inclusion Summit, Des Moines, IA.

Yoshino, K., & Smith, C. (2013). *Uncovering talent: A new model of inclusion.* Deloitte University: The Leadership Center for Inclusion.

Zarit, S. H., Todd, P. A., & Zarit, J. M. (1986). Subjective burden of husbands and wives as caregivers: A longitudinal study. *Gerontologist, 26*(3), 260–266.

Zarzycki, M., Seddon, D., Bei, E., Dekel, R., & Morrison, V. (2022). How culture shapes informal caregiver motivations: A meta-ethnographic review. *Qualitative Health Research, 32*(10), 1574–1589.

Zee, K. S., & Bolger, N. (2019). Visible and invisible social support: How, why, and when. *Current Directions in Psychological Science, 28*(3), 314–320.

In-class Activities

1. Break the class into small groups and have them come up with low, moderate, and high person-centered messages in response to one or more of the following scenarios:
   a. Your friend tells you that she's worried that she might have caught an STD.
   b. Your friend tells you that his girlfriend, who goes to tanning beds all year, has been diagnosed with melanoma.
   c. Your friend tells you that he's sick of being 30 pounds overweight and hates his body.
   d. Your friend tells you that their worried that their drinking might be getting out of hand.
2. In pairs, have students design an intervention program to provide support to caregivers. How would caregivers receive support, and what types of messages would they receive? Encourage students to be creative and detailed. Have pairs share their programs with the class.

Discussion Questions

1. In your experience, when have you found emotional, instrumental, informational, or appraisal support to be most helpful? When have you found one of these types of support to not be helpful?

2. Where have you, or someone you know, gone online to receive social support? What types of messages did you/they receive and how effective were those messages in providing the needed support?

3. Think about the levels of person-centeredness in support messages and Feng's (2009) integrated model of advice giving. Do they complement one another or possibly compete? Why or why not, and how?

The Montgomery Family
Says Goodbye

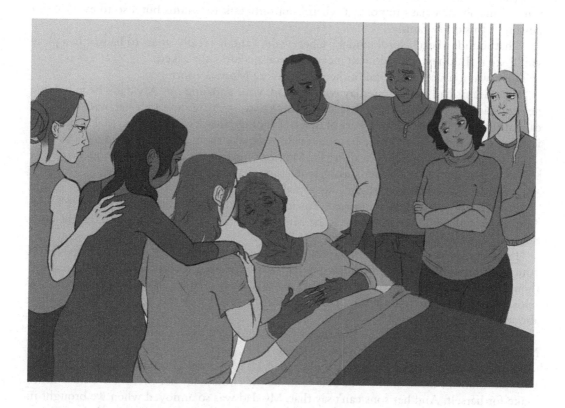

The chemo was no longer working at all for Helen. Every day Cheryl woke up being hit by the thought of her grandmother having *terminal* cancer. Cheryl's one comfort was that her cousin, Monica, had been able to serve as Helen's at-home primary caregiver for the past few months. Just like Sally, Monica was good about providing frequent updates, such as today's phone call.

"I spent years studying the intricate details of patients' bodies, but I can only recall a few lectures on what a patient personally goes through at the end of their lives. It's insane!" Monica was fuming as she spoke to Cheryl. "Now that I'm providing care for Grams, I find my training, or lack thereof, to be insanely inadequate. I never have any idea what to say to be comforting." This wasn't an entirely new conversation between Monica and Cheryl.

"I'm sure you're just being too hard on yourself. No one knows exactly what to say or do. You have a great bedside manner."

DOI: 10.4324/9781003214458-18

"If that means being nice, I don't think it's anywhere near enough," Monica lamented. "I spent almost three hours yesterday poring over all my class notes and books to see what I could find on being there emotionally and communicating with patients at the end of their lives. Do you know what I found in all that time? *Two* chapters and *one* flyer."

"Well, that's better than no flyers, I guess." Cheryl could tell she wasn't being helpful, but she wasn't entirely sure what to say.

"The flyer was pretty helpful, actually. It presented this model called the COMFORT model. It's literally designed for palliative care communication, and the communication researchers who developed it worked with nurses to do it. It's not everything I need in this moment as a family member, caregiver, decision maker, and provider all rolled into one emotionally exhausted person, but it really has been helping. I hung it on my mirror to remind me about what's important when I not only talk to Grams but also to every other person in this crazy family."

"That sounds like a helpful model," Cheryl said, "and it's really smart to hang it in a place you'll see it. But hey, what do you mean decision maker?" she asked.

There was a pause at the end of the phone before Monica continued.

"So…Grams had a talk yesterday with my dad, your dad, and me. My dad's been helping her complete her advance care directives, you know, writing down all her wishes for her care at the very end of her life. Part of that is deciding who actually gets to make the medical decisions for her should she become unable to make them for herself." Monica paused.

"Uh-huh," Cheryl replied, waiting for Monica to get to the answer to her question.

"So, Grams picked me as her surrogate decision maker," Monica stated.

"Really?" Cheryl replied, slightly surprised.

"Look, your dad is clearly annoyed. I'm actually surprised he didn't call you to tell you. And my dad absolutely expected it to be him, so he's not even speaking to me right now. So, I really need you to be on my side here."

"I'm sorry," Cheryl replied quickly. "I didn't mean to sound like I wasn't supportive. Of course, I'm on your side. I just knew my dad was expecting it to be him, but if not him, then definitely your dad, so I'm just surprised that it's not either of them. But given how selfish they both seem to be acting, I can see why she didn't pick them. How are you feeling about it being you, though?"

There was another pause, but this time Cheryl could tell by the sound of soft sniffles that Monica was collecting herself before she spoke.

"I don't want to make these decisions, Cheryl," Monica said quietly. "But I know it's what she wants. I know that I'll be able to make the choices for her that she would want to make for herself. And her sons can't say that. My dad was so annoyed when we brought in a palliative care specialist. He's an incredible pharmacist and a loving son, but he's stubborn about what he wants. If you and I hadn't snuck Grams into the doctor to meet with the palliative care specialist right away, who knows how long it would've taken to have that meeting. And that specialist has been incredible with her focus on how Grams wants to live now knowing that she'll die soon. It freed her. And me. So no, I don't want this. But I'll do it for her. And I'll make the choices that she's told me she wants."

Monica and Cheryl were now both crying.

"How do we still have any tears left after all this?" Cheryl blurted out.

"I have no idea!" Monica replied. "A medical marvel for sure," she joked rather feebly.

Monica and Cheryl spent a few more teary minutes together on the phone. After they hung up, Cheryl lay back in her bed. The past many months had sucked. But despite the family's lack of preparedness for Gram's diagnosis, they managed to get her end-of-life care plans together quickly. Cheryl couldn't help but wonder how much easier this might have been if they'd had these conversations before Grams was ever diagnosed. She knew it certainly wouldn't have made anything *easy*, but she couldn't help but feel like it would have been *easier*.

A few days later, Cheryl would receive the call she had been dreading since the day Helen was diagnosed. Helen was being moved into hospice care, and Cheryl needed to come home. Over the last year, Helen had made it clear that she wanted to be surrounded by her family at the end of her life. And to everyone's comfort, they were able to do that for her. Helen took her last breath surrounded by the people that loved her most.

8 End-of-Life Communication

If you're one of those people who don't like to talk about death, you'll be happy to know that it's not entirely your fault—you can partially blame your parents. Research shows that attitudes and beliefs about death, as well as the willingness to talk about death, are transmitted across generations within families (Freytag & Rauscher, 2017). But it's not entirely your parents' fault, either, or even your grandparents' fault. Despite the universality of death, aversion to talking about it often is baked into cultures, making death a taboo subject around the world. Indeed, fear of the unknown surrounding death causes most people discomfort and leads them to avoid the subject altogether (Ruíz-Fernández et al., 2021). But just like procrastinating on a class paper, no good comes from waiting to prepare until the last minute.

Fortunately, over the last few decades, communication researchers have been studying ways to improve end-of-life communication and demonstrating how effective end-of-life communication can enhance healthcare experiences, normalize talking about death, and support families through difficult times. This chapter will highlight this growing body of literature. We'll begin with a focus on end-of-life medical decision making and advance care planning, which involves surrogate decision makers and advance care directives. Next, we'll review the research on palliative care communication and the COMFORT model, a framework used nationwide to facilitate effective end-of-life communication between patients and their providers, decision makers, and loved ones. Following that, we'll address three challenging contexts for end-of-life conversations: parents of terminally ill children, adult children of aging parents, and healthcare providers treating dying patients. We'll conclude the chapter with information on death with dignity acts and organ donation.

End-of-Life Medical Decision Making

Let's start with a difficult, but important, question: How would you describe a good death? From the philosophical perspective of Confucianism, which is found in many Asian cultures, the criteria for a good death include having minimal physical discomfort, completing personal and family duties, not causing financial or emotional burden for the family, and passing away surrounded by loved ones (see Cha et al., 2021). Other philosophical perspectives may emphasize different criteria, of course. Regardless, a person's ability to have a good death depends in part on their willingness to communicate or document their wishes to others. To do that, they must answer the question, "What do I want for my end-of-life care?" The answer to that question typically reflects a balance between quality and quantity of life.

Finding a balance between **quality of life** and **quantity of life** is an important personal decision. For some people, time is everything, and more is always better. For others, *how* they spend their time is everything, so the quality of that time is what matters. Regardless of where people fall, they're entitled to the right to live out the final days of their lives

DOI: 10.4324/9781003214458-19

consistent with that balance. But if people never talk about their end-of-life wishes, how are those around them supposed to know? As hard as it can be, it's essential that people clearly communicate their end-of-life preferences to those closest to them, including their health-care providers. That way, if they ever find themselves unable to communicate their own wishes—either because they're physically or mentally incapacitated—someone else will know their priorities, and those priorities have a better chance of being followed. Deciding on and documenting these wishes is called advance care planning.

Advance care planning refers to the conversations people have about their medical care preferences surrounding the end of their lives. Typically, these conversations occur with people who might in some way be involved in the person's end-of-life decision making, such as healthcare providers, family members, caregivers, chosen family, and faith advisors (Butler et al., 2014). Research shows that communicating advance care planning wishes can improve end-of-life care, as well as patient and family satisfaction, and can reduce stress, anxiety, and depression among surviving relatives (Detering et al., 2010). But having such conversations is not always easy. Let's look at a study that can shed some light on why this might be.

In a focus group study involving 63 people aged 65 years and older (57% white) and 30 caregivers (90% white), Terri Fried and colleagues (2009) identified five benefits and 10 barriers to engaging in advance care planning. The benefits were managing affairs while still capable, ensuring personal wishes are met, having peace of mind, decreasing burden on loved ones, and keeping peace within the family. The barriers were difficulties with thinking about dying, lack of knowledge, inability to plan for an unknown future, seeing planning as unnecessary because family members know what to do, seeing one's future in the hands of another force, preferring physicians to make decisions, feeling as though there are no additional medical options, not having an available surrogate decision maker, fear that putting things in writing would potentially lead to treatment being withdrawn too soon, and loved ones unable or unwilling to discuss advance care planning. Because participants perceived twice as many barriers as benefits, the researchers suggested that readiness to engage in advance care planning could be improved through stage-based efforts that approach advance care planning as manageable steps (as opposed to having a conversation that addresses everything everywhere all at once). Two of those steps are determining surrogate decision makers and creating advance directives.

Surrogate Decision Makers

The Centers for Disease Control and Prevention (CDC; 2011) defines a **surrogate decision maker** as "a designated individual, legally empowered to make decisions related to the health-care of an individual, or declarant, in the event that he or she is unable to do so" (p. 1). Ideally, the surrogate will make the same choices for the patient that the patient would make for themselves. Unfortunately, though, research has shown a lack of consistency between a person's end-of-life wishes and the decisions a surrogate decision maker would make. In a review of 16 studies involving 151 hypothetical scenarios and 2,595 patient–surrogate pairs, David Shalowitz and colleagues (2006) found that surrogates predicted patient treatment preferences with only 68% accuracy. Predictions were most accurate for scenarios involving current health conditions and antibiotics (both at 72% accuracy). Predictions were least accurate for dementia and stroke (both at 58% accuracy). In a more recent study that asked 172 patients undergoing dialysis and their surrogates about end-of-life preferences, Fahad Saeed and colleagues (2021) found similar results, concluding that "there was, at best, modest agreement between responses to a range of questions about end-of-life care" (p. 1635).

Table 8.1 Theoretical Frameworks in End-of-Life Communication

Theory/Model	Brief Summary	Citation
Bystander Intervention Model	The decision to become an organ donor occurs along a causal chain whereby the potential donor first notices an event, then interprets the event as an emergency in need of an intervention. Potential donors then accept responsibility to help and must be willing to learn how to help.	Latane and Darley (1968)
COMFORT Model	This model details a set of seven competencies to assist practitioners with delivering palliative care: connect, options, making meaning, family caregivers, openings, relating, and team.	Wittenberg et al. (2019)
Model of Surrogate Decision Making	The perspective of the surrogate decision maker will fall into one of four categories: egocentric, projected, benevolent, and simulated. The perspective taken will depend on the factors of intent, significance, accountability, calibration, and empathy.	Tunney and Ziegler (2015)
Organ Donation Model	The decision to become an organ donor is a product of individual knowledge and attitudes toward organ donation, as well as noncognitive factors.	Morgan et al. (2002)
Vested Interest Theory	Individuals who hold positive attitudes toward organ donation and perceive themselves to be vested in the issue of organ donation are more likely to register as an organ donor. Factors influencing whether a person is vested include holding a high *stake* in the decision, believing in the *salience* of the issue, and having *self-efficacy* for overcoming barriers to organ donation.	Sivacek and Crano (1982)

Note. See *Supplemental Online Theory Table* for additional theories/models.

To understand the discrepancies between what a patient would want and what a surrogate decision maker thinks the patient wants (and would ultimately decide for the patient), Richard Tunney and Fenja Ziegler (2015) suggest that it's important to consider the perspective of the surrogate decision maker. In their **model of surrogate decision making** (see Table 8.1), the perspective of the surrogate falls into one of four categories. The first category is *egocentric,* where surrogates "simply fail to model the recipient's wishes and instead make a decision on the recipient's behalf that maximizes the surrogate's own, rather than the recipient's, outcome" (p. 881). Second, a *projected* surrogate "decides what he or she would do, or prefer, if he or she were in the recipient's situation" (p. 881). Third, a *benevolent* surrogate "decides what he or she thinks is best for the recipient irrespective of the recipient's...goals or desires" (p. 881). Finally, a *simulated* surrogate, the most ideal type of decision maker, "attempts to model the goals and desires of the recipient" (p. 881). Tunney and Ziegler note that the perspective a surrogate takes will depend on the factors of intent, significance, accountability, calibration (i.e., the relationship between decision maker and patient), and empathy. Considering the often-heard adage to "treat others the way you want to be treated," it's not surprising that surrogate decision makers would have a hard time making decisions for others when the decisions are different from what they would want for themselves. This model suggests that end-of-life conversations should include explicit discussion of surrogates' perspectives and how those perspectives do or do not align with the patients' wishes. Unfortunately, such explicit and detailed conversations don't always happen.

Indeed, in an older but still very relevant study, Stephen Hines and colleagues (2001) found that of 242 pairs of patients and surrogates who had engaged in at least five conversations about end-of-life decisions, many had still not discussed some of the most controversial topics in end-of-life care, including tube feeding and cardiopulmonary resuscitation (CPR). Fortunately, communication research has been testing ways to enhance patient–surrogate communication about end-of-life wishes. For example, Karin Kirchhoff and colleagues (2010) recruited 313 patient–surrogate pairs to participate in a randomized controlled trial across six outpatient clinics in Wisconsin. In the intervention group, a trained facilitator helped patients and their surrogates talk about end-of-life decisions to ensure a high-quality conversation that focused on the patient's goals for end-of-life care, factors or experiences that had affected the patient's goals for future medical decision making, and the need for engaging in future discussions as situations and preferences changed. Patient–surrogate pairs in the control group didn't meet with a facilitator. After engaging in the conversation, the patients and surrogates separately completed a questionnaire that asked them both about the patient's end-of-life preferences in four different medical situations that varied by chance of survival (low or high) and cognitive and functional impairment (low or high). The researchers found that in all four situations, surrogates in the intervention group had a significantly better understanding of the patient's wishes than surrogates in the control group. In other words, having intentional and focused conversations centered on a patient's wishes can improve a surrogate's ability to make decisions consistent with what the patient wants.

This study and others demonstrate the value of considering not only the frequency of conversations but also the quality of conversations about end-of-life decisions. (Recall our discussion of Lauren Van Scoy and Allison M. Scott's interdisciplinary research on end-of-life conversations from Chapter 2.) As Feixia Wu and colleagues (2020) note, including end-of-life preferences, as well as communication styles, into end-of-life care planning is an important first step for empowering surrogate decision makers. Another important step is for patients to prepare an advance directive for their surrogate decision makers.

Advance Directives

Advance directives are

> documents through which an individual known as a declarant, expresses personal preferences regarding health care treatment, including end-of-life care, and/or names a proxy to act on his or her behalf in the event the declarant is without decision making capacity.

> (CDC, 2011, p. 1)

The primary purpose of advance directives is to allow people the dignity of being treated the way they want at the end of their life. In the United States, following the passing of the **1991 Patient Self-Determination Act**, whenever an adult patient is admitted to a healthcare facility, the facility is mandated to offer them the opportunity to complete an advance directive (Patient Self-Determination Act, 1990). Advance directives have been praised as being central to patient-centered care. In addition, having an advance directive has been shown to reduce the decision-making burden of surrogate decision makers (Hickman & Pinto, 2013). Yet, most experts estimate the percentage of U.S. adults with an advance directive is somewhere under 40% (e.g., Yadav et al., 2017). Sadly, even if an advance directive is completed, that doesn't guarantee that a patient's wishes will be followed. Let's look at findings from an experimental test of advance directives to see why this might be.

Advance Directives

Advance directives are documents through which an individual can express personal preferences regarding healthcare treatment, including end-of-life care, and name a proxy to act on their behalf in the event they're no longer able to make decisions for themselves. In the United States, whenever an adult patient is admitted to a healthcare facility, the facility is mandated to offer them the opportunity to complete an advance directive.

Jane Schubart and colleagues (2018) wanted to see what factors influenced whether a patient's advance directive was followed. Over a five-year period, they recruited 121 patients from the Penn State Milton S. Hershey Medical Center to participate in their study. All had late-stage cancer and an anticipated life expectancy of less than two years. As part of the study, patients were required to complete an advance directive (even if they already had one). Patients in the control group completed their advance directive using standard resources, whereas patients in the experimental group completed theirs using an interactive educational decision aid. Schubart et al. monitored the role of the advance directive through patient charts and, following the patient's death, through phone interviews with the physicians and family members. They found no effect for their intervention. What they did find, though, was that patients' advance directives were followed only 65% of the time. They postulated two main reasons for this. The first reason was missing documentation. For instance, although all of the participants had created an advance directive, the researchers found that only 70% of participant electronic health records indicated the existence of one and only 35% contained a copy. Another reason that advance directives weren't followed was a lack of provider awareness. For instance, only 59 of the 113 (52%) physicians providing the end-of-life care reported knowing that the patient had an advance directive. It's important to note that "In many instances, this physician did not have an ongoing relationship with the patient but rather was on call or cross-covering at the time of death" (p. e68). Schubart et al. believe that their findings highlight "the real-world challenges of communication about and dissemination of one's wishes in complex health care systems" (p. e68). It's important to note that this study did not report the extent to which patients verbally communicated their end-of-life wishes to their providers, family, or surrogate decision makers. Given the intervention findings from Kirchhoff et al. (2010) that we discussed earlier, it's possible that quality conversations could have improved provider awareness of patient advanced directives.

    Although it may be discouraging to know that identifying a surrogate decision maker and creating an advance directive don't guarantee that your end-of-life wishes will be followed, doing so certainly increases the likelihood that your wishes will at least be known. To further increase that likelihood, patients should actively communicate their wishes to their family members and providers on an ongoing basis. For instance, occasionally remind your surrogate decision maker, close family, and provider about your end-of-life wishes and that you have an advance directive. These conversations are especially important for patients receiving palliative care.

Palliative Care

Whether from personal experience or media coverage, most people are familiar with hospice care. **Hospice** is interdisciplinary medical care to help the terminally ill live as comfortably as possible in the time they have left. It's typically implemented when a patient has an estimated life expectancy of less than six months, is rapidly declining, and is ready to forego life-prolonging treatments. What people may not be aware of, though, is palliative care. **Palliative care** is broader than hospice, focused on achieving the highest and most desirable quality of life for patients while they are seriously ill regardless of prognosis. More specifically, "palliative care permits patients to receive curative, life-prolonging treatment simultaneously with receiving care that enhances quality of life. It is holistic care that treats the whole person—not merely the disease" (Wittenberg & Goldsmith, 2022, p. 120). Although palliative care can be delivered at any stage of any diagnosis, most patients who consider palliative care are often navigating a complicated diagnosis or a complicated stage in their diagnosis. For this reason, palliative care is typically achieved through a team of practitioners working on the patient's case (as opposed to a single provider creating a treatment plan). This team not only includes traditional medical professionals, such as primary care providers, specialists, and nurses, but also includes professionals outside of the medical community who might also be working on the patient's case, such as social workers, psychologists, and religious or spiritual advisors. Together, palliative care teams work to prioritize the whole patient: mind, body, and spirit. Doing so leads to important benefits. For example, in a state-of-the-science review on palliative care in oncology, David Hui and colleagues (2018) note that compared to oncologic care alone, "concurrent palliative care improves quality of life, symptoms, and patient–clinician communication" and "enhances mood, patient satisfaction, quality of end-of-life care, survival, and caregiver outcomes" (p. 357).

Hospice Care and Palliative Care

Hospice care is typically implemented when a patient has an estimated life expectancy of less than six months. It helps terminally ill patients live as comfortably as possible during what time they have left.

Palliative care is holistic care that treats the whole person, not merely the disease, permitting patients to receive curative, life-prolonging treatment simultaneously with receiving care that enhances quality of life.

The CDC (2011; see also World Health Organization [WHO], 2020) lists the following eight characteristics of palliative care:

- Provides relief from pain and other distressing symptoms
- Affirms life and regards dying as a normal process
- Doesn't hasten or postpone death
- Integrates psychological and spiritual aspects of patient care
- Offers a support system to help patients live as actively as possible and to help the family cope
- Uses a team approach to address the needs of patients and their families, including bereavement counseling
- Enhances quality of life
- Is applicable early in the course of illness

To achieve optimal palliative care, effective communication is essential. In a review of 52 qualitative studies examining palliative care use in oncology and hematology-oncology, Marco Bennardi and colleagues (2020) identified four qualities of effective palliative care communication: (a) asking for the preferred degree of family involvement in medical decision making, (b) involving providers who have received communication skills training, (c) employing language appropriate for low health literacy levels, and (d) providing information about the medical condition and treatment options. Surprisingly, despite palliative care including comprehensive goals of care, current use of these services is relatively low.

Indeed, according to WHO (2020), despite an estimated 40 million people who are in need of palliative care, only about 14% of them will actually receive it. In the United States, nearly one-third of hospitals with 50 or more beds do not have any palliative care service (Dumanovsky et al., 2016). However, awareness and consideration of palliative care practices are growing. This growth stems from the 2014 World Health Assembly Resolution on Palliative Care (2014), which urged countries to strategically and thoughtfully invest in incorporating palliative care practices into their standard healthcare systems. Clearly, palliative care services are seen as a critical aspect of patient care, in part because these services include much-needed attention to end-of-life needs.

There are many reasons that palliative care has received praise inside and outside of the medical community, but there are two reasons that are particularly important. First, patients don't have to wait until their illness has reached difficult or unexpected stages to discuss end-of-life care wishes. Instead, palliative care emphasizes the importance of engaging in these precautionary conversations at diagnosis, which reduces the chance of their having to happen during moments of heightened stress, anxiety, and uncertainty (Anderson et al., 2019). Second, palliative care meets ill patients and their caregivers where they are, centered around their medical and personal goals. Although the wishes of the patient are typically the priority, family and caregiver needs, perspectives, and opinions are still given space to be heard. This is so much the case that palliative care has been referred to as not just patient-centered but also family-centered communication (Wittenberg & Goldsmith, 2022).

Despite medical and communication research strongly supporting the practice of palliative care for producing positive outcomes (Hui et al., 2018; WHO, 2020; Wittenberg & Goldsmith, 2022), there is some resistance to it within the medical community. In a review of the literature, Pippa Hawley (2017) found four main reasons providers do not recommend or request palliative care services on behalf of their patient. The first is a lack of available palliative care resources, particularly in community hospitals and rural or underdeveloped areas. Second is not knowing what palliative care is or that it exists. This could be because residents aren't required to do palliative care rotations or because palliative care facilities may not be located in the hospital or clinic (i.e., they may be offsite). Third, there can be a reluctance to refer patients for palliative care out of a fear of upsetting the patient, a worry of perceived patient abandonment, or seeing referral as an admission of failure. Last is the belief that once palliative care gets involved, the primary provider won't be needed or allowed to continue treating the patient. These hesitancies are important to note because unless practitioners specifically request palliative care consultations, most patients won't receive palliative care or will receive it at a very late stage, reducing its benefits.

To reduce provider hesitancy, as well as support the growing demand for palliative care, additional resources are needed. One such resource is the COMFORT model. This model serves to provide a palliative care-based set of competencies to help providers communicate competently with patients and their caregivers. It is to this model that we now turn.

The COMFORT Model

The **COMFORT model** consists of a set of evidence-based competencies designed to assist practitioners with delivering palliative care (see Table 8.1). The seven competencies of COMFORT—each represented by a letter in the acronym—are understood as interdependent and ongoing. In other words, how one competency is enacted affects the others, and providers need to continuously consider the competencies, not just enact each one once. What makes the COMFORT model especially useful is that it is a tangible communication tool that teaches providers how to use the competences in their practice. The COMFORT model, originally proposed by Melinda Villagran and colleagues (2010) as a model of bad news delivery, has been extensively revised by Elaine Wittenberg and colleagues (2019) to focus exclusively on palliative care. The following paragraphs review each competency as revised by Wittenberg and her team.

In the COMFORT approach, the "C" refers to connect. It signifies a need for practitioners to not just communicate difficult information with patients but to use narratives and person-centered messages to truly build meaning through their conversations. Connection is created not just through words (verbal communication) but also through action (nonverbal communication). People connect with others when they face each other, make eye contact, and provide appropriate touch. In addition, to build connection, practitioners should not only share their stories with patients, they should also encourage patients to tell their own stories—and then listen to them.

The first "O" stands for options. Options reflect the social, cultural, and personal constraints, including a patient's health literacy level, that influence their ability to process difficult information about their health. In general, providers should remember that each patient is unique and, therefore, their medical care wishes and communication needs will also be unique. When practitioners excel in this competency, palliative care communication is more likely to feel relevant to patients and their families (Wittenberg et al., 2019).

The "M" refers to making meaning, or the need to be physically, psychologically, and emotionally present during healthcare conversations. This includes a consideration of the meaning of suffering, an enactment of relational listening, and the acknowledgment of spirituality. When practitioners seek to make meaning with the patients for whom they are providing palliative care, they're creating space for them to cognitively and emotionally process information about their health. For instance, in some religions, a terminal diagnosis means an end to life. But in other religions, death is the next stage of a journey or the beginning of a new life. Providers who are aware of the religious beliefs of their patients can use those beliefs to help contextualize what a terminal diagnosis could mean to the patient.

The "F" stands for family caregivers. This competency applies the previous "C-O-M" competencies to family members and caregivers (who might be chosen family), recognizing that how practitioners communicate with them is essential for them to effectively deliver palliative care to the patient. Although practitioners need to be careful to center the patient, they should not ignore or push away those seeking to support the patient. In addition, practitioners should be cognizant of the fact that decision-making processes will vary from family to family.

The second "O" refers to openings, or the recognition that ongoing communication requires openings for discussion, options, and input. More specifically, openings provide an essential opportunity for providers to involve and educate patients, family members, and caregivers in palliative care. Without openings, opportunities for important discussions are limited.

The "R" stands for relating, which recognizes that the language for talking about palliative care will—and should—change as new information emerges and as the people involved adapt and change throughout the palliative care process. As patients and their caregivers process information, make decisions, and adjust to illnesses, their needs will change. The competency of relating recognizes those changes and seeks to meet people where they are at every stage as opposed to where they were at the initial diagnosis.

Finally, the "T" stands for team. This competency recognizes that when a patient is at the point of receiving palliative care, they most likely have already been navigating the health-care system and working with multiple teams of care providers to manage various aspects of their health. Palliative care is more effectively delivered when communication among team members is strong. As you learned in Chapter 6, there are different types of healthcare teams, each with their own unique communication challenges. Competent members of palliative care teams will seek to recognize potential challenges, create space for differing perspectives, and focus on the team's purpose for working together.

The COMFORT model has been translated into practice by end-of-life experts and model developers Elaine Wittenberg and Joy Goldsmith and their colleagues. Based in Los Angeles, the COMFORT Communication Project, LLC (n.d.) is a national health communication program intended to improve palliative care communication in health-care. On the website, practitioners can find evidence-based resources and programs for learning about and enacting the COMFORT model. There's also a smartphone app available to help healthcare providers and students follow the COMFORT principles in practice. The COMFORT model has been taught to more than 10,000 providers across the United States, so it's having a clear translational impact. In addition, ongoing research by Wittenberg, Goldsmith, and their colleagues continues to improve the helpfulness of the competencies for enhancing communication during one of the most challenging times of a person's life.

Difficult End-of-Life Conversations

We've established that people generally have a hard time talking about the end of life, but some people may have an even harder time given the complexity of their situations. In particular, parents of terminally ill children, adult children of aging parents, and healthcare providers face especially complex communication challenges when discussing end-of-life concerns. The following paragraphs will explore the dilemmas of talking about death for each of these groups and will include evidence-based guidelines for navigating these difficult conversations.

Parents of Terminally Ill Children

Parents of terminally ill children must face the reality that children lack the cognitive ability to fully understand what's happening to them. Their ability will vary based on their age, of course, with older children having more of a grasp of what it means to die. But the fact remains that human brains don't fully mature until a person is in their mid-20s (see Arain et al., 2013), so no matter what the child's age, talking about their death will be especially challenging. In addition, parents are confronted with their own feelings of betrayal stemming from the expectation that parents are not supposed to outlive their children. These challenges, coupled with the already taboo nature of discussing death, make talking about a child's death even more difficult. In a survey of 86 Dutch parents whose children died of cancer, Ivana van der Geest and colleagues (2015) found that most parents (64%) didn't talk with their terminally ill children about death. Importantly, of the 31 parents who did talk to their children about death, none regretted it. However, about 25% of those who did not talk with their children about death regretted not doing so. What parents need are guidelines to help them have these difficult conversations with their children. Fortunately, such guidelines exist.

One such set is called the "6 Es" (Beale et al., 2005). To follow the 6 Es, parents first should *establish* that death will be a recurring topic of discussion between the child and their loved ones. Second, parents and children should *engage* in conversations about death at opportune times, such as a change in medical status, symptoms, or the child's attitude. Third, parents need to *explore* what the child already knows about their illness and what they want to know. Fourth, parents should *explain* medical information to their children and answer medically related questions. Fifth, they should *empathize* with their child's emotional reactions, allowing the child to be upset and express feelings while providing physical comfort and validation. Finally, parents should *encourage* their child by reassuring them that the parents will be there to listen and support them. These six strategies may not make conversations about death easy, but they can guide parents through them, which can reduce uncertainty for the child and potential regret for the parents.

Adult Children of Aging Parents

Although children are supposed to outlive their parents, conversations about death are also challenging for adult children of aging parents. In an open-ended survey with 75 adults employed by the University of South Florida, Lori Roscoe and Philip Barrison (2019) identified four main communication dilemmas for advance care planning conversations with aging parents: (a) the desire to make parents feel wanted while talking to them about not being alive, (b) the ability to be gentle but direct, (c) the need to designate a decision maker without provoking family conflict, and (d) the desire to reduce the burden on the designated decision maker through informational support. The researchers called for communication efforts to recognize the reality of these dilemmas and promote strategies for navigating them.

In the first edition of this textbook, Allison Scott and Nick Iannarino (2015) provided strategies for improving the effectiveness of end-of-life conversations between children and their aging parents/parental figures. First, they suggested using another person's experience with end-of-life decision making to introduce the topic and then transition to how the adult children and their parents feel in relation to that person's experience. Second, adult children and parents should talk in general about end-of-life values to facilitate an open conversation that provides a foundation for sharing personal beliefs and making future end-of-life decisions. Third, family members need to keep their relationships in mind as they navigate any differences in perceptions and beliefs because supporting each other is essential to leaving the conversation with a relationship just as strong, if not stronger, than when the conversation began. Finally, conversations should happen sooner rather than later to avoid the stresses associated with the end of life, and they should happen periodically because circumstances can change. Knowing that parents will likely die during an adult child's lifetime doesn't make their impending death easy, but having advance care planning conversations early can reduce stress and uncertainty when the time comes.

Healthcare Providers

There are numerous unique communication challenges that can emerge for healthcare providers when a patient is navigating the end of their life. We'll highlight three of the most frequent. First, providers are required to manage multiple goals when treating a dying patient. For example, they need to deal with their own emotions without becoming emotionally disconnected while also providing emotional support for the patient (Ruíz-Fernández et al., 2021). They also need to be honest about the prognosis while still maintaining hope (e.g., Curtis et al., 2008). Providers are also responsible for answering questions about whether procedures will work or how long someone has left to live when this information is often mostly unknown and can only be estimated.

A second challenge comes when providers must honor their patient's decision when they disagree with that decision or it goes against their values (Marcus & Mott, 2014). Although a provider has as much of a right to their own beliefs as anyone else, they're responsible for actively engaging in mindful communication that recognizes when their beliefs, values, or preferences are putting undue pressure on a patient. In addition, a provider who prioritizes their own beliefs, values, and preferences over their patient's violates the foundations of patient-centered care.

The third challenge involves navigating complicated communication triangles between providers, their patients, and the patient's loved ones. Although prioritizing the patient comes first, family requests can create uncertainty about the patient's best interests. For example, in some cultures, it's seen as inappropriate to inform a patient of their terminal status (Galanti, 2008). From the family's perspective, doing so is believed to hinder the patient's will to live, reduce their quality of life, and hasten their impending death. But for the provider, not informing the patient brings about a host of ethical questions surrounding informed consent and patient autonomy (Hallenbeck & Arnold, 2007; see Chapter 11). This sets up a lose–lose situation: Either tell the patient and the family loses or do not tell the patient and the provider loses. But James Hallenbeck and Robert Arnold (2007) suggest a middle ground for providers who find themselves in such a predicament. Specifically, they recommend the following actions: do not overreact, attempt to understand the family's point of view, be flexible, respond empathically, have a conversation with the family that centers what the patient would want, contextualize your views as your personal views, and propose a negotiation where the patient is given enough information to decide whether or not they want more information. Even with these actions, more research needs to be translated into medical training and education programs to assist practitioners with developing the skills needed to support their dying patients, including talking to them about death and dying. More integration of the COMFORT program into medical school education and training could certainly help.

Death with Dignity

A holistic approach to end-of-life care recognizes that some terminally ill patients may desire medical treatments that humanely end their life. These treatment options are classified as either physician-assisted suicide or active euthanasia. **Physician-assisted suicide** occurs when a physician prescribes lethal medication for a patient to self-administer. **Active euthanasia** occurs when a physician administers a lethal dose of medication to a patient. Neither treatment option is legal in every state, and both require extensive communication and careful decision making. In the United States, legislation (typically referred to as a death with dignity act) is required before physicians can legally provide either form of treatment.

Death with dignity acts outline a set of criteria that must be met before a terminally ill person can legally choose to end their life. The criteria typically include independent terminal diagnoses from at least two clinicians and a documented request from the patient. In addition, Death with Dignity (n.d.), a nonprofit organization dedicated to promoting and supporting death with dignity legislation, specifies that to qualify under such statutes, patients must be an adult resident of a state where such a law is in effect; capable of making and communicating their own healthcare decisions; diagnosed with a terminal illness that will lead to death within six months, as confirmed by qualified clinicians; and, for physician-assisted suicide, capable of self-administering and ingesting medications without assistance. To date, these laws do not permit death with dignity requests as part of advance directive documentation. Under a death with dignity act, a patient's death isn't classified as a suicide (Death with Dignity, n.d.). This means that the patient and their families avoid suicide-related stigma and other possible complications. But what does it mean to die with dignity?

Like the subjective balance of quality versus quantity of life and the subjective preferences for a good death, what it means to die with dignity will look different for every person. To some, dignity comes from living as long as physically possible, no matter what the circumstances. To others, dignity comes from the ability to function as "normally" possibly. For most, dying with dignity will fall somewhere in between these two endpoints. In a qualitative study involving 20 nursing home residents in Germany, Sabine Pleschberger (2007) found that the perceived dignity of dying was a combination of factors that included the ability to be active; the extent to which there was respect for the patient's wishes, including the wish to be allowed to die; the option to not be in pain; and the ability to be among close friends and family. From these findings, the author concluded that "the understanding of dignity is not simply individual and personal, but is closely related to social ideas of value, which ultimately influence the basic requirements of institutions in which 'frail old people' must live" (p. 201). Partially due to the challenging nature of what a dignified death means, death with dignity acts have been exceptionally controversial pieces of legislation.

Proponents of death with dignity argue that such laws empower the sickest members of society to have control over the inevitable end of their lives. Their arguments typically center on respect for patient autonomy (the patient's ability to make their own medical decisions for themselves) and relief of patient suffering (Dugdale et al., 2019). In addition, death with dignity acts provide a medically-supported option for patients who might otherwise seek to end their life in more painful, chaotic, or dangerous ways. On the other side of the coin, opponents of death with dignity typically engage in arguments centered on philosophical or religious stances, the potential of suicide contagion (spikes in suicide after a suicide is reported), risks of assisted suicide or euthanasia being a slippery slope for hasty medical decision making, and the risk that depression could lead patients to make decisions they wouldn't make if they were in a sound state of mind (although laws include provisions to avoid this; Dugdale et al., 2019). In addition, families may feel uncomfortable with assisted suicide or euthanasia. Given these competing arguments, few states and countries have enacted death with dignity legislation. Those that have done so typically used **Oregon's 1994 Death with Dignity Act** as a model.

Death with Dignity: Definition and Perspectives

Death with dignity acts outline a series of criteria that must be met before an ill person can legally choose to end their life. Proponents of death with dignity acts argue that such laws empower the sickest members of society to have control over the inevitable end of their lives. They typically engage in arguments centered on respect for patient autonomy, relief of patient suffering, and provision of medically-supported alternatives to more painful, chaotic, or dangerous ways of ending one's life. Opponents of such bills typically engage in arguments centered on philosophical or religious stances, the potential of suicide contagion, risks of these behaviors being a slippery slope for hasty medical decision making, and depression, which could lead patients to make decisions they wouldn't make if they were in a sound state of mind.

The first U.S. state to pass death with dignity legislation was Oregon. On October 27th, 1997, the act was officially implemented, allowing terminally ill residents to end their lives through the voluntary self-administration of lethal medications, expressly prescribed by a physician for that purpose (Oregon Health Authority, 2020). Implementation of the law sparked numerous controversies and many lawsuits, one of which made its way to the U.S. Supreme Court. The case culminated in a 2006 6-3 Supreme Court ruling that upheld the state law and paved the way for similar laws to be implemented in other states (Charatan, 2006). According to World Population Review (2023), there are now seven additional U.S. states, plus Washington D.C. (see Table 8.2), that have passed death with dignity legislation. In addition, a handful of countries have national death with dignity policies that allow euthanasia or assisted suicide for terminally ill patients. These countries include Belgium, Canada, Luxembourg, the Netherlands, New Zealand, Spain, and Switzerland (Rada, 2021). To demonstrate the benevolence of these acts, let's look at the story of Brittany Maynard.

In January 2014, Brittany Maynard, a 29-year-old California native, was diagnosed with a rare brain cancer known as astrocytoma. Almost immediately after her diagnosis, she became a spokesperson and advocate for the legalization of death with dignity, working as a volunteer advocate for *Compassion and Choices*, one of the leading end-of-life organizations in the United States. In an op-ed published by CNN days before her scheduled death, Maynard (2014) shared her heartbreaking diagnosis and journey with the world, including the rationale for her decision to move to Oregon where she could end her life with dignity. She shared the following (n.p.):

> After months of research, my family and I reached a heartbreaking conclusion: There is no treatment that would save my life, and the recommended treatments would have destroyed the time I had left. I considered passing away in hospice care at my San Francisco Bay-area home. But even with palliative medication, I could develop potentially morphine-resistant pain and suffer personality changes and verbal, cognitive and motor loss of virtually any kind. Because the rest of my body is young and healthy, I am likely to physically hang on for a long time even though cancer is eating my mind. I probably would have suffered in hospice care for weeks or even months. And my family would have had to watch that... I do not want to die. But I am dying. And I want to die on my own terms.

Brittany's story personifies the complexities of end-of-life decision making. She reported living out the last few months of her life happily, advocating to make a difference that

Table 8.2 Death with Dignity Acts in the United States

Location	Act	Year Approved and Enacted
California	End of Life Option Act	Approved 2015, enacted 2016
Colorado	End of Life Options Act	Approved and enacted 2016
Hawaii	Our Care, Our Choice Act	Approved 2018, enacted 2019
Maine	Death with Dignity Act	Approved and enacted 2019
Oregon	Death with Dignity Act	Approved 1994, enacted 1997
New Jersey	Aid in Dying for the Terminally Ill Act	Approved and enacted 2019
Vermont	Patient Choice and Control at the End of Life Act	Approved and enacted 2013
Washington	Death with Dignity Act	Approved and enacted 2008
Washington D.C.	Death with Dignity Act	Approved 2016, enacted 2017

Note. Based on World Population Review (2023).

would be felt long after she was gone. And she did. According to Lydia Dugdale and colleagues (2019), Brittany's well-publicized decision to move to Oregon and schedule her death for November 2014 influenced her home state of California to pass their death with dignity act in 2015.

Organ Donation

For many people, **organ donation** will play an important role in end-of-life experiences and decision making. Not only can organ donation be an important part of conversations about advance care planning but also, for the organ recipient, it can be a decision that saves their life. In the United States, organ donation needs, intentions, and perceptions are monitored by the U.S. Department of Health and Human Services (USDHSS) in collaboration with the **United Network for Organ Sharing (UNOS)**. UNOS (2023) was founded in 1977 and serves under federal contract as the management group for the **Organ Procurement and Transplantation Network (OPTN)**. USDHHS (n.d.) describes OPTN as a unique public–private partnership that links all professionals involved in the U.S. organ donation and transplantation system. It is important to note that in the United States, as well as in several other countries such as Australia, Canada, Israel, and Japan, organ donation practices run on an **opt-in system**, or a system in which people aren't organ donors until they document their desire to be a donor. Other countries, however, such as Spain, Sweden, Columbia, and Poland, run their organ donation practices on an **opt-out system**, or a system in which people are assumed to be organ donors unless they document their desire to not be a donor. Research is mixed on which system more successfully meets organ donation needs. For our purposes, we'll focus on the U.S. system as a way to understand the role of communication in meeting organ donation needs.

As of January 2023, USDHHS (2023) reported that there were more than 104,000 people on the organ donation wait list in the United States, more than 85% of whom were waiting for a kidney transplant. Sadly, the majority of those individuals won't receive a transplant due to demand outpacing the rate of organ donation. In an analysis of 10,000 survey responses from U.S. adults, USDHHS (2020) reported that despite 94% of surveyed adults supporting organ donation, only about 50% were registered organ donors. There are many reasons that people might support the idea of organ donation but not want to be organ donors themselves. Let's look at a few of those reasons.

Susan Morgan and colleagues (2008) recruited 78 family dyads (73% of whom were white) to participate in a qualitative study examining how family members perceive and discuss organ donation. The researchers identified seven factors influencing the decision to become an organ donor: religion/spirituality, altruism, mistrust of the medical system, belief in a black market for organs, issues of recipient deservingness, family perceptions of organ donation, noncognitive reasons (such as being able to feel pain in death and thinking of organ donation as "gross"), and other personal reasons, such as "the belief that 'they wouldn't want my organs,' that there was no rush to decide to become a donor, and not feeling knowledgeable enough about donation" (Morgan et al., 2008, pp. 25–26). To supplement these findings from a mostly white participant sample, we'll share the results of a more recent study that centered African American perceptions of organ donation.

Amber Reinhart and Amanda Lilly (2020) sought to examine unique barriers that African Americans face regarding organ donation. In their discussions with 50 Black adults, they found that the most prominent barriers included a lack of knowledge, religious objections, mistrust of the medical community, and myths about donation, such as the existence of a black market for organ donation, media mis-portrayals, and medical professionals not providing life-saving measures if they know you're an organ donor. Interestingly, all of these reasons overlap with Morgan et al.'s (2008) findings. In addition to exploring barriers, though, Reinhart and Lilly also asked participants what strategies they would recommend for promoting organ donation within the Black community. The most common recommendations included reducing perceived barriers through educational efforts and taking steps to make the donation process as transparent as possible. Participants also recommended using personal testimony and involving community partners, such as religious leaders. The authors note that "By utilizing these strategies and overcoming the stated barriers an educational campaign would be well on its way toward increasing not only the number of African American donors, but also rebuilding trust and connection to the community" (pp. 199–200).

In addition to exploring perceptions about becoming an organ donor, communication researchers have tested frameworks for understanding the communicative processes underlying the decision to become an organ donor. In a comparison of such frameworks, Brian Quick and colleagues (2016) provided an overview of three models and assessed their ability to predict organ donor registration behaviors. We'll first present the model summaries from Quick et al. and then share what they found about each model's predictive power. To begin, the **organ donation model** (Morgan et al., 2002) approaches the decision to become an organ donor as a product of individual knowledge and attitudes toward organ donation, as well as a product of noncognitive factors, such as the barriers found by Morgan et al. (2008) and Reinhart and Lilly (2020). Second, the **bystander intervention model** (Latane & Darley, 1968) suggests that the decision to donate "is more likely to occur along a causal chain whereby bystanders first notice an event, then interpret the event as an emergency (i.e., requiring intervention); next, bystanders accept responsibility to help, and finally have knowledge of how to help" (Quick et al., 2016, p. 266). (It's important to note that the bystander model typically is used to guide research on violence prevention.) Lastly, **vested interest theory** (**VIT**; Sivacek & Crano, 1982) posits that individuals who hold positive attitudes toward organ donation and perceive themselves to be "vested" in the issue of organ donation are more likely to register as an organ donor. In the case of organ donation, being vested means an individual holds a high *stake* in the decision, believes in the *salience* of the issue, and has *self-efficacy* for overcoming barriers to organ donation (Quick et al., 2016).

To test the ability of these three models to predict organ donation registration behaviors, Quick et al. (2016) surveyed 688 adults aged 50–64 years. Using participant responses, the authors built statistical models of each of the three frameworks. They found that all three models reasonably explained organ donation behaviors, with VIT having the strongest explanatory power, followed by the bystander intervention model and the organ donation model. Quick et al. conclude that "From a promotion standpoint, then, if the goal is to increase the number of registered donors, the recommendation of using VIT is clear: Campaigns should strive to elevate salience, self-efficacy, and stake in targeted individuals" (p. 272). They further explain that campaigns can do this by emphasizing the altruism of organ donors, countering myths presented in the media, presenting information about the registration process, and drawing attention to the increasing shortage of organs. As we'll learn in Chapter 12, this can be a lot to ask of a single campaign, but each campaign that makes progress brings society one step closer to organ donation registration goals.

Conclusion

Benjamin Franklin said that nothing is certain in life except death and taxes. Although some unscrupulous people worm their way out of paying taxes, no one can evade death. Because of that, and because end-of-life care wishes vary from person to person, making your wishes known through advance care planning is essential. Having advance care planning conversations isn't always easy, and such planning doesn't come with guarantees, but designating a surrogate decision maker and completing an advance directive are among the best ways to ensure that your end-of-life medical care wishes are followed. It's also important to remind healthcare providers and close friends and family about advance care plans. Fortunately, growth in the use of palliative care services is providing additional opportunities for patients to engage in advance care planning conversations. But more work is needed to increase public and provider awareness of such services. More work is also needed on how to facilitate end-of-life conversations for parents of terminally ill children, adult children of aging parents, and healthcare providers, as are efforts to increase death with dignity legislation and organ donation. Although accepting the inevitability of death isn't easy, openly communicating about end-of-life wishes in a competent manner can lead to reduced stress, uncertainty, and burden, which in turn supports sound decision making, all of which makes the hardest thing a little less hard.

References

Anderson, R. J., Bloch, S., Armstrong, M., Stone, P. C., & Low, J. T. (2019). Communication between healthcare professionals and relatives of patients approaching the end-of-life: A systematic review of qualitative evidence. *Palliative Medicine, 33*(8), 926–941.

Arain, M., Haque, M., Johal, L., Mathur, P., Nel, W., Rais, A., Sandhu, R., & Sharma, S. (2013). Maturation of the adolescent brain. *Neuropsychiatric Disease and Treatment, 9,* 449–461.

Beale, E. A., Baile, W. F., & Aaron, J. (2005). Silence is not golden: Communicating with children dying from cancer. *Journal of Clinical Oncology, 23*(15), 3629–3631.

Bennardi, M., Diviani, N., Gamondi, C., Stussi, G., Saletti, P., Cinesi, I., & Rubinelli, S. (2020). Palliative care utilization in oncology and hemato-oncology: A systematic review of cognitive barriers and facilitators from the perspective of healthcare professionals, adult patients, and their families. *BMC Palliative Care, 19*(1), Article 47.

Butler, M., Ratner, E., McCreedy, E., Shippee, N., & Kane, R. L. (2014). Education materials for advance care planning: An overview of the state of the science. *Annals of Internal Medicine, 161*(6), 408–418.

Centers for Disease Control and Prevention. (2011). *Advanced care planning: An introduction for public health and aging services professionals (Version 1.0).* https://www.cdc.gov/training/ACP/

Cha, E., Kim, J., Sohn, M. K., Lee, B. S., Jung, S. S., Lee, S., & Lee, I. (2021). Perceptions on good-life, good-death, and advance care planning in Koreans with non-cancerous chronic diseases. *Journal of Advanced Nursing, 77*(2), 889–898.

Charatan, F. (2006). US Supreme Court upholds Oregon's death with dignity act. *British Medical Journal, 332,* 195.

Comfort Communication Project. (n.d.). https://www.communicatecomfort.com/.

Curtis, J. R., Engelberg, R., Young, J. P., Vig, L. K., Reinke, L. F., Wenrich, M. D., McGrath, B., McCown, E., & Back, A. L. (2008). An approach to understanding the interaction of hope and desire for explicit prognostic information among individuals with severe chronic obstructive pulmonary disease or advanced cancer. *Journal of Palliative Medicine, 11*(4), 610–620.

Death with Dignity. (n.d.). *Frequently asked questions.* https://deathwithdignity.org/resources/faqs/

Detering, K. M., Hancock, A. D., Reade, M. C., & Silvester, W. (2010). The impact of advance care planning on end of life care in elderly patients: Randomised controlled trial. *British Medical Journal, 340,* Article c1345.

Dugdale, L. S., Lerner, B. H., & Callahan, D. (2019). Pros and cons of physician aid in dying. *The Yale Journal of Biology and Medicine, 92*(4), 747–750.

Dumanovsky, T., Augustin, R., Rogers, M., Lettang, K., Meier, D. E., & Morrison, R. S. (2016). The growth of palliative care in US hospitals: A status report. *Journal of Palliative Medicine, 19*(1), 8–15.

Freytag, J., & Rauscher, E. A. (2017). The importance of intergenerational communication in advance care planning: Generational relationships among perceptions and beliefs. *Journal of Health Communication, 22*(6), 488–496.

Fried, T. R., Bullock, K., Iannone, L., & O'Leary, J. R. (2009). Understanding advance care planning as a process of health behavior change. *Journal of the American Geriatrics Society, 57*(9), 1547–1555.

Galanti, G.-A. (2008). *Caring for patients from different cultures* (4th ed.). University of Pennsylvania Press.

Hallenbeck, J., & Arnold, R. (2007). A request for nondisclosure: Don't tell mother. *Journal of Clinical Oncology, 25*(31), 5030–5034.

Hawley, P. (2017). Barriers to access to palliative care. *Palliative Care: Research and Treatment, 10.* https://doi.org/10.1177/1178224216688887

Hickman, R. L., Jr., & Pinto, M. D. (2013). Advance directives lessen the decisional burden of surrogate decision-making for the chronically critically ill. *Journal of Clinical Nursing, 23*(5–6), 756–765.

Hines, S. C., Glover, J. J., Babrow, A. S., Holley, J. L., Badzek, L. A., & Moss, A. H. (2001). Improving advance care planning by accommodating family preferences. *Journal of Palliative Medicine, 4*, 481–489.

Hui, D., Hannon, B. L., Zimmermann, C., & Bruera, E. (2018). Improving patient and caregiver outcomes in oncology: Team-based, timely, and targeted palliative care. *CA: A Cancer Journal for Clinicians, 68*(5), 356–376.

Kirchhoff, K. T., Hammes, B. J., Kehl, K. A., Briggs, L. A., & Brown, R. L. (2010). Effect of a disease-specific planning intervention on surrogate understanding of patient goals for future medical treatment. *Journal of the American Geriatrics Society, 58*, 1233–1240.

Latane, B., & Darley, J. M. (1968). Group inhibition of bystander intervention in emergencies. *Journal of Personality and Social Psychology, 10*, 215–221.

Marcus, J. D., & Mott, F. E. (2014). Difficult conversations: From diagnosis to death. *Ochsner Journal, 14*(4), 712–717.

Maynard, B. (2014, November 2). *My right to death with dignity at 29.* https://www.cnn.com/2014/10/07/opinion/maynard-assisted-suicide-cancer-dignity/index.html

Morgan, S. E., Harrison, T. R., Afifi, W. A., Long, S. D., & Stephenson, M. T. (2008). In their own words: The reasons why people will (not) sign an organ donor card. *Health Communication, 23*(1), 23–33.

Morgan, S., Miller, J., & Arasaratnam, L. (2002). Signing cards, saving lives: An evaluation of the worksite organ donation promotion project. *Communication Monographs, 69*(3), 253–273.

Oregon Health Authority. (2020). *Oregon Death with Dignity Act: 2019 Data Summary.* https://www.oregon.gov/oha/PH/PROVIDERPARTNERRESOURCES/EVALUATIONRESEARCH/DEATHWITHDIGNITYACT/Documents/year22.pdf

Patient Self-Determination Act H.R. 4449. (1990). https://www.congress.gov/bill/101st-congress/house-bill/4449

Pleschberger, S. (2007). Dignity and the challenge of dying in nursing homes: The residents' view. *Age and Ageing, 36*(2), 197–202.

Quick, B. L., Anker, A. E., Feeley, T. H., & Morgan, S. E. (2016). An examination of three theoretical models to explain the organ donation attitude–registration discrepancy among mature adults. *Health Communication, 31*(3), 265–274.

Rada, A. G. (2021). Spain will become the sixth country worldwide to allow euthanasia and assisted suicide. *British Medical Journal, 372*, 147.

Reinhart, A. M., & Lilly, A. E. (2020). Uncovering barriers and strategies for African Americans and organ donation. *Howard Journal of Communications, 31*(2), 187–203.

Roscoe, L. A., & Barrison, P. (2019). Dilemmas adult children face in discussing end-of-life care preferences with their parents. *Health Communication, 34*(14), 1788–1794.

Ruíz-Fernández, M. D., Fernández-Medina, I. M., Granero-Molina, J., Hernández-Padilla, J. M., Correa-Casado, M., & Fernández-Sola, C. (2021). Social acceptance of death and its implication for end-of-life care. *Journal of Advanced Nursing, 77*(7), 3132–3141.

Saeed, F., Butler, C. R., Clark, C., O'Loughlin, K., Engelberg, R. A., Hebert, P. L., Lavallee, D. C., Vig, E. K., Tamura, M. K., Curtis, J. R., & O'Hare, A. M. (2021). Family members' understanding of the end-of-life wishes of people undergoing maintenance dialysis. *Clinical Journal of the American Society of Nephrology, 16*(11), 1630–1638.

Schubart, J. R., Levi, B. H., Bain, M. M., Farace, E., & Green, M. J. (2018). Advance care planning among patients with advanced cancer. *Journal of Oncology Practice, 15*(1), e65–e73.

Scott, A. M., & Iannarino, N. T. (2015). Ethical issues in health communication. In N. G. Harrington (Ed.), *Health communication: Theory, method, and application* (pp. 297–330). Routledge.

Shalowitz, D. I., Garrett-Mayer, E., & Wendler, D. (2006). The accuracy of surrogate decision makers. *Archives of Internal Medicine, 166*(5), 493–497.

Sivacek, J., & Crano, W. D. (1982). Vested interest as a moderator of attitude-behavior consistency. *Journal of Personality and Social Psychology, 43*, 210–221.

Tunney, R. J., & Ziegler, F. V. (2015). Toward a psychology of surrogate decision making. *Perspectives on Psychological Science, 10*(6), 880–885.

United Network for Organ Sharing. (2023). *History of UNOS.* https://unos.org/about/history-of-unos/

US Department of Health and Human Services. (2020). *National survey of organ donation attitudes and practices, 2019: Report of findings.* https://www.organdonor.gov/sites/default/files/organ-donor/professional/grants-research/nsodap-organ-donation-survey-2019.pdf

US Department of Health and Human Services. (2023, January 5). *Organ procurement and transplantation network: National data.* https://optn.transplant.hrsa.gov/data/view-data-reports/national-data/#.

US Department of Health and Human Services. (n.d.). *About.* https://optn.transplant.hrsa.gov/about/

van der Geest, I. M., van den Heuvel-Eibrink, M. M., van Vliet, L. M., Pluijm, S. M., Streng, I. C., Michiels, E. M., Pieters, R., & Darlington, A. S. E. (2015). Talking about death with children with incurable cancer: Perspectives from parents. *The Journal of Pediatrics, 167*(6), 1320–1326.

Villagran, M., Goldsmith, J., Wittenberg-Lyles, E., & Baldwin, P. (2010). Creating COMFORT: A communication-based model for breaking bad news. *Communication Education, 59*, 220–234.

Wittenberg, E., & Goldsmith, J. (2022). Palliative care and end-of-life communication. In T. L. Thompson & N. G. Harrington (Eds.), *The Routledge handbook of health communication* (3rd ed., pp. 119–135). Routledge.

Wittenberg, E., Goldsmith, J. V., Ragan, S. L., & Parnell, T. A. (2019). *Communication in palliative nursing: The COMFORT model.* Oxford University Press.

World Health Assembly Resolution on Palliative Care. (2014). *Strengthening of palliative care as a component of comprehensive care throughout the life course.* WHA67.19. https://apps.who.int/gb/ebwha/pdf_files/WHA67/A67_R19-en.pdf

World Health Organization. (2020, August 5). *Palliative care: Key facts.* https://www.who.int/news-room/fact-sheets/detail/palliative-care

World Population Review. (2023). *Death with dignity states 2022.* https://worldpopulationreview.com/state-rankings/death-with-dignity-states

Wu, F., Zhuang, Y., Chen, X., Wen, H., Tao, W., Lao, Y., & Zhou, H. (2020). Decision-making among the substitute decision makers in intensive care units: An investigation of decision control preferences and decisional conflicts. *Journal of Advanced Nursing, 76*(9), 2323–2335.

Yadav, K. N., Gabler, N. B., Cooney, E., Kent, S., Kim, J., Herbst, N., Mante, A., Halpern, S. D., & Courtright, K. R. (2017). Approximately one in three US adults completes any type of advance directive for end-of-life care. *Health Affairs, 36*(7), 1244–1251.

In-class Activities

1. Split students into small groups. Assign each group a state or city from Table 8.2 or one of the following countries: Belgium, Canada, Luxembourg, Netherlands, New Zealand, and Spain. Give each group 15 minutes to research the death with dignity act governing their assigned region. Have groups plan to share characteristics of the act, including current reports of use.

2. Review the four perspectives from the model of surrogate decision making: egocentric, projected, benevolent, and simulated. Have the students go through each perspective and, as a class, answer the following questions for each perspective:

   a. What are some examples of a decision maker taking this perspective?

   b. How does this perspective align with the wishes of the ill patient?

   c. How might an observer noticing discrepancies between what the decision maker wants and what the patient wants discuss their observations with the decision maker in a way that encourages them to prioritize the wishes of the patient?

Discussion Questions

1. Why do you think so few people complete advance directives? How can communication efforts be used to promote the completion of advanced directives?
2. How would communication efforts to promote organ donation be different in an opt-out system from an opt-in system?
3. How is organ donation portrayed in the media? (Consider movies like *John Q* and *Seven Pounds* and television shows like *Grey's Anatomy* and *House.*) How do you think this affects people's organ donation behavior? Does Hollywood have a responsibility to portray organ donation in a positive light, or should entertainment media have creative license in portraying organ donation situations?

Unit IV

Health Communication Challenges

Cheryl Reaches Her Breaking Point

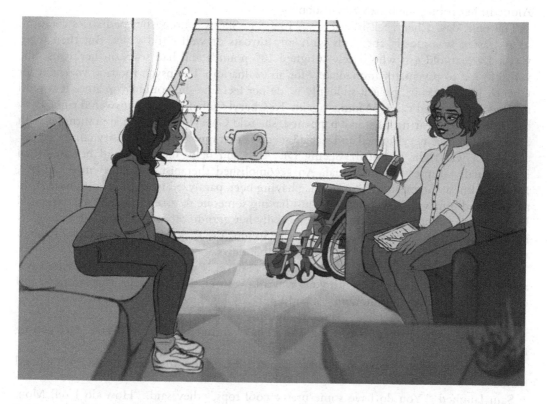

In the thick of her third year of medical school, and with the hole in her heart that wouldn't fill following Helen's passing, Cheryl was dealing with a lot of stress. Although excited about starting clinical rotations and getting to see actual patients, she'd also been anxious because it was completely different from what she was used to. There wasn't as much studying, but there was a ton of pressure going through all the rotations. She was constantly meeting new people, some of whom could be real jerks. The psychiatry rotation was coming up, and she was starting to worry about what she might see. Plus, a couple of her peers were already starting to burn out. "I just gotta get a grip," Cheryl said to herself. And then her phone rang. It was Stacey, one of her classmates.

"Hey, Stace, what's up?" There was silence. "Stace?"

"You're not gonna believe this," Stacey said. Her voice sounded like she'd been crying.

"What?" Cheryl asked, immediately concerned.

"It's Darryl." Stacey stopped.

"What about Darryl? What happened?" Cheryl felt a pit in her stomach.

DOI: 10.4324/9781003214458-21

It took a while before Stacey replied in a whisper, "He committed suicide."

"What?!" Cheryl shouted. She couldn't believe it. It made no sense. Darryl was at the top of their class. He was smart and nice to everybody. He seemed to have it all together. How could this happen? "What?" she said again, still trying to process. "What happened?"

"I don't know. I just found out. I had to call." Stacey, Cheryl, and Darryl had hung out a lot together their first two years, like Cheryl had done with Nathian and Liz in college. "I gotta go, Cher. This is just…" Stacey hung up without finishing her sentence.

Cheryl sat at her desk, her mind reeling. As she thought more about the fact that Darryl was gone—just gone—she felt tears welling. After a moment, she called Monica. There was no answer. She tried Liz. No answer. It had been years since she called Nathian, and it seemed weird to do so now. Sally, Joe, and Samuel were away for the weekend on vacation. Alone in her room, she broke down sobbing.

The next day, Cheryl felt like she was in a fog. She was doing her pediatrics rotation, so at least it was mostly cute kids with sore throats or well-child visits. But then there was a 13-year-old girl who barely weighed 100 pounds and had scars on her arms. She was referred to psychiatry immediately for an evaluation. The psych rotation was next for Cheryl. Just thinking about it suddenly made her feel like she couldn't breathe. It was all too much. She tried calling Monica again. To Cheryl's relief, Monica answered right away this time. After hearing what had happened, she told Cheryl to make an appointment with a therapist asap. Cheryl agreed and started seeing a therapist at the university clinic.

Monica was right (as usual). Seeing Dr. Ayad did help. Cheryl found her to be an exceptionally impressive individual. An accomplished therapist and Paralympic athlete, Dr. Ayad knew the meaning of resilience having been paralyzed from the waist down from a childhood injury. Cheryl found that just having someone to listen to her as she expressed her concerns about school and family, especially her grandmother and the sudden death of her friend by suicide, made a huge difference. So much so that she felt particularly prepared when her brother called her with some pretty big news.

"I'm sick of pretending, Sis," Samuel said. "I've never been a boy. I thought maybe I was a girl, you know, growing up with you. Wearing your clothes and stuff. But I'm not a girl either." They paused. "I'm nonbinary, and I'm ready for they/them pronouns."

"You got it," Cheryl replied. "Is there anything I can do to help?"

"Actually, yes. There is one thing I've been wanting to ask. Will you start calling me Sam?"

"If this means you'll leave my clothes alone, I'll call you anything you want," Cheryl teased.

Sam laughed. "You do have some pretty cool tops," they said. "How do I tell Mom and Dad?"

Cheryl thought back to their conversation almost two years ago when Sam called her about Elliot Page. "Well, I thought how you told me was great, but I can't say I have a lot of experience with this type of conversation." She thought a bit. "I have an idea. I've been seeing this therapist—"

"Are you okay?" Sam asked, worried.

"I'm fine. I was way stressed, and pretty sad, but therapy is helping. And what I was going to say before you interrupted, you little turd, was that I could ask her for advice. Would that be okay?"

"Sure," Sam said. "But you're the turd."

Cheryl exchanged a few more laughs with Sam before hanging up the phone. She thought back to a few months prior when she was worried that she'd never laugh again. This call with Sam felt like a reminder that life is worth living and that she just had to keep going.

Although she didn't think the hole she had in her heart from all the loss would ever completely close, she was noticing it now less and less.

Notes

There are numerous suicide prevention resources available.

- In the United States, 988 is the number for the *Suicide and Crisis Hotline*.
- The *American Foundation for Suicide Prevention* (https://afsp.org/) is a voluntary health organization that provides those affected by suicide with resources and a nationwide community of support.
- The CDC website *How Right Now* (www.cdc.gov/howrightnow) hosts resources to help people find support to navigate a variety of emotions, including fear, anger, grief, loneliness, and stress.

The *Real Warriors* campaign (https://www.health.mil/Military-Health-Topics/Centers-of-Excellence/Psychological-Health-Center-of-Excellence/Real-Warriors-Campaign) is dedicated to support suicide prevention among service members, veterans, and their families. Check your campus' website or ask a trusted instructor about resources available to you.

9   Mental Health and Mental Illness

In Chapter 1, you'll recall that we defined health as "a state of complete physical, mental and social well-being and not merely the absence of disease or infirmity" (World Health Organization [WHO], 1948, p. 1). In this chapter, we're going to focus specifically on the mental aspect of the definition. We're doing so for four reasons.

First, mental health has received considerably less attention than physical health from both medicine and society. For example, the Accreditation Council for Graduate Medical Education (2020–2022) lists 28 specialties (e.g., neurology, plastic surgery), only one of which is focused on mental health (psychiatry). Think, too, about how much social support people with physical illnesses receive. If you lose an appendix, people send you meals, flowers, and get well cards. If you're diagnosed with a mental illness, it's highly unlikely you'll receive any attention, in large part due to stigma.

Second, mental health has gotten worse over the past several years. From 2005 to 2017, major depression increased by 52% (from 8.7% to 13.2%) in adolescents aged 12–17 years and by 63% (from 8.1% to 13.2%) in young adults aged 18–25 years; serious psychological distress increased by 71% in young adults aged 18–25 years (Twenge et al., 2019). The impact on the economy also is getting worse. *The Lancet Global Health* (2020) reports that across all mental illnesses, the cost to the global economy was estimated at $2.5 trillion in 2010 and is predicted to increase to $6 trillion in 2030.

Third, it finally seems to be dawning on folks that good mental health is as essential to well-being as physical health—and the two are inextricably entwined. Indeed, when the U.S. government enacts legislation mandating insurance coverage for mental health (e.g., the Mental Health Parity and Addiction Equity Act, The Affordable Care Act; Mental-Health.gov, 2020), you know people are finally starting to recognize the need for mental health support.

Finally, unlike physical health, most mental health issues have a direct impact on communication. Although physical illness may be the topic of conversation and some diseases impair communication ability, mental illnesses directly influence the process of communication, so it's important for communication scholars to consider that in their research. Further, communication is central to both establishing and maintaining good mental health and preventing and treating mental illness. So, this topic certainly warrants our explicit attention.

We're covering a lot in this chapter. We begin by laying some groundwork with definitions, types, and prevalence of mental health and illness, as well as discussing stigma. Then we review mental health disparities and consider different meanings of mental health across cultures. Next, we shift our attention to suicide, providing information on prevalence, trends, and groups at risk. After that, we move to the interpersonal impact of mental illness and suicide and how they have been depicted in the media. We finish the chapter by reviewing efforts to address mental illness and prevent suicide. Because

DOI: 10.4324/9781003214458-22

good mental health is essential to well-being, we hope you find this chapter informative, meaningful, and helpful.

An Overview of Mental Health and Mental Illness

Let's begin by distinguishing between the terms **mental health** and **mental illness**. According to the Centers for Disease Control and Prevention (CDC, 2021), "Mental health includes our emotional, psychological, and social well-being. It affects how we think, feel, and act. It also helps determine how we handle stress, relate to others, and make healthy choices" (n.p.). The World Health Organization (WHO, 2022a) argues that mental health is "a basic human right" and is "crucial to personal, community and socio-economic development" (n.p.). For a definition of mental illness, we turn to the National Institute of Mental Health (NIMH, 2022a), which says mental illness is "a mental, behavioral, or emotional disorder" (n.p.). The impact of mental illness can range from no impairment to severe impairment that "substantially interferes with or limits one or more major life activities" (NIMH, 2022a, n.p.). Just as the experience of physical illness varies across individuals with the same disease, the experience of mental illness can vary across individuals with the same diagnosis.

There are more than 200 types of mental illnesses, which the American Psychiatric Association (2013) divides into 19 major categories in its *Diagnostic and Statistical Manual of Mental Disorders* (DSM-5), a manual used to diagnose mental illnesses. These categories include anxiety, depressive, and personality disorders. A person may have one or more of these disorders, and the disorders may be short or long term.

Mental illness is common. The WHO (2022b) reports that in 2019, one in eight people worldwide had some type of mental illness. The most common were anxiety and depressive disorders. The organization also reports that incidence of these disorders increased by 26% and 28%, respectively, in 2020 because of the coronavirus pandemic. The situation in the United States appears to be worse. Indeed, compiling data from several sources, the National Alliance on Mental Illness (NAMI; 2022a) reports that in any given year, one in five Americans experience a mental illness. Overall, more than half of Americans will be affected by mental illness at some point in their lives, with half of all mental illnesses beginning by the age of 14 years and three-quarters by the age of 24 years (CDC, 2021).

Mental Health and Illness: Definitions, Prevalence, and Categories of Illness

Mental health relates to emotional, psychological, and social well-being.

Mental illness is a mental, behavioral, or emotional disorder. It is common, affecting 12.5% of people worldwide and 20% of Americans in any given year, with more than 50% of Americans experiencing mental illness during their lifetime.

Select categories of mental illness include anxiety disorders, such as phobias, social anxiety, and panic attacks; depressive disorders; neurodevelopmental disorders, such as autism spectrum disorder and ADHD; psychotic disorders, such as schizophrenia; obsessive-compulsive disorders, such as hoarding and hair pulling; trauma- and stress-related disorders, such as post-traumatic stress disorder (PTSD); eating disorders, such as anorexia and bulimia; and personality disorders, such as antisocial and narcissistic personality disorder.

Stigma

Mental illness is stigmatized in our society. **Stigma** results from having a "discrediting characteristic" that is different from what society considers normal in terms of physical characteristics, personality traits, or group membership (Goffman, 1963). Rachel Smith's (2007) **model of stigma communication** (see Table 9.1) depicts how messages about mental illness can lead to social rejection, such as through microaggressions (see Chapter 2). To better understand the implications of microaggressions on communication, Lauren Gonzales and her colleagues (2015) conducted focus group interviews with formerly homeless adults with severe mental illness and undergraduate students with psychiatric disorders. They asked participants to describe a time that someone without a mental illness made them feel uncomfortable because they had one and a time when they felt subtly discriminated against because of their mental illness. The authors identified five themes of microaggressions:

- *Invalidation*: Minimizing the mental illness as not important or serious, symptomatizing behaviors that may be normal, and patronizing the person with mental illness
- *Assumption of inferiority*: Assuming the person with mental illness had lower intelligence, was incompetent, or couldn't function in everyday society
- *Fear of mental illness*: Assuming the person with mental illness was dangerous or unpredictable and therefore should be kept at a distance
- *Shaming*: Suggesting that a mental illness should be disclosed only under certain circumstances where there wouldn't be risk of a negative outcome
- *Second class citizens*: Being treated poorly when they were hospitalized or receiving psychiatric treatment

These microaggressions stigmatized those with a mental illness and led to a host of negative outcomes for the individual, including feelings of confusion, uncertainty, frustration, and anger.

Table 9.1 Theoretical Frameworks in Mental Health and Illness

Theory/Model	Brief Summary	Citation
Model of Stigma Communication	Stigmatizing messages identify and categorize people as stigmatized, suggest that stigmatized people pose risks to others, and imply that stigmatized people are responsible for their stigma. These messages lead to negative cognitive and emotional reactions, which then lead to outcomes such as perpetuating stigma messaging and isolating stigmatized persons.	Smith (2007)
Social Comparison Theory	People have an innate drive to evaluate themselves and will do so by comparing themselves with other people, either upward (comparing the self to others more well off) or downward (comparing the self to others less well off).	Festinger (1954)
Social Ecological Theory	Health behavior is influenced by individual, social, and physical environment factors and their interrelationships. To increase the likelihood of positive impact, interventions should account for multiple levels of influence as they relate to the behavior in question.	Stokels (1996)

Note. *See Supplemental Online Theory Table* for additional theories/models.

Disparities in Mental Illness

To have a complete picture of the mental health landscape, researchers need to consider **mental health disparities** in both the prevalence of mental illness and access to treatment. As shown in the column labeled "U.S. Population Data" in Table 9.2, substantial disparities exist in the United States in the prevalence of mental illness across demographic categories. (The other columns in the table will be discussed later in this chapter.) Disparities also exist in gaining equitable access to mental health treatment. Of U.S. adults experiencing a mental illness in 2020, only 46.2% received some form of mental health service. Women, older adults, and whites were the most likely groups to receive care (NIMH, 2022a). The American Psychiatric Association (2023a) notes that racial/ethnic minorities, as well as gender and sexual minorities, often suffer worse mental health outcomes because of lower access to mental health services, cultural stigma, discrimination, and knowledge gaps.

Can communication research help reduce such disparities in mental health illness? Rosalie Aldrich and Jesse Quintero Johnson (2022) use **social ecological theory** (see Table 9.1) to explore that very question, highlighting individual, social, and environmental factors to help understand disparities in mental health access and quality. Individual-level factors

Table 9.2 Prevalence and Media Representation of Mental Illness in the United States

	U.S. Population Data[*]	Depictions in Film[+]	Depictions in Television[+]
Overall Prevalence of Mental Illness	20%	1.7%	7%
Teen Prevalence of Mental Illness	49.5%	7%	6%
Mental Illness by Age Groups			
18–25 years[*]	30.6%	–	–
Young adults[+]	–	46%	62%
26–49 years[*]	25.3%	–	–
Middle aged[+]	–	33%	26%
50+ years old[*]	14.5%	–	–
65+ years old[+]	–	–	3%
Sex Ratio of Mental Illness	1.5 Female to 1 Male	1 Female to 1.5 Male	1 Female to 1 Male
Mental Illness by Race/ Ethnicity			
Mixed Race	35.8%	1%	4%
White	22.6%	80%	69%
Hispanic	18.4%	0%	5%
Black/African American	17.3%	14%	19%
Asian	13.9%	5%	4%
Prevalence of Mental Illness			
LGBTQI	40%	–	–
LGBT	–	0%	9.3%

Note. [*]Overall prevalence data from NAMI (2022a); LGBTQI prevalence data from NAMI (2022b); all other data from NIMH (2022a); [+]Data from Smith et al. (2019).

include "negative perceptions about and mistrust of mental healthcare systems and health providers" (p. 64), as well as having less access to health insurance and, for some, lower language proficiency and mental health literacy. Social factors include "systemic biases in mental health assessment, intervention tools, and mental healthcare practices resulting in discrimination that disproportionately affect poor, Asian, Black, Latinx, and Indigenous people" (p. 64). Environmental factors include "the effects of living conditions that make it difficult to offer easily accessible mental healthcare at the local and state levels" (p. 64), as well as global problems such as war and famine that lead to refugee crises. A perspective like this suggests that it's inadequate to target just one factor to effectively address the problem of mental health disparities. Researchers need to consider multilevel factors to create comprehensive approaches to promoting mental health equity.

It's important to note that mental health disparities may be exacerbated by cultural differences that lead to inadequate or inappropriate treatment or even misdiagnosis. Medical anthropologist and cultural diversity expert Geri-Ann Galanti (2015) describes some of the differences in the way mental illness is experienced, diagnosed, and treated in people from different cultures and how what may be considered abnormal behavior in some cultures may be entirely normal in others. For example, Galanti describes how belief in spirits is common among Filipinos. Claiming to see visions of dead people, then, is reasonable within this culture, but a U.S.-trained psychiatrist using the DSM-5 may diagnose such a claim as evidence of psychosis. Galanti also emphasizes how cultures differ in terms of how acceptable it is to talk to anyone outside the family about personal matters, including talking to psychiatrists or therapists about conditions like anxiety or depression. For example, people of Mexican heritage believe that personal matters should be discussed only within the family. This reduces the likelihood of seeking or accepting help from a mental health professional. Galanti also mentions how mistrust in the U.S. healthcare system may prevent members of some groups, such as Black communities, from seeking mental health services from providers who are primarily white. Finally, Galanti addresses the stigma of mental illness and how such stigma is stronger in some cultures, such as Asian cultures. Seeking and accepting treatment for mental illness among such cultures can be particularly challenging and must be navigated with great sensitivity.

Suicide

The symptoms of serious mental illness coupled with a lack of access to appropriate and effective treatment and the negative impact of stigma and shame can sometimes become so unbearable that people begin to think about ending their lives or decide to end their lives by suicide. The NIMH (2022b) defines **suicide** as "death caused by self-directed injurious behavior with intent to die as a result of the behavior" (n.p.). A **suicide attempt** is defined as "a non-fatal, self-directed, potentially injurious behavior with intent to die as a result of the behavior" (n.p.). **Suicide ideation** is "thinking about, considering, or planning suicide" (n.p.). There is a strong link between mental illness and suicide: 90% of people who died by suicide in 2020 are believed to have had a diagnosable mental illness (American Foundation for Suicide Prevention, 2020). However, suicide also can happen on impulse, in the face of major stressors such financial crises, loss of a relationship, or chronic pain or illness (WHO, 2022c).

The CDC (2023) reports that in 2020, nearly 46,000 Americans died by suicide. For every suicide committed, 275 people seriously thought about it, and 27 attempted it. Numerous disparities exist around suicide. Males were four times as likely to commit suicide as females, but females were twice as likely to attempt suicide. Suicide rates were highest among people aged 85 years or older, followed by those aged 75–84 years. Rates were lowest among those aged 10–14 years, although suicide was the second leading cause of death among youth that age. In terms of ethnicity, suicide rates were highest among American Indians, followed by whites; the lowest rate was among Asians/Pacific Islanders. The WHO (2022c) identifies refugees and migrants, indigenous peoples, LGBT and intersex persons, and prisoners at particular risk of suicide. Further, NAMI (2022b) reports that LGB high school students are four times as likely to attempt suicide as heterosexual students and 40% of transgender adults have attempted suicide compared to less than 5% of the general population. Veterans are also at higher risk, with a suicide rate 52.3% higher than the general population (U.S. Department of Veterans Affairs, 2021).

The Interpersonal Impact of Mental Illness and Suicide

So far, we've laid the groundwork on mental illness and suicide in terms of definitions, prevalence, and disparities. In this section, we'll explore influences of mental illness and suicide on interpersonal communication in families. We're taking this approach to convey the impact that mental illness and suicide have on communication, which is why it's so important to reduce stigma, encourage people to seek help, and take steps to treat mental illness and to prevent suicide.

Impact of Mental Illness on Family Communication

People's perspectives and beliefs about mental illness are predominantly learned through the conversations they have with family, and these conversations often involve storytelling. Storytelling in families is important because it helps to socialize children by conveying values, morals, norms, expectations, and life lessons (Koenig Kellas & Trees, 2022). Elizabeth Flood-Grady and Jody Koenig Kellas (2019) investigated family storytelling about mental illness and the impact that it had on younger family members. They interviewed 24 young adults who had talked about mental illness with at least one family member, finding two distinct story themes. First, families told stories of *caution*, which warned about "abnormal, destructive, and harmful actions" (p. 611) associated with mental illness. Second, families told stories of *struggle*, which "emphasized the hardships and stressors" (p. 611) that come with a family member having a mental illness. From hearing these stories, participants reported learning that it's important to be aware of mental illness and to understand it. Although the family members' stories were mostly negative, the researchers determined that the participants also learned positive lessons of empathy, caring, understanding, and helping.

Helping a loved one who's having a hard time is something people want to do. But often they don't know how to help—especially if they don't fully understand what their loved one is going through. Steven Wilson and colleagues (2015) sought to better understand this dilemma by studying how family members of U.S. military service members returning home from Iraq or Afghanistan navigate conversations about mental illness. After reading hypothetical scenarios in which a service member showed signs of mental illness (e.g., having mood swings, being anxious and withdrawn), 80 family members were asked to write what they would say to try to convince the service member to seek help, what goals they were trying to achieve, and what barriers they might face in trying to have a conversation.

Wilson et al. (2015) identified four dilemmas for having mental health-related conversations with a family member: (a) getting the family member to realize they have a problem without suggesting they aren't "normal," (b) convincing the family member to seek help without suggesting they're weak, (c) being both persistent and patient, and (d) wanting the family member to be open about their troubles without suggesting that anyone else could fully understand what they were going through. Although these findings were specific to military families, we hope you can see how their application can be relevant to many different mental health conversations.

Given these dilemmas, what can family members do to help? Wilson et al.'s (2015) findings suggest four strategies: (a) carefully consider when and how much to talk, making sure to be available when the family member is ready, (b) carefully consider how to talk about concerns, being polite and respectful, showing care and commitment, and listening without judgment, (c) frame the conversation strategically so that seeking help would be seen as a way to become healthy and happy and would be something that could be done together, and (d) turn to others for help when necessary, being sure to engage in self-care. Again, although these findings and recommendations were specific to military families, they're good advice for any family members trying to navigate conversations about mental illness.

Impact of Suicide on Siblings and Parents

Even though everyone wishes it would never happen, sometimes the unthinkable does happen, and people attempt or take their lives by suicide. In those cases, communication researchers need to consider the impact on family members so they can develop interventions to help. This section considers the impact of suicide on surviving siblings and attempted suicide on parents. It's probably no surprise that research shows that supportive communication from others can be essential for individuals coping with these situations.

Elizabeth Adams and colleagues (2019) wanted to explore the impact of having a sibling who committed suicide on the surviving sibling. Through in-depth, personal interviews with seven Australian adults who had lost a sibling to suicide, they uncovered detailed aspects of the grief process, including the role of others and how grief changed over time. One of the main themes of the analysis was *grief interactions*, which demonstrated the role of three distinct forms of interaction in navigating grief. *Interactions with family members* included protective silence and the need for better communication, as well as managing different grieving styles (e.g., expressive, restrained). *Interactions with others* included dealing with stigma and insensitive comments and seeking help from professional therapists to help manage grief and loss. Finally, *rituals* involved viewing the body and attending the funeral, both of which helped to make the death seem real. All three forms of interaction were central to the coping process for the sibling.

The ability to successfully navigate the coping process was central to participant efforts toward *meaning making and growth through grief* (another main theme of their findings). *Meaning making* included attempts to make sense of and come to peace with the death, as well as learning more about mental health and suicide. *Growing through grief* included using the sibling's death to help others in need and coming to terms with benefiting from personal growth through tragedy. In all, participants in this study revealed the overwhelming impact of their sibling's suicide on their lives and how open, supportive communication with their parents and others could serve as a protective factor as they navigated their grief and came to terms with their new reality.

Niels Buus and colleagues (2014) explored the experiences of 14 parents in Denmark whose child had attempted suicide. Attempting suicide once is a predictor of attempting it again (CDC, 2022), and so these researchers were interested in learning not only how the suicide attempt affected the family but also how parents dealt with the possibility of their child making a future attempt. Through focus groups, the researchers identified two broad themes in the parents' conversations: (a) the emotional responses and stress experienced in the family and (b) how the suicide attempt was a "double trauma," involving not only the attempt but also the negative impacts on family relationships.

In terms of the first theme, although the extent to which parents were surprised by their child's suicide attempt varied, all parents reported experiencing "panic," "horror," and an "all-consuming state of alarm" (p. 827) after the suicide attempt, believing that a second attempt could happen and they had to do everything possible to protect their child. Parents described their efforts to try to save and support their child, even while admitting that their efforts left them feeling "futile" and "with all pervasive feelings of powerlessness" (p. 827). Their feelings of futility and the ongoing problematic behavior of the suicidal child led parents to have feelings of hopelessness, anger, hate, and blame, as well as feelings of guilt for not only letting their suicidal child down but also letting down their other children who were also being affected by the trauma. They also felt isolation, shame, and ongoing, intense pressure—feelings that led two parents to admit to considering suicide themselves.

In terms of the second theme, the "double trauma," the researchers identified several negative relational effects. There were relationship problems with the suicidal child, whom parents often tried to placate, sometimes to the detriment of their family values and relationships. The parents' own relationship also was at risk. This would happen when each parent had a different opinion on the best course of action, when stereotypes led to expectations that the mother should handle all the communicative work, and when the suicidal child manipulated the parents, attempting to play them off each other. The parents' relationship with their other children was at risk as well. These children often felt neglected because the suicidal sibling was the center of attention, and this could lead to feelings of resentment toward the sibling and parents. All of this shows how crucial it is to recognize that the family of someone who attempts or dies by suicide requires support to process their emotions, communicate their needs and concerns effectively, and navigate their daily lives amid ongoing stress.

Depictions and Coverage of Mental Illness and Suicide in the Media

Knowing what researchers have learned about the interpersonal impact of mental illness and suicide in families, you might wonder whether depictions in the media come anywhere close to reflecting the lived experiences of everyday people. That's what we'll be addressing in this section: how mental illness and suicide appear or are depicted in the media. As you'll see, there's a lot that's negative, biased, and unrealistic. This is troubling because framing, priming, agenda setting, and cultivation research has established that how issues are portrayed in the media influences people's perceptions of those issues (Scheufele & Tewksbury, 2007; see also Chapter 12). Let's look and see what's being portrayed about mental illness and suicide in the media.

Entertainment Media

As you learned in Chapter 2, the **Annenberg Inclusion Initiative** at the University of Southern California Annenberg School for Communication and Journalism studies diversity and inclusion in entertainment media. One of the things they do is analyze popular film and television to assess the extent to which marginalized populations are portrayed and how accurate those portrayals are. In 2019, in collaboration with the American Foundation for Suicide Prevention, they published a report on how mental illness was depicted in the 100 top films of 2016 and the first episodes of the top 50 television shows on broadcast or basic/premium cable in 2016/2017 (Smith et al., 2019). Across the 100 films, there were 4,598 characters with speaking parts, and across the 50 TV series, there were 1,220 characters with speaking parts. A character was defined as having a mental health condition "when a *significant* and/or *persistent* negative reaction (e.g., adverse thoughts, emotions, behaviors) was evidenced by *internalizing* or *externalizing* symptoms" (p. 5).

The last two columns of Table 9.2 show the demographic characteristics of characters depicted with mental illness. As you can see, the depictions differ from real life across the board, with prevalence much lower in film and television than in real life and with gender/ethnicity ratios off the mark. But what about the kinds of mental illnesses depicted? In film and television, the top three conditions were addiction, mood disorders (e.g., depression, bipolar disorder), and anxiety/PTSD. Considering that depressive and anxiety disorders are the most prevalent mental illnesses in society and addiction is an ongoing concern, entertainment media seem to be doing a better job of representation here. But what about suicide? It was the fourth most common concern depicted in both film and television. In film, 13 characters were shown having suicide-related thoughts/behaviors, and five died from suicide (38.5%). In television, six characters were shown having suicide-related thoughts/behaviors, and two died from suicide (33.3%). In real life, the ratio of suicide ideation to suicide attempts to death by suicide is 275 to 27 to 1 (CDC, 2023), so the portrayal in film and television is extremely skewed, possibly leading viewers to lose faith in suicide prevention efforts. Smith et al. (2019) argue that this data shows that mental illness is underrepresented in popular entertainment media, with an overreliance on suicide in storytelling.

What about *how* mental illness was depicted? The authors found that 47% of the characters with mental illness in film were disparaged through name-calling (e.g., crazy, freak, weird), mostly by other characters (98%) but also sometimes by themselves (22%). In television, 38% of characters were disparaged, all by other characters (i.e., no self-disparagement). In addition, characters were stigmatized by being treated poorly, isolated, rejected, or not trusted. Sometimes characters would attempt to conceal their mental illness because of disparagement. Sometimes, however, characters with mental illness would engage in violence against other characters (46% of mentally ill characters in film and 25% in television). In real life, people with serious mental illness commit only 3–5% of violent acts but are more than 10 times as likely to be victims of violence than people in the general population (MentalHealth.gov, 2022), so these portrayals present a biased picture. There was evidence of mental illness being used for humor in both film and television, too, which the authors observe is risky because it might inhibit feelings of empathy. Smith et al. (2019) argue that this data suggests that stigma is the primary theme in mental health portrayals and that mental health is mocked in entertainment media.

Finally, is there anything positive to come out of portrayals of mental illness in film and television? Smith et al. (2019) focus on the potential to model help-seeking behavior as one benefit. In film and television, four characters and three characters, respectively, were taking some form of prescribed medication for their illness, and 19 characters and 20 characters, respectively, were in therapy. Such portrayals can contribute to normalizing help seeking and demonstrate treatment options for viewers who may have a mental illness. The authors also offer a series of questions for content creators to consider as they develop ideas for stories so that the depiction of mental illness gets a fair shake. Is mental illness just being used as a plot device? If so, perhaps the story could be better served by developing a more well-rounded portrayal of the condition. Is mental illness being used as a source of humor? If so, such "humor" would be better avoided because it may trivialize the condition and inhibit empathy. Do characters with mental illness seek and receive help? Portraying help seeking in a realistic manner is an excellent opportunity to destigmatize that behavior and provide a model for viewers with mental health conditions to follow. Finally, writers, producers, and directors should ask, "Why am I telling this story and what do I want audiences to take away?" (p. 29). The authors state their rationale for this advice poignantly (Smith et al., 2019, p. 29):

> Storytellers fill an important role in our cultural conversations about many topics. By exposing audiences to different viewpoints and perspectives, they can educate and illuminate new ideas. However, this power can come with a downside. Through portrayals

that stigmatize or disparage mental health conditions, creators may be teaching an entirely different lesson. Through critical thinking about why portrayals are needed in a story and what audiences might take away, storytellers themselves can be part of creating attitude and behavior change on the other side of the screen.

News Media

As with entertainment media, there's considerable evidence that news reporting on mental illness is skewed toward the sensational. In a study that looked at news media coverage of mental illness in the United States from 1995 to 2014, Emma McGinty and colleagues (2016) analyzed 400 news stories on mental illness, coding them for (a) *topics* covered, (b) whether *causes* and *consequences* of mental illness were addressed, (c) depictions of people with mental illness, and (d) any mention of *public policies* on mental illness. Results showed that violence was the most frequently covered topic, appearing in 55% of the stories. This violence primarily involved interpersonal gun violence and suicide. The second most frequent topic, appearing in 47% of stories, was mental health treatment, with a focus on access to, funding for, and quality of treatment. Causes of mental illness appeared in 35% of stories and emphasized stressful life events and genetics/biology. Consequences appeared in 56% of the stories and focused on involvement in the criminal justice system and stigma or discrimination. In terms of depictions of people with mental illness, they were portrayed in 47% of stories. Those stories were almost exclusively negative, however, emphasizing interpersonal violence, involvement in the criminal justice system, suicide, unsuccessful treatment, unemployment, homelessness, and discrimination. Only 7% of the stories reported successful treatment or recovery. Finally, public policy appeared in 24% of news stories and focused mostly on treatment-related issues such as expanding inpatient or outpatient services in the community. The authors conclude that media coverage of mental illness skews negative, emphasizing interpersonal violence disproportionate to actual rates of violence.

These same researchers wanted to investigate whether stories that stigmatized mental illness might result in decreased public support for funding mental health services more than stories that did not. They designed an experiment in which they randomly assigned 1,326 participants to read one of three versions of a story featuring a man who developed schizophrenia as a young adult. Story versions emphasized (a) barriers to treatment and resulting violence, (b) barriers to treatment only, or (c) successful treatment and recovery. Results showed that stories focused on barriers either with or without violence increased public support for mental health treatment, but the version with violence also increased stigma. The authors conclude that to effectively increase public support for mental health treatment without increasing stigma, news stories should emphasize barriers to treatment (McGinty et al., 2018).

The American Psychiatric Association (2023b) offers tips so that the news media can be more responsible and accurate when reporting on mental illness. They encourage reporters to ask themselves whether mental illness really is central to the story and, if not, to consider not including it. They also admonish reporters to use credible sources for their stories and not rely on hearsay, and they offer themselves as a resource for access to experts and information about mental illness conditions and treatment options. They urge reporters to be exquisitely careful in their language choices, avoiding stigmatizing and derogatory language, mentioning specific diagnoses instead of making broad reference to mental illness, and emphasizing people over conditions (e.g., say "a person with schizophrenia" instead of "a schizophrenic"). Responsible reporting is particularly important when it comes to suicide because of **suicide contagion**, or the likelihood that vulnerable people will attempt suicide after reading media reports of such deaths (Ortiz & Khin, 2018). This effect is well established, but it can be reduced with responsible reporting. Guidelines include avoiding the use of "suicide" in the headline, avoiding sensational language, and avoiding the creation of suicide role models, especially in the case of celebrity suicides, and providing information on where to seek help (Ortiz & Khin, 2018). These are all simple, clear guidelines that, if followed, have the potential to increase public understanding of mental illness, reduce stigma, and reduce the likelihood of copycat suicides.

Social Media

In day-to-day conversations, it's not uncommon to hear people wonder about the extent to which their social media use is good for their mental health. Communication scholars have dedicated much research effort exploring this very question. Although there are some mixed results, most studies suggest that there are reasons to be concerned about social media's impact on mental health. For instance, one study found that the introduction of Facebook across college campuses had a negative impact on college student mental health, which in turn had a negative impact on academic performance (Braghieri et al., 2022). Another study found that social media use was associated with increased depression, problems with behavioral conduct, and alcohol consumption (Brunborg & Andreas, 2019). These findings are just the tip of the iceberg. In this section, we'll focus specifically on three key areas of social media research: social media's influence on mood, body image, and attitudes toward mental health.

Social Media Use and Mood

There is a plethora of factors that influence mood, from biological ("I'm hangry!") to interpersonal ("He really ticks me off!") to socio-political (we won't even go there). Can the information you're exposed to on social media also affect your mood? You betcha! We have Facebook to thank for that knowledge. In 2012, for a one-week period, Facebook ran an experiment in which they manipulated the emotional tone of 689,003 users' newsfeeds (Kramer et al., 2014). They did this by reducing the number of friends' posts that were positive or negative by 10%, so a person would see relatively fewer positive or fewer negative posts than they ordinarily would. The researchers calculated the percentage of positive and negative words that were posted by users whose news feeds had been manipulated. They were interested in determining whether there was evidence of **emotional contagion**, or the extent to which the tone of what users were seeing on their newsfeeds would subsequently influence the tone of their posts. That's exactly what they found. Users whose positive content had been reduced posted status updates with a larger percentage of negative words and a smaller percentage of positive words. Users whose negative content had been reduced showed the opposite effect, posting status updates with a larger percentage of positive words and a smaller percentage of negative words. Although the effect sizes were modest, modest effects on a large scale (hundreds of thousands or millions of people) can be consequential. The authors conclude that their study provided experimental evidence that "emotional states can be transferred to others via emotional contagion, leading people to experience the same emotions without their awareness" (p. 8788). When you consider the implications of this finding, whether negative information is increased through manipulation or simply through the nature of platforms people frequent, the potential for negative impact on mood and mental health is unsettling to say the least. (We'll revisit this study in Chapter 11, so stay tuned.)

Social Media and Body Image

Also unsettling is the impact of social media use on body image. (Sorry for the spoiler alert.) Research has established that there's a negative impact from traditional media exposure and body image in both women (Grabe et al., 2008) and men (Barlett et al., 2008). Body images on television programs, movies, and commercials are carefully curated to be as attractive as possible, meeting or exceeding sociocultural standards for beauty and body composition. So social comparison, the central focus of **social comparison theory** (Festinger, 1954; see Table 9.1), almost always results in the viewer being worse off from seeing and comparing themselves to these images. The same thing happens with social media, where millions of people (influencers and regular folk alike) carefully curate their own images to show themselves in the best light. So, is the impact of social media on body image similar to that found for traditional media? Two recent studies say yes.

Alyssa Saiphoo and Zahra Vahedi (2019) conducted a meta-analysis of 56 studies (with 63 independent samples) involving 36,552 people and found that there was a relationship between social media use and negative body image. They also found this effect was stronger for younger users than older users and that studies investigating "appearance-focused" social media use showed stronger effects than studies investigating general social media use. Speaking of "appearance-focused" social media, Mary Sherlock and Danielle Wagstaff (2019) did a study looking at the effects of Instagram on 129 women aged 18–35 years. They found that frequency of Instagram use was correlated with symptoms of depression, low self-esteem, anxiety about physical appearance, and body dissatisfaction. To explore causal relationships, the researchers conducted an experiment by exposing their participants to four types of photos: beauty, fitness, travel, and no-image (control). They found that photos of beauty and fitness led to a negative impact on outcome variables, with women in those conditions reporting a decrease in self-rated attractiveness. This decrease was exacerbated by lower self-esteem and greater anxiety, depression, and body dissatisfaction.

Not to pile on, but what makes these studies even more unsettling is that Meta©, the parent company for both Facebook and Instagram, knew that Instagram use was harmful to the mental health of teenagers, particularly young girls, *and they hid it from the public.* In September 2021, *The Wall Street Journal* published leaked internal documents from the company showing that it had known for years that Instagram use was harming the mental health of its users, particularly around perceptions of body image and among girls (Wells et al., 2021). Through a series of internal studies, the company found that about 20% of young female users reported that Instagram made them feel worse about themselves. For teens already struggling with their mental health, these studies showed that teens felt Instagram harmed their mental health further through (a) pressure to conform to social stereotypes, (b) pressure to match the body shapes of influencers, (c) the need for validation through views, likes, and followers, (d) friendship conflicts, bullying, and hate speech, (e) oversexualization of girls, and (f) inappropriate advertisements targeted to vulnerable groups. The leaked studies flew in the face of years of rhetoric from Meta© officials arguing that their platforms are not negatively harming the mental health of users. Although the company states that it's working to reduce mental health harms for users, particularly teens, the fear over losing one of the world's most profitable markets has made the implementation of these changes small and slow (see Jean Twenge's commentary as reported for *Time* by Perrigo, 2021). In addition, the company's efforts to hide what it knew about its platforms from the public provide solid ground for skepticism.

Social Media and Attitudes toward Mental Health

So that everything isn't doom and gloom, let's consider an example of mental illness depiction in social media that may have a positive impact: celebrity disclosures of their struggles with mental illness. One such study comes from Diane Francis, who studied Black men's Twitter conversations after the hip-hop artist Kid Cudi disclosed that he had depression. As you know from statistics presented earlier, mental illness disproportionately affects the

Black community, and because of stigma and cultural communication norms, Black men, in particular, are affected. Francis (2019) analyzed 1,482 tweets in response to the hashtag #YouGoodMan, which was created by influencer Dayna Lynn Nuckolls to encourage conversation about Kid Cudi's disclosure among Black men. Francis identified three themes in the conversations. *Advocating for mental health disclosure* involved tweets through which the men disclosed their own troubles with mental illness and/or how they were seeking help through medical treatment or therapy. *Providing online and offline support* involved demonstrations of emotional support (e.g., showing empathy and concern), network support (e.g., emphasizing that help was available through Twitter and interpersonal channels), and informational support (e.g., sharing mental health resources or offering services). *Acknowledging the role and impact of culture and society* addressed topics such as how mental health issues are stigmatized in the Black community, how religion and prayer provide insufficient help, how masculine norms inhibit disclosure and help seeking, and how rap and hip-hop that address mental health have a positive influence. Francis shared one tweet that captured the spirit of the Twitter conversations: "Twitter is really therapeutic at times" (p. 453).

The landscape of social media continues to evolve at a rapid pace, and understanding its influence on mental health and illness from a socioecological perspective is a tall order. As with nearly everything in life, there are bad aspects and good aspects. The goal for health communication researchers is to develop as comprehensive an understanding as possible of this landscape (even as it grows and changes) to recognize how and why it has both positive and negative effects so that, ultimately, researchers can develop policy recommendations and interventions to improve mental health outcomes for users across diverse communities.

Media and Mental Health

Extensive research documents the extent to which persons with mental illness and aspects of mental illness are portrayed in entertainment, news, and social media. People with mental illness typically have been portrayed as violent and dangerous. However, they're more likely than members of the general public to be victims of violence. Communication campaigns can have positive effects on reducing stigma and encouraging people to seek help.

Approaches to Treating Mental Illness and Preventing Suicide

Given the prevalence of mental illness and suicide and the stigma surrounding both, it is morally and ethically imperative that everyone work together to reduce barriers and promote access to effective treatment to improve mental health outcomes. Effective treatment doesn't only help the individual and their families. It can also improve societal well-being and economic prosperity. Indeed, *The Lancet Global Health* (2020) reports that for every dollar invested in treating depression and anxiety, there is a four-dollar return in terms of improved health and increased productivity. Let's take a quick look at approaches to treatment and then a more detailed look at the communication campaigns developed to address mental health and illness.

Treatment Approaches

There are different approaches to treating mental illness, depending in part on the diagnosis and severity of the illness. **Medical treatment** from either primary care physicians or psychiatrists is one option (e.g., prescription medications, hospitalizations). Another option is **psychotherapy**, which is "any psychological service provided by a trained professional that primarily uses forms of communication and interaction to assess, diagnose, and treat dysfunctional emotional reactions, ways of thinking, and behavior patterns" (American Psychological Association, 2023, n.p.). These days, therapy may be offered in person or online. Regardless of channel, *communication* is at the center of therapy, where people talk through and work through the psychological and psychosocial factors that lie at the heart of their mental illness. In doing so, people and their therapists are using communication in its constitutive sense, where the meaning of mental health and illness is "co-constructed and experienced in interaction with the other" (Hall & Miller-Ott, 2020, p. 5). Such therapeutic-focused communication helps people understand and make sense of their illness experience, possibly finding ways to reframe it and move forward.

If people don't want to work with a therapist, there are a vast number of **self-help resources** available. Steven Chan and colleagues (2019) completed a comprehensive review of self-help and automated tools available for mental health care. Obviously, there are good old-fashioned books. However, there is also a plethora of mediated resources available, including interactive media, online courses and articles, mobile apps, chatbots, videos, podcasts, blogs, and internet sites—all dedicated to mental health. The benefits of such self-help resources include their reach and lower cost. The concern is whether the resource has been evaluated and found effective, or whether it's just "out there" with no basis in evidence whatsoever. Research evaluating self-help programs for depression and anxiety (e.g., Cuijpers et al., 2010), for example, does suggest that such programs can be effective, but there's a lot more work to do.

Let's take a closer look at mental health support available through smartphone apps. Such apps can substantially improve access to mental health support given that smartphones are owned by 85% of the U.S. population (Pew Research Center, 2022) and many apps are free. Akash Wasil and colleagues (2021) examined the six most popular apps in meditation and mindfulness, journaling and self-monitoring, and AI chatbots. They documented the apps' content and features and the differences between free and paid versions. The authors observed that the apps could function as standalone interventions or be used in conjunction with therapy. They also noted that although the six apps they studied accounted for 83% of mental health app users, there are literally thousands of other apps available, and there's a serious "research-to-retail gap," meaning that most apps go on the market without ever being evaluated for effectiveness.

But what about the evaluations that have been done? Mindfulness-based apps have been of particular interest to researchers. For example, Jayde Flett and colleagues (2019) conducted a randomized controlled trial in which they assigned 208 college students to one of three conditions: Headspace, Smiling Mind, and Evernote (a control condition). Participants needed to use their app for 10 minutes/day for 10 days. After that, they could use it as much or as little as they wanted over the subsequent 30 days. After the first 10 days, Headspace and Smiling Mind users showed improvements in depressive symptoms and college adjustment. Effects for depressive symptoms remained 30 days later, but effects for college adjustment did not. It seems there is some promise in using mindfulness-based apps to help with some aspects of mental health. Importantly, two recent systematic reviews and meta-analyses have shown promising effects for people of color (Sun et al., 2022) and military veterans (Goldberg et al., 2020), two historically marginalized groups. Such impact is essential for reducing disparities in mental health.

Public Communication Campaigns and Mental Health

There is a multitude of public communication campaigns that have been launched to encourage people to seek help for mental illness and to prevent suicide, as well as to reduce stigma around those issues. These campaigns utilize both traditional and social media channels. You can also find examples of such campaigns in many countries (e.g., England, France, Ireland, Australia, Sweden, India). They range from large-scale, government-run campaigns, such as the U.S. Department of Labor campaign to promote mental health at the workplace (Safety Matters, 2022), to smaller-scale, local community- or school-based campaigns, such as *Look Around Boone* (e.g., Thompson et al., 2021), and they run the gamut from targeting general audiences (e.g., employees: Safety Matters, 2022) to specific groups (e.g., military service members: Randall, 2021; older Asian American women: Cao, 2015).

Although many campaigns are never adequately evaluated, those that have been tended to show positive effects. For example, Clara González-Sanguino and colleagues (2019) reported on *Time to Change*, a program designed to raise awareness about the prevalence of mental illness, reduce stigma, and encourage helping and help-seeking behaviors among people in England. Evaluations of this campaign, which included general and targeted audiences, led to improvements in knowledge, attitudes, and stigma, as well as increases in mental health awareness among segmented audiences. In addition, certain segments showed improvements in the belief that recovery is possible, knowledge of professional help resources, and willingness to live with someone with mental illness.

Although this and many other campaigns use awareness, knowledge, or attitude as their primary outcome variable, some campaigns go the extra mile and assess influence on behavior. Anna Ross and Bridget Bassilios (2019) report on the Australian suicide prevention campaign *R U OK?*, an initiative that's been in place since 2009 and includes an *R U OK?*Day each September. The campaign encourages people to identify others who may be undergoing particularly stressful events or hard times and to talk to them by (a) asking how they're doing, (b) listening without being judgmental, (c) encouraging help seeking as needed, and (d) checking on them later to see how things are going. The latest campaign evaluation showed positive effects on awareness of the campaign and self-reported general participation in *R U OK?*Day. It also showed that people who were exposed to the campaign were two to three times more likely to have greater intentions to help a friend who "might be troubled" or was "obviously troubled," and more than six times as likely to actually engage in a helping behavior (e.g., ask a friend if something was troubling them, contact a support service for them). That is an impressive effect.

Campaigns can be highly effective in influencing the attitudes and behaviors of large numbers of people, but they only work if they reach their audience. Therefore, we want to launch a mini-campaign of our own right here to raise your awareness of resources for mental health because there are numerous resources available to help anyone in need of support. In July of 2022, the United States adopted **988** as the number to call for its **Suicide and Crisis Hotline**. The CDC has a website called **How Right Now** (www.cdc.gov/howrightnow) that helps people find resources that can help them navigate a variety of emotions, including fear, anger, grief, loneliness, and stress. There are many support groups through social media, including those run by advocacy groups like **The You Rock Foundation**, which uses the power of music to reach those suffering from depression, and **Real Warriors**, dedicated to service members, veterans, and their families. And never forget campus resources. College and university administrators are extremely aware of the importance of mental health for the success and well-being of their students, and they devote resources to support student needs. Check your campus' website or ask a trusted instructor about resources available to you. The information is out there for you.

Approaches to Treating Mental Illness

Mental illness can be treated in a variety of ways, including through medication, psychotherapy, and self-help. Help is available in person and online. The National Institute of Mental Health (https://www.nimh.nih.gov/health/find-help) lists how to get help in an immediate crisis and how to find a healthcare provider or treatment. It also offers free publications on mental disorders.

In the United States, 988 is the number for the *Suicide and Crisis Hotline.* You can also check with your instructor or your college or university website to find out where on campus students can go for mental health services.

Conclusion

We told you that we were going to cover a lot in this chapter, and we have. We provided definitions and statistics on the prevalence of mental health and illness, and we discussed how mental illness is stigmatized. We covered disparities in the diagnosis and treatment of mental illness, and we considered how the meaning of mental illness varies across cultures. We addressed suicide, providing information on prevalence, trends, and groups at risk. We also covered the influence of mental health and suicide on families and how the topics are covered in entertainment, news, and social media. We wrapped up the chapter by presenting approaches to mental health treatment and reviewing awareness/prevention campaigns, organizations, and resources to help promote mental health and prevent suicide.

To ensure that people don't suffer needlessly and get access to the help they need, it's incumbent upon everyone to play a role in reducing stigma and promoting good mental health. At the heart of diagnosis and treatment is communication. In the words of Fred Rogers, "Anything that's human is mentionable, and anything that is mentionable can be more manageable. When we can talk about our feelings, they become less overwhelming, less upsetting, and less scary." We hope that you will be willing to talk about your feelings, listen to other people talk about theirs, and take good care of your mental health.

References

Accreditation Council for Graduate Medical Education. (2020–2022). *Specialties.* https://www.acgme.org/specialties/

Adams, E., Hawgood, J., Bundock, A., & Kõlves, K. (2019). A phenomenological study of siblings bereaved by suicide: A shared experience. *Death Studies, 43*(5), 324–332.

Aldrich, R. S., & Quintero Johnson, J. (2022). Mental health, mental illness, and suicide. In T. L. Thompson & N. G. Harrington (Eds.), *The Routledge handbook of health communication* (pp. 63–76). Routledge.

American Foundation for Suicide Prevention. (2020). *Suicide statistics: Suicide facts & figures national fact sheet.* https://afsp.org/suicide-statistics/

American Psychiatric Association. (2013). *DSM-5 table of contents.* https://www.psychiatry.org/File%20Library/Psychiatrists/Practice/DSM/APA_DSM-5-Contents.pdf

American Psychiatric Association. (2023a). *Mental health disparities: Diverse populations.* https://www.psychiatry.org/psychiatrists/diversity/education/mental-health-facts

American Psychiatric Association. (2023b). *Words matter: Reporting on mental health conditions.* https://www.psychiatry.org/newsroom/reporting-on-mental-health-conditions

American Psychological Association. (2023). *APA dictionary of psychology.* https://dictionary.apa.org/psychotherapy

Barlett, C. P., Vowels, C. L., & Saucier, D. A. (2008). Meta-analyses of the effects of media images on men's body-image concerns. *Journal of Social and Clinical Psychology, 27,* 279–310.

Braghieri, L., Levy, R., & Makarin, A. (2022, February 24). *Social media and mental health.* Discussion Paper, No. 320. Ludwig-Maximilians-Universität München und Humboldt-Universität zu Berlin, Collaborative Research Center Transregio 190- Rationality and Competition, München und Berlin. https://rationality-and-competition.de/wp-content/uploads/2022/02/320.pdf

Brunborg, G. S., & Andreas, J. B. (2019). Increase in time spent on social media is associated with modest increase in depression, conduct problems, and episodic heavy drinking. *Journal of Adolescence, 74,* 201–209.

Buus, N., Caspersen, J., Hansen, R., Stenager, E., & Fleischer, E. (2014). Experiences of parents whose sons or daughters have (had) attempted suicide. *Journal of Advanced Nursing, 70*(4), 823–832.

Cao, K. O. (2015). Preventing suicide among older Adult Asian women. *Generations, 38*(4), 82–85.

Centers for Disease Control and Prevention. (2021). *About mental health.* https://www.cdc.gov/mentalhealth/learn/index.htm

Centers for Disease Control and Prevention. (2022). *Risk and protective factors.* https://www.cdc.gov/suicide/factors/index.html

Centers for Disease Control and Prevention. (2023). *Suicide data and statistics.* https://www.cdc.gov/suicide/suicide-data-statistics.html

Chan, S., Li, L., Torous, J., Gratzer, D., & Yellowlees, P. M. (2019). Review and implementation of self-help and automated tools in mental health care. *Psychiatric Clinics of North America, 42*(4), 597–609.

Cuijpers, P., Donker, T., van Straten, A., Li, J., & Andersson, G. (2010). Is guided self-help as effective as face-to-face psychotherapy for depression and anxiety disorders? A systematic review and meta-analysis of comparative outcome studies. *Psychological Medicine, 40*(12), 1943–1957.

Festinger, L. (1954). A theory of social comparison processes. *Human Relations, 7,* 117–140.

Flett, J., Hayne, H., Riordan, B., Thompson, L. M., & Connor, T. S. (2019). Mobile mindfulness meditation: A randomised controlled trial of the effect of two popular apps on mental health. *Mindfulness, 10*(2), 863–876.

Flood-Grady, E., & Koenig Kellas, J. (2019). Sense-making, socialization, and stigma: Exploring narratives told in families about mental illness. *Health Communication, 34*(6), 607–617.

Francis, D. B. (2019). "Twitter is really therapeutic at times": Examination of Black men's Twitter conversations following hip-hop artist Kid Cudi's depression disclosure. *Health Communication, 36*(4), 448–456.

Galanti, G.-A. (2015). *Caring for patients from different cultures.* University of Pennsylvania Press.

Goffman, E. (1963). *Notes on the management of spoiled identity.* Prentice Hall.

Goldberg, S. B., Riordan, K. M., Sun, S., Kearney, D. J., & Simpson, T. L. (2020). Efficacy and acceptability of mindfulness-based interventions for military veterans: A systematic review and meta-analysis. *Journal of Psychosomatic Research, 113,* 110232.

Gonzales, L., Davidoff, K. C., Nadal, K. L., & Yanos, P. T. (2015). Microaggressions experienced by persons with mental illnesses: An exploratory study. *Psychiatric Rehabilitation Journal, 38*(3), 234–241.

González-Sanguino, C., Potts, L. C., Milenova, M., & Henderson, C. (2019). Time to Change's social marketing campaign for a new target population: Results from 2017 to 2019. *BMC Psychiatry, 19*(1), 417.

Grabe, S., Ward, L. M., & Hyde, J. S. (2008). The role of the media in body image concerns among women: A meta-analysis of experimental and correlational studies. *Psychological Bulletin, 134*(3), 460–476.

Hall, R. D., & Miller-Ott, A. E. (2020). Communicating about mental health: What we know, what we need, and what we give. In L. R. Lippert, R. D. Hall, A. E. Miller-Ott, & D. C. Davis (Eds.), *Communicating mental health: History, contexts, and perspectives* (pp. 3–10). Lexington Books.

Koenig Kellas, J., & Trees, A. R. (2022). Family stories and storytelling: Windows into the family soul. In A. L. Vangelisti (Ed.), *The Routledge handbook of family communication* (3rd ed., pp. 359–374). Routledge.

Kramer, A. D. I., Guillory, J. E., & Hancock, J. T. (2014). Experimental evidence of massive-scale emotional contagion through social networks. *PNAS, 111*(24), 8788–8790.

McGinty, E. E., Goldman, H. H., Pescosolido, B. A., & Barry, C. L. (2018). Communicating about mental illness and violence: balancing increased support for services and stigma. *Journal of Health Politics, Policy and Law, 43*(2), 185–228.

McGinty, E. E., Kennedy-Hendricks, A., Chosky, S., & Barry, C. L. (2016). Trends in news media coverage of mental illness in the United States: 1995–2014. *Health Affairs (Millwood), 35*(6), 1121–1129.

MentalHealth.gov. (2020). *Health insurance and mental health services*. https://www.mentalhealth.gov/get-help/health-insurance

MentalHealth.gov. (2022). *Mental health myths and facts*. https://www.mentalhealth.gov/basics/mental-health-myths-facts

National Alliance on Mental Illness. (2022a). *Mental health by the numbers*. https://www.nami.org/mhstats

National Alliance on Mental Illness. (2022b). *LGBTQI*. https://www.nami.org/Your-Journey/Identity-and-Cultural-Dimensions/LGBTQI

National Institute of Mental Health. (2022a). *Mental illness*. https://www.nimh.nih.gov/health/statistics/mental-illness

National Institute of Mental Health. (2022b). *Suicide*. https://www.nimh.nih.gov/health/statistics/suicide

Ortiz, P., & Khin, E. K. (2018). Traditional and new media's influence on suicidal behavior and contagion. *Behavioral Sciences & the Law, 36*(2), 245–256.

Perrigo, B. (2021, September 16). Instagram makes teen girls hate themselves. Is that a bug or a feature? *Time*. https://time.com/6098771/instagram-body-image-teen-girls/

Pew Research Center. (2022). *Mobile fact sheet*. https://www.pewresearch.org/internet/fact-sheet/mobile/

Randall, T. S. (2021). Mired in shadows: The U.S. Army's campaign to encourage mental health treatment. *Visual Communication Quarterly, 28*(2), 112–125.

Ross, A. M., & Bassilios, B. (2019). Australian R U OK?Day campaign: Improving helping beliefs, intentions and behaviours. *International Journal of Mental Health Systems, 13*, Article 61.

Safety Matters. (2022). DOL launches campaign on mental health in the workplace. *Professional Safety, 67*(7), 6.

Saiphoo, A. N., & Vahedi, Z. (2019). Meta-analytic review of the relationship between social media use and body image disturbance. *Computers in Human Behavior, 101*, 259–275.

Scheufele, D. A., & Tewksbury, D. (2007). Framing, agenda setting, and priming: The evolution of three media effects models. *Journal of Communication, 57*(1), 9–20.

Sherlock, M., & Wagstaff, D. L. (2019). Exploring the relationship between frequency of Instagram use, exposure to idealized images, and psychological well-being in women. *Psychology of Popular Media Culture, 8*(4), 482–490.

Smith, R. A. (2007). Language of the lost: An explication of stigma communication. *Communication Theory, 17*(4), 462–485.

Smith, S. L., Choueiti, M., Choi, A., Piper, K., & Moutier, C. (2019). *Mental health conditions in film and TV: Portrayals that dehumanize and trivialize characters*. USC Annenberg Inclusion Initiative and American Foundation for Suicide Prevention. https://assets.uscannenberg.org/docs/aii-study-mental-health-media_052019.pdf

Stokols, D. (1996). Translating social ecological theory into guidelines for community health promotion. *American Journal of Health Promotion, 10*(4), 282–298.

Sun, S., Goldberg, S. B., Loucks, E. B., & Brewer, J. A. (2022). Mindfulness-based interventions among people of color: A systematic review and meta-analysis. *Psychotherapy Research, 32*(3), 277–290.

The Lancet Global Health. (2020). Mental health matters. *The Lancet Global Health, 8*(11), E1352.

Thompson, A., Hollis, S., Herman, K. C., Reinke, W. M., Hawley, K., & Magee, S. (2021). Evaluation of a social media campaign on youth mental health stigma and help-seeking. *School Psychology Review, 50*(1), 36–41.

Twenge, J. M., Cooper, A. B., Joiner, T. E., Duffy, M. E., & Binau, S. G. (2019). Age, period, and cohort trends in mood disorder indicators and suicide-related outcomes in a nationally representative dataset, 2005–2017. *Journal of Abnormal Psychology, 128*(3), 185–199.

U.S. Department of Veterans Affairs. (2021). *2021 national veteran suicide prevention annual report*. https://www.mentalhealth.va.gov/docs/data-sheets/2021/2021-National-Veteran-Suicide-Prevention-Annual-Report-FINAL-9-8-21.pdf

Wasil, A. R., Palermo, E. H., Lorezno-Luaces, L., & DeRubeis, R. J. (2021). "Is there an app for that?": A review of popular apps for depression, anxiety, and well-being. *Cognitive and Behavioral Practice*. doi:10.1016/j.cbpra.2021.07.001

Wells, G., Horwitz, J., & Seetharaman, D. (2021, September 14). The Facebook files: Facebook knows Instragram is toxic for teen girls, company documents show. *The Wall Street Journal*. https://www.wsj.com/articles/facebook-knows-instagram-is-toxic-for-teen-girls-company-documents-show-11631620739

Wilson, S. R., Gettings, P. E., Hall, E. D., & Pastor, R. G. (2015). Dilemmas families face in talking with returning U.S. military service members about seeking professional help for mental health issues. *Health Communication, 30*(8), 772–783.

World Health Organization. (1948). *Constitution of the World Health Organization.* http://apps.who.int/gb/bd/PDF/bd47/EN/constitution-en.pdf

World Health Organization. (2022a). *Mental health: Strengthening our response.* https://www.who.int/en/news-room/fact-sheets/detail/mental-health-strengthening-our-response

World Health Organization. (2022b). *Mental disorders.* https://www.who.int/news-room/fact-sheets/detail/mental-disorders

World Health Organization. (2022c). *Suicide.* https://www.who.int/news-room/fact-sheets/detail/suicide

In-class Activities

1. In small groups, have students discuss their experiences seeing posts about mental health issues on social media. What are some positives? What are some negatives?
2. In small groups, have students discuss movies or TV shows they remember seeing that dealt with mental illness. Have them list ways the depictions seemed realistic or unrealistic, either in positive or negative ways. Assess whether the depictions influenced how they think about mental illness.

Discussion Questions

1. What issues in this chapter are consistent with your expectations about mental health and illness? What issues are different from your expectations?
2. What stories have you heard other people tell about experiences with mental illness? To what extent have these stories shaped your attitudes and beliefs?
3. Thinking back to the findings from the Annenberg Inclusion Initiative study, does the entertainment industry "owe" anything to its patrons in terms of depicting mental illness more accurately? What about the news industry?

Monica Prepares for an Adventure Abroad

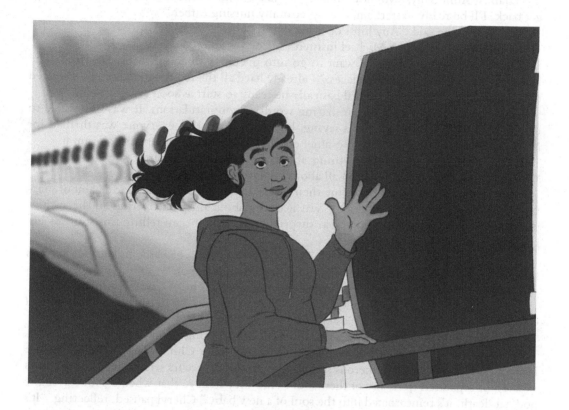

One by one, each member of the Montgomery family found a way to cope with Helen's death. Sally started painting again, which she knew would make Helen happy. Joe started a program in his school district to help kids cope with loss. Every two weeks, he and volunteer counselors met with students who needed a place to talk and grieve. Anytime he heard laughter during the sessions, Joe felt he was making his mother smile from above. Monica, however, seemed to need the biggest change.

"Okay, but how confident are you that you'll be able to find Wi-Fi?" Cheryl asked Monica on the family Zoom, which was still happening each week.

"Reasonably confident," Monica replied. "I might not be able to Zoom every week, but I'll do my best."

In chorus, everyone started grumbling, wishing Monica would be able to join more consistently.

DOI: 10.4324/9781003214458-23

"Really, you all are going to lay on a guilt trip this thick?" Monica asked jokingly. "I'm joining Doctors Without Borders. It's not like I'm going to be off galivanting. And the Wi-Fi challenges are because I'll be in rural Ethiopia, not because I can't be bothered to join you."

"True. You might not be on vacation, but I still want a souvenir!" Cheryl interjected.

"Me, too! And make sure it's bigger than Cheryl's," Sam joked.

Everyone started laughing. The complaining and teasing were a front for the worry they felt about Monica heading overseas. Although they were very proud of her and knew she needed this change, no one knew exactly what she might face during her assignment.

"We're so proud of you, sweetie," Sally said. "We're just going to miss you so much."

"Thanks, Aunt Sally," Monica replied. "It's just going to be a few months. And when I get back, I'll be ready to start a new chapter of my nursing career."

"Oh, yeah," Joe said. "Any hints on what that will be?"

"Go on, share the plan," Michael insisted.

"Okay, okay. I decided that I want to go into oncology nursing," Monica shared. The Zoom screen filled with smiling faces. "I already have all the required credentials. I'll need to shadow for a little while, but I'll basically be ready to start as soon as I get back."

Simultaneously, everyone began sharing words of congratulations. It was impossible to decipher exactly what anyone was saying, but it was clear that everyone was thrilled for Monica. As the celebration began to quiet down, Cheryl found a moment to jump in.

"I just can't wait to hear everything about the Ethiopian culture," she told Monica. "Speaking of culture, did I tell you all about my Hmong patient from last week?"

Everyone on the call started shaking their heads. Lately, Cheryl had made a habit of sharing different cultural perspectives she was learning about through treating all the various patients at her hospital. So no one was surprised when she began telling this story of her latest patient.

"So, my patient had pain in her back," Cheryl began, "and she came in because her legs started to go numb. We ran some tests and found a spinal tumor."

"Is this a sad story, because we might need a rain check if it is," Savannah interrupted.

"No, Aunt Savannah. It's just interesting," Cheryl replied. "So anyway, her father did *not* want her to have the surgery because he's a Hmong elder."

"Wait, what does that mean?" Savannah asked, interrupting again.

"Hmong are an ethnic group of people originally from China. They believe that the human body is a host for numerous souls and that disease occurs when the body becomes isolated or separated from any of their souls. And they believe that when a soul leaves the body at death, it's reincarnated into the soul of a new baby." Cheryl paused, reflecting. "It's really quite a beautiful perspective on death when you think about it. I mean, when you consider all the different cultural—"

Cheryl was interrupted again, but this time by Sally, who knew that if she let Cheryl lecture them on cultural perspectives on life and death, they'd be there all day. "So what happened with your patient, sweetie?" Sally asked politely.

"Okay, okay," Cheryl replied, recognizing the gentle reminder to get back on track. "So without this surgery, my patient would eventually be paralyzed. But her father was adamantly against it and believed that her sickness was caused by one of her souls being missing. And my poor patient was stuck between everyone's opinion about what she should do."

"Sad, getting sad," Savannah chimed in.

"No, I'm almost done. Not sad," Cheryl continued. "So I reached out to hospital administration, and they invited the patient and her father to sit down with a team of providers and discuss what they felt would be a reasonable solution. And as it turns out, a Hmong shaman was not far away. The father agreed to have him come to the hospital and complete a healing ritual for his daughter that would bring the missing soul back to her. After that, he let us take her into surgery, which went great. I found the whole thing just a wonderful example of competent intercultural medicine."

"That must have been very special to see," Monica replied. "And now you have me even more excited for what I might see on my trip!"

And again, in unison, everyone started talking at once about how excited they were for Monica. Cheryl, however, sat quietly, smiling. It had been really hard for her to join the family Zooms without her grandmother. But if her patient's father was right, it's possible that her grandmother's soul might have lived on in someone else. She found that to be a comforting thought.

Notes

Doctors Without Borders is an international organization that provides emergency medical assistance around the globe. There are several volunteer opportunities available. Learn more here: https://www. doctorswithoutborders.org/

Cheryl's Hmong patient's experience is based on a story portrayed in an episode of *Grey's Anatomy*. You can read more about the episode here: https://greysanatomy.fandom.com/wiki/Anna_Chue

Learn more about the Hmong culture here: https://www.pbs.org/splithorn/shamanism1.html

10 Intercultural Health Communication

The now classic book *The Spirit Catches You and You Fall Down* by Ann Fadiman (1997) tells the story of Lia Lee, a Hmong child who had epilepsy. Lia had her first seizure when she was three months old. Her parents thought it was caused by Lia's soul leaving her body after being startled by a slamming door. Her parents sought medical care, but Lia's diagnosis of epilepsy was delayed because there was a lack of interpreters at the community medical center. Even after diagnosis, there were challenges to Lia's treatment. The treatment was complicated and difficult for her parents to follow, the medication caused unpleasant side effects, and her parents may not have fully understood the purpose of the medication. These factors led to noncompliance with the western medical regimen. At the same time, Lia's parents were also following traditional Hmong healing practices, including calling on a shaman to help retrieve Lia's soul. Eventually, Lia had a massive seizure and developed septic shock, resulting in brain death. The doctors allowed her parents to take her home, thinking she would die soon. She lived for another 26 years.

Lia's story highlights some of the challenges inherent in intercultural health communication, such as different beliefs about the causes of a health condition, delays in diagnosis because there are limited interpreter services, and noncompliance with treatment recommendations because of a lack of understanding. It's important to recognize, though, that each culture has its own health beliefs, and what it means to be healthy can vary considerably from culture to culture, with race/ethnicity, religion, socioeconomic status, age, and gender (to name a few) all influencing perceptions of health and healthy behaviors. So awareness is absolutely essential.

In a review of how different cultures see health and illness, Renata Schiavo (2014) presented findings from across the literature on cultural beliefs surrounding health for different racial/ethnic, religious, and age groups. Regarding perceptions of "good health," Korean cultures saw it as a balance between organic and inorganic elements, mind, and body. Hindus, on the other hand, saw it as the result of good karma. In another example, Brazilian children defined good health as positive feelings. Regarding illness, Vietnamese communities defined it as an indication that the body was out of balance, whereas Muslims saw it as a punishment or way of washing away sins. Elderly Mexican adults, however, saw illness as a normal part of aging but a negative side effect of decisions made when younger. Although some individuals within these cultures may not share these definitions, they serve as exemplars of the ways in which different groups of people can vary in how they see, understand, and experience health and illness.

We hope that at this point in the textbook, you've come to realize the numerous ways in which health communication inherently intersects with intercultural communication—and that you cannot fully consider health without also considering culture. Although we believe that every topic covered by the discipline of health communication should be considered through an intercultural lens, in essence eliminating the need for the traditional

DOI: 10.4324/9781003214458-24

"cultural chapter," there are some essential elements of health communication that fall exclusively under the purview of intercultural communication. Thus, our inclusion of a "culture chapter" is intended as a supplement to the ways culture is considered throughout all the other chapters. This chapter will begin with a deeper dive into how we conceptualize culture. Then, we'll explore the importance of cultural competency within healthcare settings and the theoretical approaches that help guide culture-centered health communication research and practice. Finally, we'll conclude with a recognition of the limitations of taking a western perspective in health communication research.

What Is Culture?

Pop quiz! What is the definition of culture? Unless you've already taken an intercultural communication course (which we highly recommend doing before you graduate), this might seem like an odd question. But stop reading for a second and really try to find the words to define culture. (We'll wait.) ... Okay, for most of you, trying to define culture was probably harder than you expected. Despite culture being something engrained into people's identities—something that influences people whether they realize it not—it's hard to capture a succinct definition that fully encompasses what the term means. For this book, we're going to follow the lead of the U.S. Office of Minority Health (OMH; 2013), which defines **culture** as "the integrated pattern of thoughts, communications, actions, customs, beliefs, values, and institutions associated, wholly or partially, with racial, ethnic, or linguistic groups, as well as with religious, spiritual, biological, geographical, or sociological characteristics" (p. 10). Although people from the same culture will have many similarities, it's important to remember that they won't have the same exact cultural experiences. Geri-Ann Galanti (2000) notes that health professionals often "think that if they just treat each patient with respect, they will avert most cultural problems. But that isn't always the case. Some knowledge of cultural customs can help avoid misunderstandings and enable practitioners to provide better care" (p. 335). This is especially important because there are numerous ways that culture influences health.

According to the Centers for Disease Control and Prevention (CDC; 2014), culture and language can influence a host of health-related experiences, including beliefs surrounding health, healing, and wellness; perceptions of illness, disease, and their causes; behaviors when seeking healthcare, including attitudes toward clinicians; and the delivery of services by providers, who view the world through their own particular cultural lenses. For example, Galanti (2003) explored how traditional Hispanic familial expectations, such as family dynamics and gender roles, could influence health outcomes. She concluded that the combined cultural factors of male dominance, female modesty, and the practice of keeping problems within the family perpetuated health risks, such as heavy drinking, risky sexual behaviors, and acts of domestic violence. However, she noted that healthcare professionals who were aware of these cultural factors could work to build a personal relationship with Hispanic community members as a way to earn their trust and confidence, therefore reducing the health risks. In order for providers to be prepared to build such relationships, however, they must be culturally competent communicators.

Cultural Competency and Health Communication

Over the last few decades, public health and health communication efforts have been devoted to highlight the role of culture in the prevalence of health disparities and health inequalities. Simultaneously, political tensions have risen around the world surrounding discussions of race, ethnicity, and culture. Most of these tensions are fueled by a fear of the "other" or a loss of something you think you'll have to give to an "other." From a communication perspective, these tensions obscure the personal growth that can come with a respect for, and understanding of, other cultures. Instead of seeing intercultural communication as something we *have* to navigate out of political correctness or required policy, health communication scholars see intercultural communication as something we have the *honor* of navigating in an effort to promote positive health outcomes for all people and groups. One way we show respect to others is by being culturally literate, or working to build a culturally competent skillset.

Cultural competency is commonly defined as "a set of congruent behaviors, attitudes, and policies that come together in a system, agency, or among professionals that enables effective work in cross-cultural situations" (Cross et al., 1989, p. 11). By this definition, to be culturally competent communicators, people must not only positively value different cultures but also behave in a fashion that shows respect for other cultures. Competent communicators also must exercise their ability to support policies that recognize the existence of cultural differences, including the ways in which barriers to healthcare can be different for different cultures. These barriers could include a lack of racial/ethnic minority healthcare employees, insufficient interpreter services, and limited access to healthcare. This definition is an important foundation that many scholars have used to build a more specific understanding of what it means to be a culturally competent communicator. Two such scholars are Rukhsana Ahmed and Benjamin Bates.

Cultural Competency

Cultural competency is a set of congruent behaviors, attitudes, and policies that come together in a system, agency, or among professionals that enables effective work in cross-cultural situations.

Ahmed and Bates (2012) proposed four key characteristics of culturally competent health communication. First, cultural competency is a *process*. Becoming culturally competent isn't a series of items on a checklist where once you check them all off, you can officially consider yourself culturally competent. Instead, cultural competency requires intermittent evaluations of existing systems, policies, and personal perspectives. Through these evaluations, culturally competent skills can be strengthened and improved. Second, cultural competency *considers the perspective of both healthcare providers and patients*. Effective communication occurs when the beliefs, values, and perspectives of both sides of the communication exchange are considered. An individual's self-awareness is key to recognizing their communication habits and preferences that may not be culturally sensitive and inclusive. Third, cultural competency is an *intentional* effort to advance and promote knowledge, awareness, and recognition of individual differences and differences across cultures. This ongoing work manifests in the form of advocacy, education, and structural change. If people aren't actively enriching their understanding of unique cultural experiences and challenges, then they're not being culturally competent. Finally, healthcare providers and organizations engage in cultural adaptation where they're beginning to *recognize and embrace* the cultural nuances, differences, and perspectives of the patients they care for. It bears repeating that different doesn't mean better or worse. It's just different. Differences need to be understood so they can be respected, not feared.

Often when the expression "cultural competency" is used, it evokes thoughts of communication between people of different races or people who speak different languages. But being culturally competent means having not only racial and ethnic communication competency but also communication competency surrounding non-race-based cultural groups, such as gender identities, physical abilities, cognitive abilities, and regional communities. For instance, to examine cultural competency surrounding the LGBT community, Smita Banerjee and colleagues (2018) surveyed more than 1,200 providers working at a cancer center, including oncologists, cardiologists, geriatricians, physician assistants, nurse practitioners, and registered nurses. Most of the respondents identified as white, female, and Christian. In the survey, they were asked about their knowledge, beliefs, and behaviors surrounding the LGBT community. Although the results showed that providers had relatively low knowledge about LGBT healthcare needs, they also showed that more knowledge was associated with more positive beliefs and behaviors, such as open communication with transgender patients and perceived importance of LGBT sensitivity and communication skills training. Although based on cross-sectional data, these findings suggest that efforts to improve cultural competency may lead to more positive health outcomes for members of the LGBT community. These findings exemplify the gaps in cultural competency for non-race-based groups, as well as the potential for improved cultural competency to strengthen healthcare delivery. One way to improve cultural competency in healthcare is by offering communication guidelines and interventions to providers.

In the United States, the leading cultural competency guidelines come from OMH (2013) and are called the National **CLAS (culturally and linguistically appropriate services) standards**. Following the National Center for Cultural Competence (Goode & Dunne, 2003), the OMH (2013) identified the following six reasons that cultural competency is essential in U.S. healthcare services:

1. The continuously diversifying demographic make-up of the nation has resulted in more multicultural healthcare interactions.
2. Cultural competency has been shown to improve health disparities commonly associated with the social determinants of race, ethnicity, and culture.
3. Cultural competency improves the quality of services and primary care outcomes.
4. Cultural competency trainings meet mandates by legislative, regulatory, and accrediting agencies.
5. Cultural competency skills increase the "competitive edge" in the U.S. capitalist healthcare system.
6. When organizations and healthcare providers embrace cultural competency, the likelihood of liability/malpractice claims decreases.

CLAS provides 15 action steps to help healthcare providers and organizations enact culturally competent practices. Table 10.1 lists these steps, beginning with the overarching *principal standard*: provide effective, equitable, understandable, and respectful quality care and services that are responsive to diverse cultural health beliefs and practices, preferred languages, health literacy, and other communication needs. The remaining 14 steps are distributed across the three themes of (a) *Governance, Leadership, and Workforce*, (b) *Communication and Language Assistance*, and (c) *Engagement, Continuous Improvement, and Accountability*. Each theme encompasses multiple goals for enacting culturally competent healthcare.

These themes reflect the broad and comprehensive reach of the impact of culture across the entire healthcare experience. The central integration of culture into healthcare systems and practices improves patient healthcare experiences. Likewise, considering culture in

Table 10.1 U.S. Culturally and Linguistically Appropriate Services Standards (CLAS)

Principal Standard

1. Provide effective, equitable, understandable, and respectful quality care and services that are responsive to diverse cultural health beliefs and practices, preferred languages, health literacy, and other communication needs.

Governance, Leadership, and Workforce
2. Advance and sustain organizational governance and leadership that promotes CLAS and health equity through policy, practices, and allocated resources.
3. Recruit, promote, and support culturally and linguistically diverse governance, leadership, and workforce that are responsive to the population in the service area.
4. Educate and train governance, leadership, and workforce in culturally and linguistically appropriate policies and practices on an ongoing basis.

Communication and Language Assistance
5. Offer language assistance to individuals who have limited English proficiency and/or other communication needs, at no cost to them, to facilitate timely access to all healthcare and services.
6. Inform all individuals of the availability of language assistance services clearly and in their preferred language, verbally and in writing.
7. Ensure the competence of individuals providing language assistance, recognizing that the use of untrained individuals and/or minors as interpreters should be avoided.
8. Provide easy-to-understand print and multimedia materials and signage in the languages commonly used by the populations in the service area.

Engagement, Continuous Improvement, and Accountability
9. Establish culturally and linguistically appropriate goals, policies, and management accountability, and infuse them throughout the organization's planning and operations.
10. Conduct ongoing assessments of the organization's CLAS-related activities, and integrate CLAS-related measures into measurement and continuous quality improvement activities.
11. Collect and maintain accurate and reliable demographic data to monitor and evaluate the impact of CLAS on health equity and outcomes and to inform service delivery.
12. Conduct regular assessments of community health assets and needs and use the results to plan and implement services that respond to the cultural and linguistic diversity of populations in the service area.
13. Partner with the community to design, implement, and evaluate policies, practices, and services to ensure cultural and linguistic appropriateness.
14. Create conflict and grievance resolution processes that are culturally and linguistically appropriate to identify, prevent, and resolve conflicts or complaints.
15. Communicate the organization's progress in implementing and sustaining CLAS to all stakeholders, constituents, and the general public.

Note. From the U.S. Office of Minority Health (2013).

theoretical frameworks enhances researchers' abilities to understand communication strategies and practices that are the most effective and relevant for diverse communities.

Culture-Centered Theories for Studying Health Communication

Although culture is always relevant, it isn't always prioritized. In order to emphasize the importance of culture, communication theorists have developed and adapted numerous theoretical frameworks that center the role of culture in the healthcare experience. Table 10.2 presents some of these theories. Two of the more common theories, the PEN-3 model and the culture-centered approach (CCA), will be explored further in the following paragraphs.

Table 10.2 Theoretical Frameworks in Intercultural Health Communication

Theory/Model	Brief Summary	Citation
Cultural Sensitivity	Extent to which ethnic/cultural characteristics, experiences, norms, values, behavioral patterns, and beliefs of a target population, as well as relevant historical, environmental, and social forces, are incorporated in the design, delivery, and evaluation of targeted health promotion materials and programs. Programs are evaluated by considering surface and deep structures.	Resnicow et al. (1999)
Culture-centered Approach	The process of creating communicative spaces and sites in which marginalized communities can co-create their theoretical frameworks, have these frameworks be heard in ways that matter, and develop solutions based on the frameworks. Efforts are examined through constructs of structure, culture, and agency.	Dutta (2008)
Deficit Model of Cultural Differences	The process of culturalism occurs when healthcare providers attribute a patient's healthcare-related behaviors, such as adherence habits, communication preferences, and health practices, to less acceptable cultural customs and traditions instead of to influences from larger systemic forces.	Johnson et al. (2004)
PEN-3 Model	An intervention framework for understanding and evaluating culture through the three domains of (1) relationships and expectations, where behaviors are a function of perception (knowledge, beliefs, values), enablers (power from resources, institutional support, wealth), and nurturers (influences of family and friends); (2) cultural empowerment, where culture is considered positive (promoting good health), existential (having no impact on health), or negative (promoting poor health); and (3) cultural identity, as reflected by the person (multiple, complex identities), extended family (generational differences), and neighborhood (community capacity for health promotion).	Airhihenbuwa (1995)

Note. See *Supplemental Online Theory Table* for additional theories/models.

PEN-3 Model

The **PEN-3 model**, proposed by Collins Airhihenbuwa (1995), was developed following evidence that the health promotion ideas from "the West" were not working in non-Western countries. Specifically, Airhihenbuwa felt that the inclusion of culture in health promotion programs appropriated cultures by predominantly emphasizing cultural barriers without considering systemic barriers or positive cultural practices. Following these concerns, he developed the PEN-3 model to provide researchers and practitioners with a tool to understand and evaluate culture from multiple dimensions and to aid with the development of equitable health programs, such as behavior change interventions and educational programs.

The model centers three domains for understanding and evaluating culture. The first is *relationships and expectations*, where behaviors are a function of perception (knowledge, beliefs, values), enablers (power from resources, institutional support, wealth), and nurturers (influences of family and friends). The second is *cultural empowerment*, where culture is considered positive (promoting good health), existential (having no impact on health), or negative (promoting poor health). The third is *cultural identity*, which is reflected by the person (multiple, complex identities), extended family (generational differences), and neighborhood (community capacity for health promotion). Across the three domains of the model, the goal is for developers of health interventions and programs to recognize that behavior is often a product of culture by highlighting what behaviors are healthy and considering individual identity as the intersection of multiple cultures, or intersectionality.

The PEN-3 was originally studied in the context of developing HIV/AIDs prevention and awareness programs in Africa (Airhihenbuwa, 1995; Airhihenbuwa & Webster, 2004). More recent research has sought to broaden the application of the model. For instance, Kimberly Kline (2007) applied the PEN-3 model as a lens for examining the cultural appropriateness of breast cancer education materials targeting African women. Study results showed that although the materials clearly targeted African women, they fell short of the priorities laid out in the PEN-3 model. Such shortcomings included a focus on negative behaviors instead of unique cultural elements, prioritizing personal values over cultural values, and a lack of emphasis on barriers to performing preventative behaviors. In an extended application of the PEN-3 model, Victoria Orrego Dunleavy and colleagues (2018) sought to develop a gender and culturally specific empowerment-based HIV intervention targeting indigenous Mayan women in Guatemala. The authors analyzed interview and focus group data through the lens of the PEN-3 model. In other words, information provided by their participants was organized into the nine priorities of the model. That information was used to design a campaign unique to the gender, religion, and sexual orientation of their target audience. These example studies demonstrate how applying the PEN-3 model can center culture as a way to develop effective health promotion programs and interventions.

Culture-Centered Approach

The **culture-centered approach (CCA)** recognizes that the relationship between *neoliberal policies* (e.g., capitalism, deregulation, limited government involvement) and *globalization* (i.e., the increasing interconnectedness of the world) have influenced the creation and experience of health disparities (Dutta, 2008). Mohan Dutta (2018) explains that the "predominant emphasis of culture-centered processes is on creating communicative spaces and sites in which subaltern communities can co-create their theoretical frameworks, have these frameworks be heard in ways that matter, and develop solutions on the basis of this framework" (p. 240). In other words, the CCA was designed to prioritize the voices of members of marginalized communities, creating space for sharing their experiences with health inequities. More specifically, the framework looks at how the three constructs of structure, culture, and agency interact to create spaces where the voices of those who are traditionally not heard can now not only be considered in conversations but also become part of the dialogue.

Dutta (2008) provides further elaboration of these three constructs. First, *structure* refers to the elements in society that either constrict or facilitate a person's ability to engage in health behaviors, such as accessing medical services, transportation, food, and shelter. Structures such as limited healthcare access constrict, whereas structures such as public transportation facilitate. Second, *culture* can be understood as a reflection of shared practices, values, and meanings, rooted in the idea that communities are diverse sites of meaning making and conversation. Finally, *agency* refers to the capability that members of a culture have to challenge current structures while at the same time navigating these structures to find healthcare options. Communicatively, structure, culture, and agency are interdependent constructs that actively operate simultaneously while individuals navigate everyday life.

The CCA has been used to explore the health experiences of marginalized groups in regions around the world. These explorations include the health experiences of international domestic workers in Singapore (Dutta et al., 2018), Ethiopian immigrants in

Israel (Guttman et al., 2013), undocumented U.S. students (Ortiz Juarez-Pas, 2017), and Bangladeshi migrant workers in the Middle East (Kumar & Jamil, 2020). The CCA has also been used for applied communication efforts. For instance, Jennifer Horner and colleagues (2008) used the qualitative narratives from African American adolescents not only to highlight unheard voices but also to design broadcast messages for HIV prevention.

Findings from all these studies have revealed the unique ways in which culture, structure, and agency emerge from healthcare experiences of marginalized communities. For instance, Raihan Jamil and Mohan Dutta (2012) found that structural constraints such as limited access to economic opportunities that were experienced by those living at the margins of Bangladeshi society further reinforced the potential perpetuation of poverty. Anna Ortiz Juarez-Pas (2017) found that "the undocumented student movement has created a culture in which an immigration story is something powerful, a tool used to communicate resistance, perfectly normal and even necessary to share with friends and strangers" (p. 171). Finally, Rati Kumar and Raihan Jamil (2020) noted that agency was demonstrated through prioritizing spiritual and mental strength in the face of physical and structural exploitation experienced by Bangladeshi migrant workers. These explorations, among many others, highlight the health narratives of the marginalized groups and shed light on the often-overshadowed experiences that perpetuate health disparities, such as protective policies not being enacted as intended and a lack of compliance with regulations.

Health Communication and Culture in Practice

Culture is ingrained in some fashion into all our health communication exchanges, and there are countless strategies for exploring the influence of culture on the practice of health communication. The following sections will highlight two such approaches: exploring cultural sensitivity and studying the experiences of medical interpreters.

Cultural Sensitivity

Within the discipline of health communication, **cultural sensitivity** is an applied framework (see Table 10.2) for creating culturally appropriate health communication materials, programs, and interventions. Ken Resnicow and colleagues (1999) defined cultural sensitivity as the extent to which "ethnic/cultural characteristics, experiences, norms, values, behavioral patterns, and beliefs of a target population as well as relevant historical, environmental, and social forces are incorporated in the design, delivery, and evaluation of targeted health promotion materials and programs" (p. 11). They saw cultural competency as the capacity of an individual to enact cultural sensitivity in interpersonal communication contexts. But for mediated content, such as printed materials, educational programs, and interventions, cultural sensitivity was a muti-dimensional construct with two key dimensions: surface structure and deep structure.

First, *surface structure* is the matching of messaging, whether for printed material, verbal delivery, or digital content, to the observable characteristics of a particular culture. For instance, a public health program working to reduce obesity-related health disparities might create videos of healthy food recipes that feature dishes commonly consumed by the culture of the target community. Other surface-level messaging characteristics include featuring people of a particular culture, using music created by that culture, and highlighting geographic areas connected to the culture. Historically, surface structures are the culturally-targeted components of messages that health communication and health promotion scholars have done well. Problematically, these are often the only cultural components of messages that have been considered.

The second dimension of cultural sensitivity is *deep structure*. Generally, messaging efforts to encompass this dimension have not been as successful as efforts based on surface structure characteristics. This dimension requires a deeper understanding of the target culture, including social norms, history, environmental impacts, and unique psychological feelings that members of the culture experience. Messages that leverage deep structures will call out misperceptions, show respect for cultural values, and demonstrate a comprehensive understanding of the culture. This level of work requires a true and authentic investment into getting to know the culture that the researchers are working with to promote positive health outcomes. It also includes learning whether the targeted health outcome actually is valued by members of the culture. Research has shown that the extra effort to address deep structures typically pays off in the long run. In a meta-analysis of 36 studies of culturally-tailored cancer prevention messages, Yan Huang and Fuyuan Shen (2016) found that when deep tailoring occurred, such as integrating cultural values, norms, and religious beliefs of the target ethnic group, there were significantly stronger positive outcomes than for surface tailoring, which might only consider language, diet, and risk statistics. Consistent with Huang and Shen's study, other research has found considerations of cultural sensitivity to more effectively educate target audiences, as we describe next.

In an experimental test of oral health promotion pamphlets targeting Spanish-speaking Mexican heritage mothers, Theodore Singelis and colleagues (2018) developed messages intentionally varying the two dimensions of cultural sensitivity. Results showed that participants who received culturally sensitive pamphlets had higher knowledge about oral health after the intervention than those who did not receive culturally sensitive pamphlets. Researchers have also examined cultural sensitivity in video-, audio-, and digitally-based content. For example, Kline et al. (2016) sought to examine the cultural sensitivity of an interactive entertainment-education program for improving diabetes self-management among Hispanic audiences. The 123 recruited participants watched the intervention telenovela entitled *Sugar, Heart, and Life*. Through analysis of participant surveys and open-ended feedback, the researchers concluded that the intervention was successful at creating a user-friendly program that depicted realistic, culturally sensitive characters and storylines that resonated with Hispanic audiences. Most importantly, they found exposure to the program improved self-efficacy to engage in healthy lifestyle changes for improved diabetes self-management.

In sum, cultural sensitivity is an applied health communication framework used for connecting with audiences from different cultures. As you can tell from the last few paragraphs, the majority of this work has focused on African American or Hispanic/Spanish-speaking populations. Although these populations are important cultures for health communication research, there are many more cultures around the world receiving health promotion materials with unknown degrees of culturally sensitivity.

Medical Interpreters

According to the 2020 U.S. census, 21.5% of people speak a language other than English at home. This means that seeking medical assistance may be particularly challenging for a significant number of people with limited English proficiency (LEP) living in the United States. It's so much of a challenge that in 2000, former President Clinton signed executive order 13166, Improving Access to Services for Persons with Limited English Proficiency, requiring that "Federal agencies work to ensure that recipients of Federal financial assistance provide meaningful access to their LEP applicants and beneficiaries" (U.S. Department of Justice, 2000, p. 50121). For many health systems, this order has taken the form of hiring medical interpreters. In the following paragraphs, we'll review different types of medical interpreters, including what roles they can serve for improving patient care. In addition, we'll explore how technology has enhanced access to medical interpreters.

What Are Medical Interpreters?

Medical interpreters traditionally have been viewed as conduits of information, serving as strictly "word-for-word" **translators** between healthcare providers and patients (Dysart-Gale, 2007; Hsieh, 2006). The metaphor of the **conduit** reflects an overly simplistic model of communication: The healthcare provider sends a message, the interpreter translates the message to the patient, the patient replies, and the interpreter translates a patient's reply back to the healthcare provider. However, given the complexities of communication (e.g., indirect questions, tone, humor), the conduit model has been found to inadequately reflect the experiences of medical interpreters (Dysart-Gale, 2005). And as communication scholars, we know that in practice, communicative interactions can never be that simple. To that end, Maria-Paz Beltran Avery (2001) identified three additional roles medical interpreters serve.

First, medical interpreters can serve as **clarifiers** in that they may have to stray from the direct translation and add information to convey the correct meaning. Words and phrases don't always directly translate to the same meaning. Thus, medical interpreters might make adjustments to ensure that the receiver comprehends the message, often prefacing their words with "the interpreter would like to state..." (Juckett et al., 2014, p. 478). Second, medical interpreters can act as **culture brokers** in that they may draw on their unique knowledge of the patient's culture to situate the healthcare provider's message within the patient's cultural context. For example, in an analysis of 12 recorded medical encounters in Germany that involved a medical interpreter for patients of Turkish or Albanian origin, Michaela Albl-Mikasa and colleagues (2015) found that culturally specific communication hedges and phatic tokens (i.e., small talk) were essential for trust building and positive interactions between the provider and the patient. However, these moments were rarely translated by the interpreter, missing an opportunity to participate as a culture broker to the detriment of the patient's care.

Finally, medical interpreters can also serve as **patient advocates** by considering the quality of the patient's experience, including care and communication. Accordingly, the interpreter may do more than translate between the healthcare provider and patient. For example, in an autobiographic analysis of her experience serving as a chance interpreter (defined shortly) for her father, a Canadian immigrant who had recently moved to Israel, Dr. Rhona Seidelman reflects on a moment where she decided it was in her father's best interest for her *not* to translate something the doctor said (Seidelman & Bachner, 2010, p. 390):

> I don't recall exactly what it was that Dr. Abu said, but my immediate response to him was, "Okay, that I won't translate." He had said something about there being too many questions, or something about him needing to go...knowing my parents, I knew that response of his would have broken through the appearance of calm they were barely maintaining, and as their daughter, censorship of the doctor seemed to be my only option.

Such advocacy behavior is meant to facilitate better care for the patient.

To add to the four previous roles, Elaine Hsieh (2007) proposed a fifth role for medical interpreters: **co-diagnostician**. In this role, medical interpreters may seek to improve the healthcare interaction through strategies of asking the patient questions without prompting from the provider, asking follow-up questions, editing patient responses, and even examining the patient. In this role, they may also give the patient medical advice without direction from a medical provider. The interpreter roles added by Beltran Avery and Hsieh extend the responsibilities and duties of a medical interpreter beyond providing translations as a mere conduit.

In addition to roles that interpreters might play, there are also different categories, or types, of medical interpreters. Hsieh (2006) proposed five types: chance interpreters, untrained interpreters, bilingual healthcare provider, on-site interpreters, and telephone interpreters. Although each type of interpreter can serve all five roles, they vary in their experience, training, and location. The first two, chance and untrained interpreters, are the least preferred type of medical interpreter. **Chance interpreters** are individuals who happen to be nearby during a medical exchange, such as Dr. Seidelman when she served as a medical interpreter for her father. These interpreters have not undergone medical interpreter training and are generally called on because either they know the patient well (e.g., friend, family) or are nearby at the time (e.g., bilingual speaker in the room). Although family or friends may be very helpful because the patient may feel comfortable with them in the room, a chance interpreter may negatively influence the patient's care due to not knowing medical terminology, providing inaccurate interpretations, or behaving inappropriately for the role (e.g., answer for the patient, not maintain confidentiality). Healthcare providers can also be hesitant to use chance interpreters. In a qualitative analysis of 69 Australian providers, Rachyl Pines and colleagues (2020) found most of them to only prefer chance-type medical interpreters when the information that needed to be translated was not medically serious or confidential. They did, however, make an exception in emergency situations.

An **untrained interpreter** refers to bilingual support staff in the healthcare organization, such as an HR staff person or technician, who has not been trained as an official medical interpreter. Unlike a chance interpreter who is most likely a family member or friend, an untrained interpreter can maintain a professional distance from the patient (i.e., they can maintain more emotional distance). Although these types of interpreters are convenient and may know healthcare settings and medical terminology, they may not be able to spend much time with a patient. For example, a technician serving as an untrained interpreter may be able to sit in during the diagnosis but not have time to accompany the patient to the receptionist or pharmacist following the discussion with the physician. Similar to chance interpreters, untrained interpreters may also interpret information incorrectly or behave inappropriately for the role because they haven't received training. Given the limitations of chance and untrained interpreters, bilingual healthcare providers, on-site medical interpreters, and telephone interpreters are typically the more preferred types.

A **bilingual healthcare provider** is a clinician who speaks more than one language and is therefore able to serve as both the provider and the medical interpreter. Bilingual healthcare providers are able to communicate directly with the patient, which can build rapport and increase the comfort of patients to ask questions and engage in the conversation. Although this type of interpreter may seem like an efficient option, they're not without their challenges. First, bilingual healthcare providers can be bilingual without being bicultural. This means they may have studied the language but might not know cultural beliefs or values or have other background information that could influence language choices or behaviors. This, in turn, limits their ability to serve as a culture broker. Second, bilingual healthcare providers may overestimate their language skills, perceiving themselves as more competent at interpreting and communicating medical information than they actually are. Although trainings could help overcome these challenges, bilingual healthcare providers are a relatively rare form of medical interpreter.

The most preferred type of medical interpreter is an **on-site medical interpreter**. This type of interpreter is a professionally employed, bilingual individual who has received specific training as a medical interpreter. In addition to the benefit of being specially trained, on-site interpreters bring with them cultural and medical experiences pertinent to the healthcare environment. This background makes them more likely to be actively engaged during a medical encounter. Because these interpreters are on-site, they can be in the room with patients, increasing patient comfort and more clearly observing nonverbal interactions that could be important to the translation. But of course, on-site medical interpreters have their limitations. For one, they're expensive. This extra cost is compounded by the fact that hiring multiple on-site medical interpreters may be necessary to cover a variety of different languages that patients may speak. One way to overcome these challenges is to use the last type of medical interpreter, a telephone interpreter.

Like on-site interpreters, **telephone interpreters** are professionally trained medical interpreters. This means they, too, have the medical and cultural background needed for medical encounters. Telephone interpreters can be especially helpful for rare or less commonly spoken languages. Thus, they're often a more accessible and affordable option for healthcare organizations. However, because the interpreters are part of a telephone service, they work offsite. This means they're unable to consider nonverbal cues during the medical interaction. Similarly, patients are unlikely to build the same rapport with a telephone interpreter as they would with an on-site interpreter. Modern technologies have helped reduce some of these concerns, allowing interpreters to virtually join cases via video. To that end, it might be more accurate to call them *virtual* or *distance* interpreters. Although video allows interpreters to observe nonverbal behavior, the information is still limited by distance, and building rapport is still challenging. Regardless of the role or type of medical interpreter, research shows that medical interpreters play a central part in an LEP patient's healthcare experience.

Roles and Types of Medical Interpreters

Medical interpreters serve one of five roles:

Translator (Conduit): Provides word-for-word translation
Clarifier: Adds information to convey the correct meaning
Culture broker: Draws on knowledge culture to contextualize a message
Patient advocate: Considers the quality of the care and communication experience
Co-diagnostician: Expands healthcare interaction through involvement

There are five types of medical interpreters:

Chance: Individuals who happen to be nearby during a medical exchange, often family members or friends
Untrained interpreter: Bilingual support staff who are not official medical interpreters
Bilingual healthcare provider: Clinicians who speak more than one language
On-site medical interpreter: Professionally employed medical interpreters
Telephone interpreters: Trained medical interpreters available through a telephone service

---

How Has Technology Affected Medical Interpretation Practices?

Technological advancements have continued to equip patients and providers with translation tools that improve patient care. There are two types of technologies that have particularly advanced the medical interpretation research over the last decade: translation apps and video conferencing. First, translation apps, such as iTranslate©, Google Translate©, and Microsoft Translator©, provide immediate translation services on mobile and internet-based platforms. Reliance on such services is typically met with caution, however, because of the limited vocabulary and varying accuracy of the algorithm-based translations. For instance, Xuewei Chen and colleagues (2016) compared the accuracy of the Google Translate© app to educational materials about diabetes that had been professionally translated into Spanish and Chinese. Although they found that the Spanish translations were comparable to that of a professional translator, the Chinese translation done by the app was substantially less accurate than the professional interpreter's translation. Despite these limitations, many people still advocate for the benefit of translation apps in healthcare interactions given accessibility, cost-effectiveness, and immediacy of translation (e.g., Birkenbeuel et al., 2021).

Second, although video conferencing already had been a growing trend in healthcare services, the COVID-19 pandemic pushed the adoption of the technology into high gear. Video conferencing services such as Zoom©, Skype©, Slack©, and BlueJeans© can make telephone-based translation services more engaging for patients, as well as for the medical interpreter and clinician. In a study of Spanish-speaking LEP parents using medical interpretation services during their child's pediatric emergency room visit, Casey Lion and colleagues (2015) found the perceived quality of care was equal for parents in both the telephone- and video-based medical interpreter conditions. However, parents in the video-based condition were more likely to name the child's diagnosis correctly and less likely to report that providers attempted to communicate with them outside of using the interpreter services. Interestingly, in further analysis of this data, Lion et al. (2021) analyzed factors surrounding provider use of medical interpreter services. They found that all providers were able to initiate video-based medical interpreting services more quickly than telephone-based services. In addition, providers were more likely to initiate video-based medical interpreting services than telephone-based services, although this effect was not found among nurses. These results are similar to findings from Craig Locatis and colleagues (2010), who found that although their sample of Hispanic patients equally favored in-person, phone, and video interpreting, providers and interpreters preferred video conferencing over in-person or telephone interpreting.

Research on technological advancements in medical interpretation consistently shows positive ways that technology can improve patient outcomes for LEP patients. However, what's also clear is that these advancements don't eliminate the need for trained professional medical translators to be available during medical encounters. Additional research in this area is needed to enhance equitable care opportunities for LEP patients.

Limitations of the Lens of Western Medicine

Western medicine refers to a system of healthcare in which "medical doctors and other healthcare professionals (such as nurses, pharmacists, and therapists) treat symptoms and diseases using drugs, radiation, or surgery. [It is] also called allopathic medicine, biomedicine, conventional medicine, mainstream medicine, and orthodox medicine" (National Cancer Institute [NCI], n.d.). For many people in westernized nations, this form of medicine is so standard and seems so normal that they assume it's the primary form of medicine everywhere. This perspective is called **Eurocentrism**, or "an attitude, conceptual apparatus, or set of empirical beliefs that frame Europe as the primary engine and architect of world history, the bearer of universal values and reason, and the pinnacle and therefore model of progress and development" (Sundberg, 2009, p. 638). But there are many other ways in which medicine is practiced around the world, such as homeopathic, ayurvedic, complementary/alternative, naturopathy, siddha, and unani. These practices vary in the extent to which their conclusions are supported by clinical research evidence, but most have longstanding traditions that are important to acknowledge.

Similar to a western bias in the practice of medicine, social science researchers studying human behaviors have predominantly recruited participants from overwhelmingly western, educated, industrialized, rich, and democratic, or **WEIRD**, countries (Henrich et al., 2010). This practice has resulted in published research studies whose limitations sections include brief statements acknowledging that cultural variations in study findings may be possible but were "beyond the scope" of the particular study. Elaine Hsieh and Eric Kramer (2021) refer to this treatment of culture as a *caveat*. They argue that this approach to studying culture ignores how the contextual nature of culture serves as both a resource and a product of individuals' health behaviors, shapes communities' responses in offering support for some members while silencing suffering for others, and supports institutional structures and policies that reinforce disparities. Recognizing these limitations in studying culture is important because "in culturally diverse societies, the dominant culture, which is expressed through social institutions, including the health care system, regulates what sorts of problems are recognized and what kinds of social or cultural differences are viewed as worthy of attention" (Kirmayer, 2012, p. 149).

WEIRD Research

Research is WEIRD when research participants are predominantly western, educated, and from industrialized, rich, and democratic countries.

By assuming all individuals practice western medicine or behave like WEIRD participants, people unintentionally "other" marginalized and underserved ethnic groups. According to Joy Johnson and colleagues (2004), **othering** occurs when the culture of a dominant group, including its characteristics, beliefs, and practices, is considered the general norm and any deviations from that norm are considered "less than." In their analysis of interactions between healthcare providers and South Asian immigrant women, Johnson et al. found three distinct forms of othering that can occur during conversations. First, *essentializing explanations* are broad overgeneralizations, or stereotypes, pulling from cultural characteristics such as race, geography, social background, and healthcare practices. For example, a healthcare provider assuming someone is overweight because of the standard diet within their culture would be employing an essentializing explanation. Second, *culturalist explanations* are those that overlook the effects of systemic barriers on health and, instead, attribute health outcomes to cultural characteristics. For example, a provider assuming a patient is always late because time management is different in their culture is overlooking the chance that the patient might have social determinant-based barriers for getting to their appointment, such as relying on public transportation or having inflexible work hours. Finally, *racializing explanations* are references to racial differences that don't directly verbalize a race-related term. For instance, Johnson et al. reported that a nurse referred to "normal" waiting room behaviors as those done by white women, such as knitting or reading, and that waiting room behavior by South Asian women, such as lying down or sleeping, was less acceptable.

These examples reflect the limitations of standardizing the beliefs and practices of a dominant culture, most often a white European culture, as the unquestioned norm. This can create a **deficit model of cultural differences** (Johnson et al., 2004). According to this model (see Table 10.2), a process called **culturalism** can occur when providers attribute a patient's health-related behaviors, such as adherence habits, communication preferences, and health practices, to less acceptable cultural customs and traditions instead of to influences from larger systemic forces. Although most research has focused on othering and culturalism as they relate to race, these experiences can be enacted toward any marginalized or underserved group. For example, in a discourse analysis of health policy documents in New Zealand, Jo Ann Walton and Mariana Lazzaro-Salazar (2016) found that, as written, the policies other the chronically ill. In particular, they found that the documents blamed the chronically ill for being a burden to themselves, their families, and society, as well as overly emphasizing economic concerns surrounding the chronically ill population. Walton and Lazzaro-Salazar argue that othering is most likely when people treat all cultures and groups, especially minority groups, as a monolith. Large generalizations mask the nuances that make people unique. And it's a recognition of those unique characteristics that will allow people to support each other in living their healthiest lives.

Before we end this chapter, we want to leave you with one example of an organization working to break barriers to healthcare on a global scale: Doctors Without Borders. **Doctors Without Borders** was founded in France in 1971 as Médecins Sans Frontières (MSF). Now, more than 50 years later, MSF has become a global movement with "more than 63,000 staff providing over 10 million medical consultations in more than 70 countries every year" (Doctors Without Borders, "Our History," para. 3). The organization's mission is to bring "medical humanitarian assistance to victims of conflict, natural disasters, epidemics and health care exclusion" (Doctors Without Borders, "Our Work," n.p.). In 1999, MSF won the Nobel Peace Prize for their medical humanitarianism (Redfield, 2013). As a nonprofit organization dependent on volunteers and donations, MSF oversees numerous healthcare teams working around the globe to respond to the world's most pressing needs. In an ethnographic reflection on MSF, Peter Redfield (2013) writes that "MSF knows it can't save the world. Nonetheless, it operates within a wider field of expectations, inspiring hope" (p. 6). In our estimation, MSF symbolizes the best of what globalized healthcare can be, with multiple health disciplines coming together to care for patients in need around the world. Bravo, MSF!

Conclusion

Although we hope culture has been in the forefront of your mind throughout all of our chapters, the intention of this chapter was to put a spotlight on intercultural health communication research. In doing so, we reviewed the definition of culture and what it means to be a culturally competent communicator. We presented the frameworks of the PEN-3 model and the CCA to demonstrate ways in which researchers can center culture in health communication research. In addition, we explored the applied areas of cultural sensitivity and medical interpreters to understand the challenges surrounding intercultural communication in practice. Finally, we acknowledged that Westernized medicine has its limitations in meeting the healthcare needs of all people. Although intercultural communication practices face less resistance than they did in past decades, there's still much more work to do be done on this front.

In a 1989 report for the National Institute of Mental Health's Child and Adolescent Service System Program, Terry Cross and colleagues proclaimed that for a healthcare system to be culturally competent, the organizations, institutions, agencies, and professionals within it must value diversity, have the capacity for cultural self-assessment, be conscious of the dynamics inherent when cultures interact, have institutionalized cultural knowledge, and have developed adaptations to diversity (Cross et al., 1989). Despite the many years that have passed since this report, systems around the world still struggle to meet the daily goal of providing culturally competent healthcare to all who need it. Some advocates have called for required community-engaged clinical experiences as a way to prepare graduate students in health disciplines to engage with culturally diverse populations (Taliancich-Klinger et al., 2022). What we know for sure is that more research and training are needed to enhance healthcare providers' ability to engage in culturally competent health communication. When that can happen, patients, families, and providers from diverse cultural perspectives can come together to achieve mutual understanding and make the most effective, appropriate, and informed decisions, and no one may ever again have to endure the tragic experience of Lia Lee.

References

Ahmed, R., & Bates, B. R. (2012). Development of scales to assess patients' perceptions of physicians' cultural competence in health care interactions. *Journal of Transcultural Nursing, 23*(3), 287–296.

Airhihenbuwa, C. O. (1995). *Health and culture: Beyond the western paradigm.* Sage.

Airhihenbuwa, C. O., & Webster, J. D. (2004). Culture and African contexts of HIV/AIDS prevention, care and support. *Sahara-J: Journal of Social Aspects of HIV/AIDS, 1*(1), 4–13.

Albl-Mikasa, M., Glatz, E., Hofer, G., & Sleptsova, M. (2015). Caution and compliance in medical encounters: Non-interpretation of hedges and phatic tokens. *Translation & Interpreting, 7*(3), 76–89.

Banerjee, S. C., Walters, C. B., Staley, J. M., Alexander, K., & Parker, P. A. (2018). Knowledge, beliefs, and communication behavior of oncology health-care providers (HCPs) regarding lesbian, gay, bisexual, and transgender (LGBT) patient health care. *Journal of Health Communication, 23*(4), 329–339.

Beltran Avery, M. (2001). The role of the health care interpreter: An evolving dialogue *Department of Health and Human Services Office of Minority Health.* http://www.tararogersinterpreter.com/uploads/1/0/3/7/103709790/the_role_of_the_healthcare_interpreter_avery_011_1_.pdf

Birkenbeuel, J., Joyce, H., Sahyouni, R., Cheung, D., Maducdoc, M., Mostaghni, N., Sahyouni, S., Djalilian, H., Chen, J., & Lin, H. (2021). Google Translate in healthcare: Preliminary evaluation of transcription, translation and speech synthesis accuracy. *BMJ Innovations, 7*(2), 422–429.

Centers for Disease Control & Prevention. (2014). *Practical strategies for culturally competent evaluation.* https://www.cdc.gov/dhdsp/docs/Cultural_Competence_Guide.pdf

Chen, X., Acosta, S., & Barry, A. E. (2016). Evaluating the accuracy of Google translate for diabetes education material. *JMIR Diabetes, 1*(1), e5848.

Cross, T., Bazron, B., Dennis, K., & Isaacs, M. (1989). *Towards a culturally competent system of care.* Washington, DC: National Technical Assistance Center for Children's Mental Health, Georgetown University Child Development Center. https://files.eric.ed.gov/fulltext/ED330171.pdf

Dutta, M. J. (2008). *Communicating health: A culture-centered approach.* Polity Press.

Dutta, M. J. (2018). Culture-centered approach in addressing health disparities: Communication infrastructures for subaltern voices. *Communication Methods and Measures, 12*(4), 239–259.

Dutta, M. J., Comer, S., Teo, D., Luk, P., Lee, M., Zapata, D., & Kaur, S. (2018). Health meanings among foreign domestic workers in Singapore: A culture-centered approach. *Health Communication, 33*(5), 643–652.

Dysart-Gale, D. (2005). Communication models, professionalization, and the work of medical interpreters. *Health Communication, 17*(1), 91–103.

Dysart-Gale, D. (2007). Clinicians and medical interpreters: Negotiating culturally appropriate care for patients with limited English ability. *Family & Community Health, 30*(3), 237–246.

Fadiman, A. (1997). *The spirit catches you and you fall down.* Farrar, Straus and Giroux.

Galanti, G.-A. (2000). An introduction to cultural differences. *Western Journal of Medicine, 172*(5), 335.

Galanti, G.-A. (2003). The Hispanic family and male-female relationships: An overview. *Journal of Transcultural Nursing, 14*(3), 180–185.

Goode, T. D., & Dunne, C. (2003). *Policy brief 1: Rationale for cultural competence in primary care.* Washington, DC: National Center for Cultural Competence, Georgetown University Center for Child and Human Development. https://nccc.georgetown.edu/documents/Policy_Brief_1_2003.pdf

Guttman, N., Gesser-Edelsburg, A., & Aycheh, S. (2013). Communicating health rights to disadvantaged populations: Challenges in developing a culture-centered approach for Ethiopian immigrants in Israel. *Health Communication, 28*(6), 546–556.

Henrich, J., Heine, S. J., & Norenzayan, A. (2010). Most people are not WEIRD. *Nature, 466*(7302), 29.

Horner, J., Romer, D., Vanable, P., Salazar, L., Carey, M., Juzang, I., & Valois, R. (2008). Using culture-centered qualitative formative research to design broadcast messages for HIV prevention for African American adolescents. *Journal of Health Communication, 13*(4), 309–325.

Hsieh, E. (2006). Understanding medical interpreters: Reconceptualizing bilingual health communication. *Health Communication, 20*(2), 177–186.

Hsieh, E. (2007). Interpreters as co-diagnosticians: Overlapping roles and services between providers and interpreters. *Social Science & Medicine, 64*(4), 924–937.

Hsieh, E., & Kramer, E. M. (2021). *Rethinking culture in health communication: Social interactions as intercultural encounters*. Wiley Blackwell.

Huang, Y., & Shen, F. (2016). Effects of cultural tailoring on persuasion in cancer communication: A meta-analysis. *Journal of Communication, 66*(4), 694–715.

Jamil, R., & Dutta, M. (2012). A culture-centered exploration of health: Constructions from rural Bangladesh. *Health Communication, 27*(4), 369–379.

Johnson, J. L., Bootorff, J. L., Browne, A. J., Grewal, S., Hilton, B. A., & Clarke, H. (2004). Othering and being othered in the context of health care services. *Health Communication, 16*(2), 253–271.

Juckett, G., & Unger, K. (2014). Appropriate use of medical interpreters. *American Family Physician, 90*(7), 476–480.

Kirmayer, L. J. (2012). Rethinking cultural competence. *Transcultural Psychiatry, 49*(2), 149–164.

Kline, K. N. (2007). Cultural sensitivity and health promotion: Assessing breast cancer education pamphlets designed for African American women. *Health Communication, 21*(1), 85–96.

Kline, K. N., Montealegre, J. R., Rustveld, L. O., Glover, T. L., Chauca, G., Reed, B. C., & Jibaja-Weiss, M. L. (2016). Incorporating cultural sensitivity into interactive entertainment-education for diabetes self-management designed for Hispanic audiences. *Journal of Health Communication, 21*(6), 658–668.

Kumar, R., & Jamil, R. (2020). Labor, health, and marginalization: A culture-centered analysis of the challenges of male Bangladeshi migrant workers in the Middle East. *Qualitative Health Research, 30*(11), 1723–1736.

Lion, K. C., Brown, J. C., Ebel, B. E., Klein, E. J., Strelitz, B., Gutman, C. K., Hencz, P., Fernandez, J., & Mangione-Smith, R. (2015). Effect of telephone vs video interpretation on parent comprehension, communication, and utilization in the pediatric emergency department: A randomized clinical trial. *JAMA Pediatrics, 169*(12), 1117–1125.

Lion, K. C., Gritton, J., Scannell, J., Brown, J. C., Ebel, B. E., Klein, E. J., & Mangione-Smith, R. (2021). Patterns and predictors of professional interpreter use in the pediatric emergency department. *Pediatrics, 147*(2), e20193312.

Locatis, C., Williamson, D., Gould-Kabler, C., Zone-Smith, L., Detzler, I., Roberson, J., Maisiak, R., & Ackerman, M. (2010). Comparing in-person, video, and telephonic medical interpretation. *Journal of General Internal Medicine, 25*(4), 345–350.

National Cancer Institute. (n.d.). *Dictionary of cancer terms: Western medicine.* https://www.cancer.gov/publications/dictionaries/cancer-terms/

Office of Minority Health. (2013). *National standards for culturally and linguistically appropriate services in health and health care: A blueprint for advancing and sustaining CLAS policy and practice.* https://thinkcultural-health.hhs.gov/assets/pdfs/EnhancedCLASStandardsBlueprint.pdf

Orrego Dunleavy, V., Chudnovskaya, E., Phillips, J., & McFarlane, S. J. (2018). Applying the PEN-3 cultural model to address HIV/AIDS prevention in rural Guatemala. *Journal of Intercultural Communication Research, 47*(1), 1–20.

Ortiz Juarez-Paz, A. V. (2017). Undocumented identity storytelling: (Re)framing public relations. *International Journal of Media & Cultural Politics, 13*(1/2), 165–178.

Pines, R. L., Jones, L., & Sheeran, N. (2020). Using family members as medical interpreters: An explanation of healthcare practitioners' normative practices in pediatric and neonatal departments in Australia. *Health Communication, 35*(7), 902–909.

Redfield, P. (2013). *Life in crisis: The ethical journey of doctors without borders.* University of California Press.

Resnicow, K., Baranowski, T., Ahluwalia, J., & Braithwaite, R. (1999). Cultural sensitivity in public health: Defined and demystified. *Ethnicity & Disease, 9*, 10–21.

Schiavo, R. (2014). *Health communication: From theory to practice* (2nd ed.). Jossey-Bass, Wiley.

Seidelman, R. D., & Bachner, Y. G. (2010). That I won't translate! Experiences of a family medical interpreter in a multicultural environment. *Mount Sinai Journal of Medicine: A Journal of Translational and Personalized Medicine, 77*(4), 389–393.

Singelis, T. M., Garcia, R. I., Barker, J. C., & Davis, R. E. (2018). An experimental test of the two-dimensional theory of cultural sensitivity in health communication. *Journal of Health Communication, 23*(4), 321–328.

Sundberg, J. (2009). Eurocentrism. In R. Kitchin & N. Thrift (Eds.), *International encyclopedia of human geography* (Vol. 3, pp. 638–643). Elsevier.

Taliancich-Klinger, C., Hernandez, N. A., & Maurer, A. (2022). Engaging graduate students in cultural experiences early: The development, implementation, and preliminary student perceptions of a community engagement clinical experience. *American Journal of Speech-Language Pathology, 31*(2), 539–551.

U.S. Department of Justice. (2000). *The President: Executive Order 13166—Improving access to services for persons with limited English proficiency.* https://www.govinfo.gov/content/pkg/FR-2000-08-16/pdf/00-20938.pdf

Walton, J. A., & Lazzaro-Salazar, M. (2016). Othering the chronically ill: A discourse analysis of New Zealand health policy documents. *Health Communication, 31*(4), 460–467.

In-class Activities

1. How do you cure hiccups? What happens if you go to sleep with your hair wet? To help students internalize the cultural nature of the illness experience, investigate a common "illness" (like hiccups) with no clear treatment or an everyday "health warning" (like avoiding sleeping with wet hair). Have students interview each other in class about the causes, treatments, consequences, and sources of information for the illness/warning. Compile all the answers to see how culturally similar or different people are.

2. Non-native speakers seeking medical attention may find the experience particularly daunting. They may be limited to nonverbal communication to describe their symptoms, receive their diagnosis, and understand next care steps. Have students pair up, designating one person as the doctor and one person as the patient.

    Patient: Pretend that you are starting to feel ill (you can pick your illness, but don't say it out loud). Explain your symptoms to the "doctor" without using English.

    Doctor: Diagnose the "patient" and present them with instructions for getting better without using English.

    After five minutes, facilitate a conversation about the experience.

Discussion Questions

1. Table 10.1 lists the 15 action steps of the U.S. *Culturally and Linguistically Appropriate Services Standards (CLAS)*. These steps are intended to enhance culturally competent healthcare practices. Where and how does communication fit in promoting these steps?

2. As a patient, what would be your biggest concerns about including a medical interpreter in your appointment? How might your concerns differ due to the type of medical interpreter included in your appointment? What might the medical interpreter say or do to help you feel more comfortable?

3. What are healthcare examples of the deficit model of communication? How are these problematic, and how can communication be used to correct these misperceptions?

The Gray Area

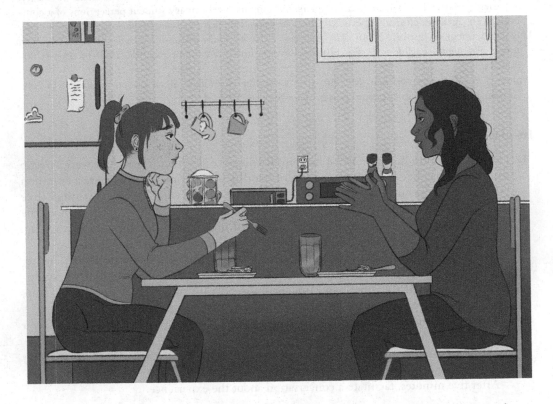

It was the luck of the Match that brought Cheryl and Liz back together for their residency. They found an apartment to share near their hospital. Their days were hectic, but they usually managed to cook dinner together, just like they had in undergrad. Cheryl called it a form of self-care. Sadly, both of them had almost entirely lost touch with Nathian.

Over lasagna one night, Liz shared a concern she was grappling with. That morning, she'd gotten test results for one of her patients, a 78-year-old woman with a large family that had been filling the waiting room day and night. The woman had started having trouble walking, was forgetting things, and was beginning to lose her vision. She'd been in excellent health up until the symptoms started. Liz had run several tests and all signs were pointing to Creutzfeldt-Jakob disease.

"Geez, Liz, that's such an awful disease," Cheryl said. CJD was a terminal neurological disease that led to rapid deterioration and death typically within a year.

"The thing is, she's from a Greek family, and all of them are adamant that I don't tell her. From the start, when she first was admitted, her husband and oldest daughter told me that

DOI: 10.4324/9781003214458-25

I should tell them first, whatever it was, and they would handle it. So, I told them. But I don't know if I should have because now they say they don't want her to know!" Liz shook her head. "But she deserves to know, right? What do I do?"

"What does Hogue say?" Cheryl asked, referring to Liz's attending.

Liz scoffed. "He said, 'She's your patient. Figure it out.'"

Cheryl thought back to one of her health communication classes that covered the ethical principles guiding physician–patient communication. "You really are supposed to tell your patients the truth. But sometimes it's not that simple, especially when strong family cultures are involved. In that case, telling her might do more harm than good."

"That's what her husband said. But how can I not tell her? She trusts me."

"This sounds like a case for our hospital ethics committee," Cheryl advised.

"That's a great idea! Why didn't I think of that?" Liz asked, more to herself than Cheryl.

"You just keep feeding me, and I'll keep solving all of your problems," Cheryl said through a mouth full of lasagna.

Although it wasn't uncommon in Cheryl's life for questions of ethics to be a point of discussion, it usually didn't happen multiple times in one month. But Cheryl was clearly just having one of those months, because a few weeks after her discussion with Liz, she found herself in another sticky situation when she made a visit home to join a family cookout. She was excited to catch up with everyone and tell them about her work. She was sitting with her Uncle Michael while her father grilled hamburgers, telling them both about a new program through her hospital where community members can volunteer to participate in clinical research. Aunt Savannah was within earshot and came over to listen.

"These researchers from the university did this study that showed when you include community members in planning, you can create really effective programs for enrolling people in clinical trials, especially people of color," Cheryl said.

"Who historically have *not* been well represented," Michael added.

"Exactly!" Cheryl agreed. "There's this new Phase I trial that's testing an HIV vaccine. So far, we..."

The "tsk" from Savannah was loud enough to stop Cheryl mid-sentence. She locked eyes with her uncle, both of them bracing for what Savannah would say next.

"If you ask me," Savannah said, "the people who stay out of this kind of research are the smart ones. There's just too many risks, and you never know what's really in those vaccines anyway." To Cheryl's dismay, Savannah made air quotes with her fingers when she said "vaccines."

"Aunt Savannah, clinical research is really important. Look at how many lives have been saved because of the COVID vaccine," Cheryl tried to explain as calmly as possible.

"COVID?" Savannah scoffed. "No way anyone's getting me to get that. It's all a hoax anyway."

"Savannah, don't get started on this again," Michael said. "I can't believe we are still going in circles on this issue. You need to quit listening to those—"

Joe cleared his voice loudly, turning from the grill. "Savannah, it looks like Sally might need help in the kitchen." He nodded toward the house.

Savannah turned to see. "She never can manage, can she?"

Alone with her dad and uncle again, Cheryl just shook her head. "She's *still* not vaccinated, is she," Cheryl asked.

"Nope," Joe replied.

"And I tried," Michael added. "'No waiting at my pharmacy,' I told her. 'The vaccine is free.' But she wouldn't budge."

"It's not like it's gonna matter," Sam said from their seat at the picnic table, where they'd been listening to the conversation.

"What do you mean?" Cheryl asked as she walked over and sat next to them.

"We're destroying our planet," Sam stated. "Didn't you hear Greta's speech last week?" Greta Thunberg was still Sam's hero.

"I did not," Cheryl said. "I'm a busy resident, remember? But you're too young to be this cynical. I thought *you* were gonna save the planet!"

"I can't even get you all to go vegan. And every time I get on Aunt Savannah for not recycling, she mocks me. How can *I* save the planet?"

"One step at a time, kiddo," Joe said. "One step at a time." Sam and Cheryl both looked at Joe, who was happily grilling away. "There are some veggie burgers on this grill, you know!" he informed them.

"It'll be you who saves us all, I know it," Cheryl said, smiling at Sam.

Sam smiled back at Cheryl while Joe put a plate of delicious-smelling burgers on the table. And like bees to honey, everyone found a seat at the table and started filling their plates. Cheryl knew that the next few weeks of residency were going to be especially hectic as a number of folks had put in for vacation. She decided it was best to eat two burgers—one regular and one veggie.

Notes

The Match refers to the residential match process, explained here: https://www.nrmp.org/

You can learn more about Creutzfeldt-Jakob Disease here: https://www.ninds.nih.gov/creutzfeldt-jakob-disease-fact-sheet

11 Ethical Issues in Health Communication

Henrietta Lacks was born on August 1, 1920, in Roanoke, Virginia. In January of 1951, she went to Johns Hopkins hospital, one of the few places that would treat poor Black patients, with symptoms of severe abdominal pain and vaginal bleeding. She was diagnosed with cervical cancer. Treatment was unsuccessful, and she died on October 4, 1951—but not before doctors removed two samples of cervical tissue and shared them with a research lab without her consent (Johns Hopkins Medicine, 2023).

To the surprise of the doctors, there was something very special about Mrs. Lacks' cells. Whereas cell samples from other patients would die in a few days, hers were powerhouses, not only living but thriving, doubling in number every day. The research physician who made this observation created a cell line (i.e., a collection of cells that can be kept alive) from Henrietta's cells. He named the line HeLa (based on the first two letters of her first and last name) and shared samples with many other research scientists. Research using the HeLa cell line revolutionized medical research:

> Today, work done with HeLa cells underpins much of modern medicine; they have been involved in key discoveries in many fields, including cancer, immunology and infectious disease. One of their most recent applications has been in research for vaccines against COVID-19.
>
> (Nature, 2020, p. 7)

Despite the revolutionary advances, the case of Henrietta Lacks and the events that followed raise many ethical issues. Although collecting and using cell samples from patients without their consent was legal back in the 1950s (Johns Hopkins Medicine, 2023), we still have to ask, was it ethical? Ethical issues are central to any activity involving human subjects, and that's why we're devoting this chapter to them. We'll begin with a review of foundational principles guiding medical and social science research, including communication research. Then, we'll address the issue of medical mistakes and how healthcare providers should admit their mistakes to patients and family members. Next, we'll address the principles of informed consent and the importance of clinical trial participation. Then we'll review ethical concerns associated with pharmaceutical advertising and marketing. Finally, we'll return to the story of Henrietta Lacks and her legacy.

Foundational Principles in Research Ethics

From developing medications to refining strategies for public health communication campaigns, medical and social science research is necessary to create new knowledge so that society can benefit. However, the history of such research reveals that human subjects can easily be mistreated and exploited if safeguards aren't in place. Prominent examples include

DOI: 10.4324/9781003214458-26

research atrocities conducted by Nazi doctors on people imprisoned in concentration camps during World War II and the U.S. Public Health Service Syphilis Study at Tuskegee, begun in 1932, in which 399 Black men who had syphilis were studied over several years to document the course of the disease and were left untreated even after penicillin was found to be an effective treatment in the mid-1940s (Centers for Disease Control and Prevention [CDC], 2021a). As a result of these and other unethical studies, several sets of research guidelines have been developed.

The first was the **Nuremberg Code**, which has been called "the most important document in the history of the ethics of medical research" (Shuster, 1997, p. 1436). The code resulted from the Nazi Doctors' Trial, during which 23 defendants were tried for "murder and torture in the conduct of medical experiments on concentration camp inmates" (p. 1437). The Code consists of 10 principles, the first of which states, "The voluntary consent of the human subject is absolutely essential." The remaining nine principles include that the protection of human subjects is paramount, experiments should be conducted only by highly qualified researchers, and the research should be necessary for the good of society. Together, principles from the Nuremberg Code provided the foundation for conducting ethical research on human subjects. As we'll see, these ethical principles have come to apply not only to research but also to medical practice.

Building on the experimental research principles outlined in the Nuremberg Code, philosophers Tom Beauchamp and James Childress (2001) developed a framework of four core moral principles to guide both medical treatment and research practice. **Respect for autonomy** means prioritizing a person's right to make their own decisions when agreeing to or refusing medical treatment or participation in a research study. **Nonmaleficence** means doing no harm. **Beneficence** means acting in a patient's best interests by restoring health and relieving suffering in the context of medical treatment or in a participant's or society's best interests by advancing knowledge in the context of research. **Justice** means ensuring equal distribution of benefits and risks, so every person receives the same access to medical treatment and research opportunities and findings, regardless of socioeconomic status, race, or sex. Sometimes these principles are easy to follow, but sometimes they conflict, which leads to ethical dilemmas. For example, you saw such a dilemma in Mrs. Lacks' story at the opening of the chapter: Although her doctors followed the principle of beneficence by attempting to treat her cancer, they violated her autonomy by not obtaining consent to use her cells for research (although, as noted, doing so was legal practice at the time). These moral principles provide the foundation for a system of ethics to guide regulations on conducting research with human subjects. One such system is presented in the Belmont Report.

Moral Principles in Medical and Research Ethics

Systems of medical and research ethics are based on four moral principles:

1. Respect for autonomy: Respecting a person's right to make their own decisions when agreeing to or refusing medical treatment or participation in a research study
2. Nonmaleficence: Doing no harm
3. Beneficence: Acting in a patient's best interests by restoring health and relieving suffering in the context of medical treatment or in a participant's or society's best interests by advancing knowledge in the context of research
4. Justice: Ensuring equal distribution of benefits and risks

The Belmont Report

Although navigating ethical dilemmas is challenging, regulations in research ethics provide guidelines—built on moral principles of research ethics—for researchers to follow. In the United States, the foundation of human subjects protection regulations is the Belmont Report. The **Belmont Report** was developed by the National Commission for the Protection of Human Subjects of Biomedical and Behavioral Research (National Commission, 1979), a commission created as part of the U.S. National Research Act. The commission was charged with identifying the basic ethical principles that should underlie the conduct of biomedical and social behavioral research involving human subjects and with developing guidelines to assure that such research is conducted in accordance with those principles.

The report has three parts. The first part distinguishes between research and practice. *Practice* refers to the medical context and the prevention, diagnosis, and treatment of disease. *Research*, on the other hand, refers to conducting studies to discover new knowledge. Although research and practice often go hand in hand, the Belmont Report does make a distinction because of important differences between the two. For example, medical treatment is typically necessary for the well-being of the patient, whereas research may not benefit a participant in the least.

The second and third parts of the Belmont Report present three ethical principles for research and discuss how the principles should be applied in research studies. Belmont's ethical principles will sound familiar to you from Beauchamp and Childress' (2001) work. The first is *respect for persons*. This principle requires that "individuals should be treated as autonomous agents" and "persons with diminished autonomy are entitled to protection" (National Commission, 1979, p. 4). In application, the principle is related to informed consent, which we'll review later in the chapter. The second is *beneficence*. This principle requires researchers to "maximize possible benefits and minimize possible harms" (National Commission, 1979, p. 5). In application, it requires researchers to analyze the risks and benefits of their research. Finally, the third principle is *justice*. The report emphasizes how justice is related to "who ought to receive the benefits of research" and who should "bear its burdens" (National Commission, 1979, p. 5). In practice, justice is aligned with the selection of research subjects. Researchers need to be sensitive to recruiting a sample that does not take advantage of marginalized or vulnerable populations, yet represents them adequately.

The Belmont Report led to the establishment of **institutional review boards (IRBs)**, which oversee biomedical and social science research conducted at universities, medical centers, and hospitals across the nation. Any institution receiving Public Health Service (PHS) funding is required to have an IRB. Clinicians and social and behavioral scientists who conduct human subjects research must have their research protocols approved by their IRBs. They're also required to undergo training in human subjects protections and responsible conduct of research. IRB reviews and researcher training are intended to prevent **research misconduct**, which is defined as "fabrication, falsification, or plagiarism in proposing, performing, or reviewing research, or in reporting research results" (PHS, 2005, Sec. 93.103). Research misconduct is taken extremely seriously. Researchers who are found guilty of engaging in misconduct face several possible consequences, including being barred from receiving federal funds to support their research, fired from their appointments, and required to either correct or retract research publications.

Perhaps the most egregious contemporary example of research misconduct comes from Andrew Wakefield, the former gastroenterologist and current anti-vaxxer who published a study in the prestigious journal *The Lancet* in 1998 that raised the possibility of a link between the MMR (measles-mumps-rubella) vaccine and autism. The data from the study supported no such link. Wakefield, however, claimed there was one in a press conference. As we mentioned in Chapter 5, this led to a media feeding frenzy and widespread public distrust of the vaccine, and it lit a fire under the anti-vaxxer movement. But the egregious ethical violations don't stop there. Come to find out, Wakefield had received £55,000 ($101,000) from the British Legal Aid board "to investigate a possible claim against the manufacturers of the vaccine—a claim involving some of the children in the study" (Mayor, 2004, para. 8). This constituted a financial conflict of interest that he should have reported when he submitted his paper for publication. Beyond that, Wakefield had applied for patents based on his research that could have generated significant profit (Deer, 2011), another financial conflict of interest.

Were there consequences to this unethical behavior? You bet. Ten of Wakefield's 12 co-authors came out against the fraudulent interpretation of the data (Mayor, 2004), and the journal retracted the paper. Furthermore, he was "found guilty of serious professional misconduct and struck off the medical register by the General Medical Council" (Kmietowicz, 2010). More important than the blow to Wakefield's reputation and career, however, are the health consequences faced by the rest of us. Measles, a serious and highly contagious disease that can cause debilitating or fatal complications, had been nearly eliminated (thanks to vaccines), but because of the anti-vaxxer movement spurred by Wakefield's research misconduct, it has seen a resurgence, reaching "emergency levels" in the United States and several other countries (Benecke & DeYoung, 2019). Gee, thanks, Wakefield.

The experimental research principles of the Nuremberg Code, the core moral principles from Beauchamp and Childress (2001), and the ethical principles presented in the Belmont Report provide overarching ethical standards for medical and/or research applications. To provide further guidance for ethical behavior in the medical context, Beauchamp and Childress provide a more specific set of principles, called moral rules, for patient–provider communication. It is to these that we now turn.

Moral Rules for Patient–Provider Relationships

Beauchamp and Childress (2001) presented four moral rules that apply to patient–provider communication in medical research and practice. **Veracity** refers to sharing "comprehensive, accurate, and objective" information, as well as striving to make sure that the patient or research subject understands the information provided (p. 284). **Privacy** entails five domains: informational, physical, decisional (personal choices), proprietary (property), and relational (family or close friends involved in decision making). **Confidentiality** is related to informational privacy and the expectation that information won't be disclosed outside the patient–provider/healthcare system relationship without permission. **Fidelity** has to do with trust, confidence, and loyalty in the patient–provider relationship because the provider is entrusted with the patient's well-being. As with all rules, there are challenges to following these four.

For example, maintaining *veracity* is especially difficult when it comes to delivering bad news. Examples of bad news about health include the diagnosis of chronic or terminal conditions. Although ethical and legal principles in the United States require that patients be given this information, there may be hesitation if family members or healthcare providers believe that sharing the news would do more harm than good, especially if a patient's culture privileges nondisclosure in bad news situations (Galanti, 2015). Regarding *privacy*, an individual's right to it needs to be balanced with public interest and policy. Although some people would argue it violates their right to privacy, testing for HIV and tuberculosis (as well as COVID-19) currently is mandatory in certain contexts, such as blood donation and employment in certain sectors, and screening of newborn babies for certain conditions is mandatory in the United States (CDC, 2021b). Although mandatory screening can reduce morbidity and mortality from many diseases, a systematic review of 42 studies investigating public perceptions of genetic testing revealed substantial concerns worldwide about possible discrimination based on genetic diseases discovered through mandatory testing, even though laws against such discrimination are in place (Wauters & Van Hoyweghen, 2016).

Confidentiality may be breached when there is a high probability of severe risk to other people, although determining probability and severity of risk invites additional challenges. Examples include clinicians disclosing genetic test results to patients' family members or therapists disclosing threats of violence to people targeted by their clients. Finally, the *fidelity* of the patient–provider relationship may be tested by several competing interests, not the least of which are conflicts of financial interest for the provider. Unfortunately, Beauchamp and Childress (2001) say these conflicts are "common" and "continue to pervade fee-for-service medicine, which provides an incentive for physicians to use additional diagnostic and therapeutic procedures, even when they would not serve the patient's interests" (p. 318).

Medical Mistakes

It's a sad fact of life that people make mistakes, and healthcare providers, being people, are not immune. Although some **medical mistakes** might not cause harm, especially if they're caught before affecting the patient, sometimes they lead to very serious outcomes, including death. In fact, a 2016 analysis by researchers from Johns Hopkins found that medical mistakes were the third leading cause of death in the United States, responsible for between 250,000 and 400,000 deaths annually (Makary & Daniel, 2016). In this section, we're going to look at how competent communication may protect healthcare providers from malpractice claims when they make mistakes and how healthcare providers should admit their mistakes to patients or their families when they happen. Keep in mind that admitting medical mistakes is an ethical issue given that principles of respect for persons, beneficence, and justice are all involved.

For decades now, research has shown that communication plays a key role in the successful navigation of medical mistakes and, in turn, reduction in malpractice claims. In a foundational article, Wendy Levinson (1994) reviewed several studies on malpractice claims and physician communication behavior, concluding that competent patient–provider communication was essential to avoiding malpractice lawsuits. Two of the studies she reviewed looked at malpractice claims against obstetricians, considering the quality of care they provided and patient satisfaction with their care. One found that there was "no demonstrable correlation between the quality of care provided by the obstetricians and their prior malpractice claims history" (p. 1619). The other found that "Patients of physicians who had frequent prior claims were significantly less satisfied than patients of physicians who had no prior claims" (p. 1619), saying that they felt rushed and ignored and didn't receive adequate information. A third study Levinson reviewed identified four communication problems associated with malpractice claims: "deserting the patient, devaluing patients' views, delivering information poorly, and failing to understand patients' perspectives" (p. 1619). A fourth study revealed that malpractice attorneys believed that 82% of lawsuits were due to communication problems. So, Houston, we have a problem.

Clearly, competent communication is essential to avoiding malpractice claims when clinicians make medical mistakes. But it's also essential when admitting those mistakes to patients and/or their families. Annagret Hannawa (2017) conducted a series of studies to identify what communication behaviors are associated with patient perceptions of competent disclosure of medical mistakes. Grounding her work in a model of communication competence (see Table 11.1), she began by conducting focus groups with Swiss patients to

Table 11.1 Theoretical Frameworks in Ethics in Health Communication

Theory/Model	Brief Summary	Citation
Cognitive-Affective Theory of Multimedia Learning	An extension of the cognitive theory of multimedia learning, this theory states that long-term memory for information learned through verbal and nonverbal channels, as well as the meaning of that information as processed by the learner, is mediated by affective, metacognitive, and individual difference factors.	Moreno (2006)
Communication Competence Model	Competent communication has two dimensions: appropriateness and effectiveness. A communicator's knowledge, skill, and motivation lead them to be able to produce messages that are perceived as appropriate and effective, thus competent.	Spitzberg and Cupach (1984)
Medical Error Disclosure Competence Model	There are four core medical error disclosure skills, use of which leads to patient perceptions of disclosure adequacy; adequacy, in turn, leads to disclosure effectiveness.	Hannawa (2017)
Social Cognitive Theory	Individual perceptions and behaviors are a product of individual experiences, observing the actions of others, and environmental factors.	Bandura (1986)
Uncertainty Management Theory	Uncertainty is a central part of human experience and interactions. The meaning of uncertainty varies by person and situation. People will try to reduce, maintain, or increase uncertainty depending on its meaning.	Brashers (2001)

Note. See *Supplemental Online Theory Table* for additional theories/models.

determine what the patients expected from their healthcare providers when disclosing a medical mistake. Results showed that patients wanted physicians (a) to be fully informed about what went wrong and to share that information clearly and honestly, (b) to acknowledge responsibility, be remorseful, and apologize, (c) to be attentive, composed, and expressive, and (d) to adapt to patients' needs. From these results, Hannawa developed a Medical Error Disclosure Competence model and tested it over a series of studies.

The model includes four core medical error disclosure skills: (a) providing a complete account of the medical error, (b) offering a sincere apology that shows regret and remorse, (c) adapting to the patient's informational and emotional needs, and (d) being nonverbally attentive, composed, coordinated, and expressive. According to the model, demonstrating these skills will lead to patient perceptions of disclosure adequacy; adequacy, in turn, will lead to disclosure effectiveness, with patients experiencing less trauma and more resilience in the face of the error and demonstrating better coping tactics. Studies have shown support for several parts of the model, particularly the importance of nonverbal skills (Hannawa, 2019; Hannawa & Frankel, 2021).

Informed Consent

We mentioned earlier that the Belmont report indicates that the ethical principle of respect for persons requires that people must give informed consent to participate in research. It further indicates that **informed consent** contains three elements: information, comprehension, and voluntariness. **Information** should be "sufficient" in terms of the purpose of the research, details of the research procedure, and anticipated risks and benefits, as well as the ability to refuse to participate without consequences or stop participation once the study is underway. **Comprehension** means that participants (or their parent or legal guardian in the case of child participants or mentally disabled adults) need to be able to understand the information provided to be able to give true informed consent. **Voluntariness** means that subjects should never be coerced into participating (this is of particular concern for vulnerable populations such as children or prisoners) and must be able to opt out of participating, even after the study has started.

Informed Consent

For medical research and practice to be ethical, participants/patients must provide informed consent. Informed consent is based on respect for a person's autonomy. It requires three elements: sufficient information, comprehension, and voluntariness. In practice, true informed consent is difficult to attain because information may not be comprehensive and patients may not fully understand it. Communication research can improve the process and procedures of informed consent.

You might be interested to know that sometimes the informed consent process is modified. This can happen when a subject's knowing the true purpose of the study would compromise results. In other words, the researcher has to deceive their participants. In this case, when participants are debriefed at the end of the study, they must be given the opportunity to withdraw their data from the study. Of course, such deception requires IRB approval. Well, it requires approval unless researchers cross the line—which has happened. We'll demonstrate.

You might recall the Kramer et al. (2014) study we presented in Chapter 9, which reported results of a Facebook experiment in which researchers manipulated the emotional tone of 689,003 users' newsfeeds and looked for effects of emotional contagion (which they found). Users whose feeds were more negative than usual made more negative posts, and users whose feeds were more positive than usual made more positive posts. After the study was published, there was quite a hullabaloo in the research community over ethical concerns regarding informed consent and voluntariness. The major concern was that Facebook users had been given no information whatsoever about the study. Although in the paper Kramer et al. wrote that their study protocol "was consistent with Facebook's Data Use Policy, to which all users agree prior to creating an account on Facebook, constituting informed consent for this research" (p. 8789), you have to wonder whether the information provided in the data use policy was either sufficient or comprehended by users. Also, "participants" in this experiment were hardly given the opportunity to opt out. Thus, the principle of voluntariness was compromised.

It's interesting to consider the affiliations of the paper's three authors. The first author, Adam Kramer, worked for Facebook on their core data science team. As a private company, Facebook is not legally required to follow federal policy concerning human subjects protections. The other authors, though, worked for Cornell University, an institution that most certainly is. Because the experiment had already been conducted by the time these authors joined the study, Cornell's IRB determined they were not engaged in human subjects research and, therefore, no IRB review was necessary. But does that make the study ethical?

In an article delving into the study for *The Atlantic*, Robinson Meyer (2014) wrote that he's "seen and heard both privacy advocates and casual users express surprise at the audacity of the experiment" (para. 5). In addition, *PNAS*, the journal that published the study, published an "Editorial Expression of Concern" about the study. In it, the editor acknowledged that "Questions have been raised about the principles of informed consent and opportunity to opt out in connection with the research" and stated that even though Facebook was not subject to those regulations, "It is nevertheless a matter of concern that the collection of the data by Facebook may have involved practices that were not fully consistent with the principles of obtaining informed consent and allowing participants to opt out" (Verma, 2014, p. 10779). Perhaps in a twist of irony, in the aftermath, the lead author made the following post to Facebook: "Having written and designed this experiment myself, I can tell you that our goal was never to upset anyone ... In hindsight, the research benefits of the paper may not have justified all of this anxiety" (Meyer, 2014, para. 9). Gee, ya think?

Clearly, informed consent is essential in health communication. It applies not only to research but also to medical treatment. In both cases, people are supposed to be fully informed about what's going to happen to them, have the opportunity to opt out, and understand the risks and benefits. You may never participate in a research study, but chances are good that you'll undergo some form of medical treatment. Unfortunately, in that context, there's plenty of evidence that most people don't understand the consent forms that they sign (National Quality Forum, 2005). This is a serious problem because it means that patients aren't protected and healthcare providers could be at risk of malpractice lawsuits if things go wrong and patients say they weren't fully informed. Therefore, health communication researchers are studying ways to improve the process and procedures for obtaining informed consent. Erin Donovan is one such scholar.

Improving Informed Consent Procedures

Donovan and her colleagues conducted a series of studies investigating how to improve existing medical consent forms so that patients' uncertainty is reduced and understanding is increased. In one study, she and her team wanted to know how health literacy and self-efficacy were related to understanding medical procedures and their risks (Donovan et al., 2012). Guided by social cognitive theory (see Table 11.1), they hypothesized that there would be a relationship between a person's health literacy and their self-efficacy to understand the risks of the procedure and make an informed decision about going through with it. In turn, self-efficacy then would be related to understanding the consent form. The researchers recruited 254 adults from Texas and randomly assigned them to read standard medical consent forms for either a cardiac catheterization procedure or gallbladder removal surgery, asking them to imagine that they were going to have the procedure themselves. Afterward, participants answered a series of questions about their health literacy and their self-efficacy, and they indicated whether they thought the consent form provided adequate information, whether various sections of the consent form might confuse people, and whether they still would want more information after reading it. As hypothesized, results showed that lower health literacy predicted lower self-efficacy, which then was related to thinking the consent form did not provide adequate information, finding the document more confusing, and saying they wanted more information about the medical procedure and its risks.

Donovan and colleagues (2013) wanted to know more about what exactly made the consent documents confusing to participants, so they did a follow-up analysis of that data. This time, they used uncertainty management theory as a guiding framework (see Table 11.1). They developed a coding scheme to analyze the participants' responses about the parts of the consent form that were confusing and identified four sources of uncertainty: language use, risks and hazards, nature of the procedure, and consent form composition and format. More specifically, participants indicated that the consent form used too much medical jargon and did not use everyday language that an average person could understand. The participants also wanted to know a whole lot more about the risks involved with the procedure: what exactly the risks entailed; how likely they would be; why they would happen; if they did happen, then what would happen next; what *other* risks might there be that weren't mentioned; and what were the risks of *not* going through with the procedure. In terms of the nature of the procedure, participants just wanted more information, saying details in the consent form were vague. They also wanted to know more about what other healthcare staff might be assisting the primary physician and what additional procedures might be necessary beyond the main procedure, including the use of blood/blood products and anesthesia—all things that were mentioned in the consent form but not adequately explained. Finally, there was added uncertainty because the way the consent form was organized and written was confusing to participants. They also said it was too long (possibly like this paragraph). The tension between wanting more information and wanting less text is one that affects many areas of communication—and one that must be handled with great care.

Armed with the knowledge of what people found confusing about consent forms, Donovan and colleagues (2014) set about revising the cardiac catheterization form to make it clearer and more comprehensible. Specifically, they worked on "simplifying complex sentences and providing explanations of medico-legal terms" (terms related to both medicine and law; p. 246). For example, instead of having "I (we) understand that no warranty or guarantee has been made to me as to result or cure" (what?!?), the revised form stated, "I understand that this procedure does not guarantee a cure to my condition." And instead of using the term "hemorrhage" on its own, the revised form had "hemorrhage (lots of bleeding)." The researchers then designed an experiment to test whether their revised consent form would perform better than the original. They recruited 278 adults (still from Texas) to participate. All were told to imagine they were to undergo a cardiac catheterization; 128 received the original consent form, and 150 received the revised form. Results of the experiment showed that people who read the revised form understood the medico-legal terms better and had less uncertainty about the procedure than people who read the original form.

Donovan and colleagues' program of research on improving informed consent documents has made a significant contribution to the discipline of health communication by advancing knowledge about how reducing sources of uncertainty can make information more comprehensible—so much so that the publication reporting the experiment (Donovan et al., 2014) was awarded the *2015 Bill Eadie Distinguished Scholarly Article Award* from the National Communication Association's Applied Communication Division. Beyond scholarly impact, her work also has had an impact on practice. Texas recently underwent a regulatory revision of consent procedures for the state. Donovan advised the Texas Medical Disclosure Panel of the Texas State Legislature on the process. The template for informed consent that she created was officially added to the Texas Administrative Code and went into effect statewide in 2020. As we mentioned in Chapter 1, this is an excellent example of translational applied health communication research having a positive impact on patients and healthcare providers alike.

Improving Clinical Trial Enrollment

Another applied area related to informed consent that has received attention from communication researchers is clinical trial enrollment. A **clinical trial** is a special kind of research study designed to "test how well new medical approaches work in people" as investigators strive to find innovative ways "to prevent, screen for, diagnose, or treat a disease" (MedlinePlus, 2018, n.p.). As of 2022, there were more than 425,000 clinical trials going on worldwide, including in all 50 U.S. states and more than 200 countries (ClinicalTrials.gov, n.d.). These studies often test a new drug, medical procedure, or intervention against either a placebo (to see if the treatment works in the first place) or the standard of care (to see if the treatment can improve health outcomes beyond current practice). As you can imagine, clinical trials are very important because they advance medical knowledge, with a goal of improving population health. Unfortunately, recruiting research subjects for these trials is challenging.

To be able to draw valid and generalizable conclusions about the safety and efficacy of the drug or procedure being tested in a clinical trial, it's essential to have a rigorous study design. That includes recruiting an adequate and diverse sample of research participants because people of different sexes, races, and ethnicities can respond differently to new treatments. Historically, however, women and members of marginalized populations have been inadequately represented in clinical trials (Clark et al., 2019; Liu & DiPietro Mager, 2016). Although the provision of ethical guidelines has reduced rates of exclusion, inadequate representation remains a problem for a variety of reasons, including concerns over past medical research abuses (e.g., the Tuskegee Syphilis Study). Health communication research has been at the forefront of understanding the factors that influence clinical trial participation and developing interventions to broaden participation.

Barriers to participation in clinical trials vary for different groups, communities, and cultures. We'll demonstrate this by presenting three studies on three communities, all exploring barriers to participating in clinical trials. First, Luther Clark and colleagues (2019) conducted an extensive literature review to understand barriers to clinical trial participation among members of historically marginalized racial and ethnic communities. They identified several barriers, including "overall mistrust of process, lack of understanding the value of clinical research, fear, stigma of participating, family members' opinions, financial burden, time commitment, and transportation" (p. 167). Such barriers show the breadth of hesitation that people can experience.

Second, Jeske van Diemen and colleagues (2021) also conducted an extensive literature search to identify barriers to clinical trial participation among women, but they ran into a barrier themselves when they found only six studies that were relevant to their goal. In reviewing those six studies, they didn't find substantial differences in the barriers to women's versus men's willingness to participate in terms of time constraints, concerns about the experimental nature of the drug/procedure, or concerns about potential harm. However, women seemed to have greater concerns over the potential for harm, as well as being more concerned about transportation. But remember, only six studies were relevant to exploring this question. Additional research is clearly needed.

Finally, Wei Peng and colleagues (2019) took a different approach to understanding barriers to clinical trial participation when they did a content analysis of discussions about clinical trials on breastcancer.org, an online discussion forum centered on breast health and breast cancer. They analyzed 270 posts made by 154 users over a six-month period (demographic data on who posted was not available). Data analysis identified barriers to, incentives for, and misconceptions about participating in clinical trials. Barriers included concerns about side effects, a lack of treatment benefit from participating, and study inclusion or exclusion criteria (i.e., the person might not qualify for the trial). The main incentive and the main misconception were identical: thinking that there would be a therapeutic benefit from participating in the clinical trial (something that is not guaranteed).

These three studies identify areas for improving understanding of the purpose and processes of clinical trials among diverse groups, which is essential to informed consent, and they identify some important attitudinal and logistical barriers. So the question now is what the next steps should be. Soroya Julian McFarlane and colleagues (2022) have some suggestions based on their 10-year systematic review of using community-based participatory research strategies to enhance participation.

Community-based participatory research (CBPR) is an approach to research that creates a partnership between community members and researchers, as well as others who might be stakeholders in the endeavor, such as public health officials or city leaders. As you can imagine, CBPR recognizes the importance of involving the people whose lives are at the center of the research, instead of letting researchers control all aspects of a project. McFarlane et al. (2022) located 104 studies that used CBPR methods to increase clinical trial participation among racial and ethnic minorities and found that 88 of the projects were successful in doing so. The authors identified several ways that the projects' researchers increased community involvement in the projects. Specifically, researchers involved community members in (a) serving on advisory boards, (b) posing research questions, (c) collecting data, (d) developing and delivering interventions, (e) recruiting participants, (f) interpreting research findings, and/or (g) disseminating study results. The success of the 88 projects in increasing clinical trial participation is credited to using these community-involved strategies.

McFarlane et al. (2022) also took a close look at the communication strategies researchers used in the successful projects. They found three broad strategies. First, researchers and community leaders had "regular and transparent communication" to ensure "shared decision making and mutual understanding" (p. 1079). Second, researchers made sure that intervention materials were clearly communicated "by validating and adapting messages based on literacy levels" (p. 1084). And third, researchers worked with community members to culturally target intervention messages and materials (following the cultural sensitivity approach presented in Chapter 10). Such targeting was done on a *surface level* by referencing religious symbols and rituals and using participants' preferred language, among other strategies. *Deep level* targeting was achieved by incorporating community beliefs, values, and lifestyle preferences into intervention messages and materials, as well as addressing misconceptions held by a community and acknowledging its sociohistorical context. Although all this work takes considerable effort, it absolutely pays off in terms of enhancing the participation of diverse populations in clinical trials, which is a win for everybody.

Technology Use to Increase Research Participation

Whether people are consenting to participate in clinical trials or other types of research studies, it's important to consider how technology may be used to promote participation. We want to touch very quickly on two studies that investigated different technology-based strategies for this purpose. One study looked at the effect of using multimedia animation to enhance knowledge of and attitudes toward clinical trials. Guided by the cognitive-affective theory of multimedia learning, Aurora Occa and Susan Morgan (2019) developed an experimental video using whiteboard animation with voiceover to convey basic clinical trial concepts (e.g., placebo, randomization) and compared it to clinical trial informational brochures either with or without visual images. The researchers recruited 1,194 cancer patients and survivors to participate in their study. They found that participants who saw the animated video had greater knowledge about and better attitudes toward clinical trials than participants who saw the brochures. With advances in technology and software, creating the animated videos didn't require a huge investment of time or resources, so using animation to enhance clinical trial participation is definitely a strategy worth considering.

Another study looked at using electronic consent forms to increase participation in research. You'll remember from Chapter 3 that clinics and hospitals these days rely on electronic health records to store patient information. With all that health information available electronically, there's great opportunity to mine it for research purposes. Therefore, patients often are asked whether researchers may access their health information for future research, and patients need to sign consent forms to say yes. Elizabeth Golembiewski and colleagues (2021) tested three versions of an electronic consent form to assess impact on participation: a *standard* version that just presented information, an *interactive* version that included hyperlinks to additional information, and a *trust-enhanced* version that included not only the hyperlinks but also information about research regulations, researcher training, and data protection. They recruited 734 patients from family medicine clinics to engage with one of the three consent forms and assessed patients' responses immediately after they'd read the consent form, one week later, and then six months later. Most participants (94%) consented to having their health data used for future research, and there were no differences between conditions on any of the outcome variables immediately after the study or one week later. However, at the six-month mark, patients in the trust-enhanced condition were more satisfied with their decision and had greater understanding than patients in the other two conditions. It's not difficult to include hyperlinks in an electronic document, nor is it difficult to add information on research regulations and data protections (although the information would need to be presented clearly). This study provides evidence that doing so will result in better research participation outcomes.

Pharmaceutical Advertising and Marketing

We can't have a chapter on ethics in health communication without addressing issues related to pharmaceutical advertising and marketing. We'll first look at direct-to-consumer advertising of prescription drugs. Then we'll look at how the pharmaceutical industry works to influence physician prescribing behavior.

Direct-to-Consumer Advertising

The marketing of prescription drugs to the public is called **direct-to-consumer advertising (DTCA)**. The United States and New Zealand are the only countries that allow drug advertising targeted to consumers (Ventola, 2011). The Food and Drug Administration (FDA) has jurisdiction over DTCA in the United States. (The Federal Trade Commission deals with over-the-counter [OTC] products, by the way.) For many years, regulations required that television ads "summarize potential adverse reactions and contraindications to drugs" (Frosch & Grande, 2010, p. 1). In 1997, the guidelines changed so that TV ads did not have to include that information but instead could tell consumers where to go to find it (e.g., a print ad, a website, their doctor). This change led to an explosion of DTCA on TV, with companies increasing spending from $2.1 billion in 1997 to $9.6 billion in 2016 (Schwartz & Woloshin, 2019). With all that advertising, one study estimated that people see more than 30 hours of prescription and OTC drug ads annually (Brownfield et al., 2004). That figure does *not* compare favorably with the amount of time most patients spend with their physicians. The question for us, then, is what the ethical implications of such advertising are, particularly in terms of the information these ads provide to consumers and the ads' impact on patient behavior and patient–provider communication.

The FDA allows three types of medication ads. **Product claim ads** provide information about the medication. **Help-seeking ads** mention medical conditions and encourage people to seek help from their doctor, but they don't mention the medication. **Reminder**

ads just mention the name of the medication. The FDA says that ads must be "truthful, accurately communicated, and balanced in presenting the drug's risks and benefits" (FDA, 2015, para. 7). Furthermore, they say an ad is misleading or false if it does any of the following (FDA, 2015, para. 8):

- Promotes the drug as being better or more effective than actually demonstrated
- Implies that a drug is safer or has fewer or less severe side effects than demonstrated
- Claims, without substantial evidence, that its product is better than a competitor's drug
- Gives a false, misleading or unbalanced presentation of risk information about a drug product
- Promotes the product as being able to treat conditions not approved by the FDA

Direct-to-Consumer Advertising

The FDA oversees prescription drug advertising. It groups ads into three categories:

Product Claim Ads: These ads name specific drugs and include information about their uses, benefits, and risks.
Help-seeking Ads: These ads present information about a disease or medical condition and encourage people to see their doctor if they think they might have it. The ads don't mention specific drugs.
Reminder Ad: These ads are designed to increase product name recognition. They don't mention the drug's uses or make any claims about its effects on diseases or medical conditions.

Probably not surprisingly, pharmaceutical companies sometimes don't follow these guidelines very well. In fact, the FDA receives numerous complaints each year about such ads from consumers, healthcare providers, and, interestingly, competing drug companies (FDA, 2015). How are pharmaceutical companies violating these guidelines? One content analysis of 97 drug ads found that whereas 25 of the ads included data about how well the drugs worked, none of the ads included data about drug risks, and 13 ads suggested "off-label uses," which violates the stipulation that ads are only supposed to address the conditions for which the drug is indicated (Klara et al., 2018). If the FDA finds that an ad violates regulations, they most often send a "warning letter" or a "notice of violation" to the company. But there can be more severe penalties. Indeed, some companies have paid billions of dollars in penalties for misleading information in DTCA (Parekh & Shrank, 2018).

Robert Shmerling (2022) discusses common examples of how the language used in DTCA can be misleading. For example, "No other treatment has been proven better" implies that the advertised drug is the best. Shmerling points out, however, that the drug actually "might be only as good as — and no better than — older, less expensive, or even over-the-counter competitors" and goes on to say that "drug ads are unlikely to mention the option of taking *nothing* for the condition in question, even though many minor ailments get better on their own" (para. 11). He also discusses how ads will use anecdotes of how a drug miraculously helped a single person, ignoring clinical studies that may show limited effects in larger groups of people. Shmerling warns consumers that the bottom line for the pharmaceutical industry is to make money, so buyers should beware.

Given First Amendment rights of commercial interests in the United States, DTCA isn't going anywhere anytime soon. So, it's good to consider the pros and cons of such advertising. Shmerling (2022) provides a handy list, which we present in Table 11.2.

Table 11.2 The Pros and Cons of DTCA

Pros	Cons
Educates people about conditions and treatments they were unaware of	Presents incomplete or biased information
Improves health by encouraging people to take needed medications	Spurs people to ask for medications they don't need
Lessens stigma surrounding certain conditions, such as mental illness or erectile dysfunction	Promotes medications before long-term safety is known
Increases detection of unrelated diseases if patients are inspired to see their doctors	Creates conflicts between patients asking for a drug and doctors who don't recommend it
Increases knowledge of possible side effects because regulations require consumers to be referred to a website, magazine, or other source for more information	Drives up healthcare costs without adding health benefits (because new drugs are much more expensive than generic drugs)

Note. Adapted from Shmerling (2022).

Dominick Frosch and David Grande (2010) offer a summary of some of the evidence that aligns with these pros and cons. On the plus side, most patients do believe that these ads improve their knowledge about diseases and treatments, many use information from the ads to make medical decisions or are prompted to seek more information, and some may even become more adherent. Physicians also agree that patients gain knowledge from the ads and participate more in shared decision making, but they have concerns that the ads encourage patients to inappropriately request certain medications and that such requests may lead to longer and even unnecessary office visits. In terms of the content of the ads, Frosch and Grande note that information may be vague or overemphasize benefits, that visual imagery and verbal messaging don't match when the ads present risk information (e.g., information about nasty side effects is overshadowed by images of happy people), and information in printed material tends to exceed the recommended 8th-grade reading level. They offer a number of recommendations for improving DTCA, including better audience targeting, more specific information about risks, and more accurate, less emotional information about drug benefits. Even if DTCA were completely accurate, balanced, and comprehensive, though, there remains the issue of pharmaceutical and medical device companies marketing directly to physicians to influence their prescribing and treatment behavior. We turn to that topic next.

Marketing to Physicians

Whereas the pharmaceutical industry spent more than $3 billion on DTCA in 2012, it spent more than $24 billion that year on marketing to physicians (PEW, 2013) and $89.5 billion on physician–pharmaceutical sales representative (PSR) interactions (Fickweiler et al., 2017). The concern is that such spending may unduly influence physician prescribing behavior. Research shows this concern is a valid one.

To learn more about how physicians might be influenced by pharmaceutical marketing practices, Freek Fickweiler and colleagues (2017) conducted a systematic review of 49 studies that included physicians from around the world (e.g., Brazil, Ethiopia, Iran, Japan, Poland, United States). The authors discovered that physicians received visits from sales reps at least once a month and received several types of gifts, including drug samples, honoraria, support for travel to conferences, money for research, and free lunches and dinners. They found that although most physicians thought that meeting with sales reps and receiving gifts would not affect their prescribing behavior, it did. For example, physicians who accepted drug samples as gifts were more likely to prescribe the brand drug than generics, physicians who accepted honoraria or research funding were more likely to ask their hospital to add the brand drug to its formulary, and physicians who received conference travel support tripled the rate at which they prescribed the brand drug.

Fickweiler and colleagues (2017) conclude that "physicians are susceptible to pharmaceutical industry and PSR interactions, which influences their clinical decision making leading to greater prescriptions of branded drugs over low-cost generic medicines and increasing healthcare costs" (p. 10). The authors recommend additional policy and educational interventions to stem the influence of pharmaceutical marketing on physician behavior. Such steps are needed because, according to Paul Thacker,

> I don't think most doctors realize the extent to which their profession has been compromised by industry. They're in the dark. The overwhelming majority [of doctors] are just trying to do their jobs—run a practice and think about patients—and they're not completely aware of the extent this has been going on.
>
> (Silverman, 2013, p. 1)

Thacker's words were more than just words: He drafted one of the first major pieces of legislation to increase transparency around physician-corporate relationships — the Sunshine Act.

To address concerns about companies influencing physician decision making, the **Physician Payments Sunshine Act** of 2010 requires companies that receive federal healthcare funding, such as through Medicare, Medicaid, or the Affordable Care Act, to collect and report data on "financial relationships" between the companies and physicians and academic medical centers. In addition, between 2006 and 2012, many academic medical centers "enacted policies restricting sales visits from pharmaceutical representatives to their practicing physicians," which resulted in some reduction in prescribing targeted medications by some of the physicians in some of the centers (Larkin et al., 2017, p. 1786). Still, there are concerns.

For example, Aaron Mitchell and Deborah Korenstein (2020) report that approximately half of the doctors in the United States each year "accept money or gifts from drug and device companies, totaling more than \$2 billion" (n.p). Physician "incentives" include free meals, medical textbooks, paid trips to conferences, and tuition for continuing medical education (PEW, 2013). The overarching goal is to get doctors to prescribe the medications being sold, even if there are other drugs on the market that are as effective yet less expensive. To really drive this point home, here's a paragraph from MedReps.com, a job site for medical salespeople, on how to influence physician behavior (MedReps.com, 2022, para. 3, emphasis added):

> In order for you to get your job done as a medical sales rep, you need to figure out just how you can influence the physicians and other prescribers that you meet with on a regular basis. Each is different, so you'll need to have a variety of approaches available to choose from. Customizing your approach is the key to success. *After all, your main goal is for all the doctors in your sales network to begin prescribing the medications that you sell.*

Kind of gives you pause.

Conclusion

We've covered a lot of ethical ground in this chapter and given you a lot to think about. We reviewed foundational ethical principles guiding medical and social science research, including principles from the Nuremberg Code and the Belmont Report. We addressed the issue of medical mistakes and strategies for healthcare providers to communicate their mistakes to patients and family members. We reviewed the principles of informed consent and discussed the importance of clinical trial participation, and we presented a review of ethical concerns associated with pharmaceutical advertising and marketing. We hope you can sense that all of these ethical issues are often challenging because of inherent conflicts among the core principles in research and treatment contexts. There's also the arguable disregard for certain ethical principles in pharmaceutical advertising and marketing contexts. However, the scientific community has developed strict regulations that are meant to provide protections to human subjects, and regulations also are in place to stem undue influence on patients and physicians from the advertising and marketing of medications and medical devices.

It's now time for us to return to the story of Henrietta Lacks. If she were being treated today, she would have had to give consent for her cells to be used in medical research. That was not the case in the '50s, though, and it was decades before her family found out about the HeLa cell line. They found out quite by accident when scientists approached some of the family members to ask them for samples of their DNA because HeLa cells had contaminated other cell samples (Gajanan, 2017). As you can imagine, this was a huge shock to the family:

> The Lacks family had lived in poverty for most of their lives—finding out about the cells and how they were instrumental in launching a multi-billion-dollar industry prompted them to launch a campaign to get the money they felt they were owed.
>
> (Gajanan, 2017, para. 5)

The family has hired the attorney who represented the families of George Floyd and Breonna Taylor and an attorney with success winning major settlements against large corporations, and they're planning to sue the many, many companies that are profiting from the HeLa cell line, beginning with Thermo Fisher Scientific (Kabbara, 2021; LeMoult, 2022). They're claiming "unjust enrichment and nonconsensual use of her cells and tissue samples" (Kabbara, 2021, para. 2). But the family doesn't just want economic justice. They want the world to know about Henrietta and her legacy. Said one of her granddaughters, "I want scientists to acknowledge that HeLa cells came from an African American woman who was flesh and blood, who had a family and who had a story" (Nature, 2020, p. 7).

The best-selling book *The Immortal Life of Henrietta Lacks* (Skloot, 2010) and an HBO movie by the same name helped bring attention to Henrietta's story. Her contributions to research will be further acknowledged with a 34,000-square-foot research facility, the Lacks Building, being built on the Johns Hopkins campus. It's important to note that Johns Hopkins never sold or profited from the HeLA cell line, and they worked closely with the Lacks family and the National Institutes of Health (NIH) "to help craft an agreement that requires scientists to receive permission to use Henrietta Lacks' genetic blueprint in NIH-funded research" (Johns Hopkins Medicine, 2022, para. 17). Still, they admit that

> Having reviewed our interactions with Henrietta Lacks and with the Lacks family over more than 50 years, we found that Johns Hopkins could have – and should have – done more to inform and work with members of Henrietta Lacks' family out of respect for them, their privacy and their personal interests.
>
> (Johns Hopkins Medicine, 2023, para. 6)

And therein lies the nature of ethics.

References

Bandura, A. (1986). *Social foundations of thought and action: A social cognitive theory.* Prentice-Hall, Inc.

Beauchamp, T. L., & Childress, J. F. (2001). *Principles of biomedical ethics* (5th ed.). Oxford University Press.

Benecke, O., & DeYoung, S. E. (2019). Anti-vaccine decision-making and measles resurgence in the United States. *Global Pediatric Health, 6,* 1–5.

Brashers, D. E. (2001). Communication and uncertainty management. *Journal of Communication, 51*(3), 477–497.

Brownfield, E. D., Bernhardt, J. M., Phan, J. L., Williams, M. V., & Parker, R. M. (2004). Direct-to-consumer drug advertisements on network television: An exploration of quantity, frequency, and placement. *Journal of Health Communication, 9*(6), 491–497.

Centers for Disease Control and Prevention. (2021a). *The Tuskegee timeline.* https://www.cdc.gov/tuskegee/timeline.htm

Centers for Disease Control and Prevention. (2021b). *Newborn screening portal.* https://www.cdc.gov/newbornscreening/index.html

Clark, L. T., Watkins, L., Piña, I. L., Elmer, M., Akinboboye, O., Gorham, M., Jamerson, B., Burroughs, A., McCullough, C., Pierre, C., Polis, A. B., Puckrein, G., & Regnante, J. M. (2019). Increasing diversity in clinical trials: Overcoming critical barriers. *Current Problems in Cardiology, 44,* 148–172.

ClinicalTrials.gov. (n.d.) *ClinicalTrials.gov is a database of privately and publicly funded clinical studies conducted around the world.* U.S. National Library of Medicine. https://clinicaltrials.gov/ct2/home

Deer, B. (2011). How the case against the MMR vaccine was fixed. *British Medical Journal, 342*(7788), Article c5347.

Donovan, E. E., Crook, B., Brown, L. E., Pastorek, A. E., Hall, C. A., Mackert, M. S., & Stephens, K. K. (2014). An experimental test of medical disclosure and consent documentation: Assessing patient comprehension, self-efficacy, and uncertainty. *Communication Monographs, 81*(2), 239–260.

Donovan-Kicken, E., Mackert, M., Guinn, T. D., Tollison, A. C., & Breckinridge, B. (2013). Sources of patient uncertainty when reviewing medical disclosure and consent documentation. *Patient Education and Counseling, 90*(2), 254–260.

Donovan-Kicken, E., Mackert, M., Guinn, T. D., Tollison, A. C., Breckinridge, B., & Pont, S. J. (2012). Health literacy, self-efficacy, and patients' assessment of medical disclosure and consent documentation. *Health Communication, 27*(6), 581–590.

Fickweiler, F., Fickweiler, W., & Urbach, E. (2017). Interactions between physicians and the pharmaceutical industry generally and sales representatives specifically and their association with physicians' attitudes and prescribing habits: A systematic review. *BMJ Open, 7,* Article e016408.

Food and Drug Administration. (2015). *From the manufacturers' mouth to your ears: Direct to consumer advertising.* https://www.fda.gov/drugs/special-features/manufacturers-mouth-your-ears-direct-consumer-advertising

Frosch, D. L., & Grande, D. (2010). Direct-to-consumer advertising of prescription drugs. *Leonard Davis Institute of Health Economics Issue Brief, 15*(3), 1–4.

Golembiewski, E. H., Mainous, A. G., III, Rahmanian, K. P., Brumback, B., Rooks, B. J., Krieger, J. L., Goodman, K. W., Moseley, R. E., & Harle, C. A. (2021). An electronic tool to support patient-centered broad consent: A multi-arm randomized clinical trial in family medicine. *Annals of Family Medicine, 19*(1), 16–23.

Gajanan, M. (2017, April 21). What to know about *The Immortal Life of Henrietta Lacks. Time.* https://time.com/4742472/henrietta-lacks-what-to-know/

Galanti, G.-A. (2015). *Caring for patients from different cultures.* University of Pennsylvania Press.

Hannawa, A. F. (2017). What constitutes "competent error disclosure"? Insights from a national focus group study in Switzerland. *Swiss Medical Weekly, 147,* Article 14427.

Hannawa, A. F. (2019). When facing our fallibility constitutes "safe practice": Further evidence for the Medical Error Disclosure Competence (MEDC) guidelines. *Patient Education and Counseling, 102,* 1840–1846.

Hannawa, A. F., & Frankel, R. M. (2021). "It matters what I think, not what you say": Scientific evidence for a medical error disclosure competence (MEDC) model. *Journal of Patient Safety, 17*(8), e1130–e1137.

Johns Hopkins Medicine. (2022, February 24). *Johns Hopkins: Local and minority-owned businesses lead design, construction contracts for building named in honor of Henrietta Lacks.* https://www.hopkinsmedicine.org/

news/newsroom/news-releases/johns-hopkins-local-and-minority-owned-businesses-lead-design-construction-contracts-for-building-named-in-honor-of-henrietta-lacks

Johns Hopkins Medicine. (2023). *The legacy of Henrietta Lacks.* https://www.hopkinsmedicine.org/henriettalacks/

Kabbara, K. (2021, October 14). Henrietta Lacks family seeks justice: Grandchildren sue biotech company. *ABC News.* https://abcnews.go.com/US/henrietta-lacks-family-seeks-justice-grandchildren-sue-biotech/story?id=80539229

Klara, K., Kim, J., & Ross, J. S. (2018). Direct-to-consumer broadcast advertisements for pharmaceuticals: Off-label promotion and adherence to FDA guidelines. *Journal of General Internal Medicine, 33*(5), 651–658.

Kramer, A. D. I., Guillory, J. E., & Hancock, J. T. (2014). Experimental evidence of massive-scale emotional contagion through social networks. *PNAS, 111*(24), 8788–8790.

Kmietowicz, Z. (2010). Wakefield is struck off for the "serious and wide-ranging findings against him." *BMJ, 340*(7757). doi: 10.1136/bmj.c2803

Larkin, I., Ang, D., Steinhart, J., Chao, M., Patterson, M., Sah, S., Wu, T., Schoenbaum, M., Hutchins, D., Brennan, T., & Loewenstein, G. (2017). Association between academic medical center pharmaceutical detailing policies and physician prescribing. *JAMA, 317*(17), 1785–1795.

LeMoult, C. (2022, May 17). Thermo Fisher seeks dismissal of Henrietta Lacks' family's lawsuit regarding sale of her cells. *GBH News.* https://www.wgbh.org/news/local-news/2022/05/17/thermo-fisher-seeks-dismissal-of-henrietta-lacks-familys-lawsuit-regarding-sale-of-her-cells

Levinson, W. (1994). Physician-patient communication: A key to malpractice prevention. *JAMA, 272*(2), 1619–1620.

Liu, K. A., & DiPietro Mager, N. A. (2016). Women's involvement in clinical trials: Historical perspective and future implications. *Pharmacy Practice, 14*(1), Article 708.

Makary, M. A., & Daniel, M. (2016). Medical error—The third leading cause of death in the US. *BMJ, 353*, Article i 2139.

Mayor, S. (2004). Authors reject interpretation linking autism and MMR vaccine. *BMJ, 328*(7440). https://www.ncbi.nlm.nih.gov/pmc/articles/PMC381161/

McFarlane, J. S., Occa, A., Peng, W., Awonuga, O., & Morgan, S. E. (2022). Community-based participatory research (CBPR) to enhance participation of racial/ethnic minorities in clinical trials: A 10-year systematic review. *Health Communication, 37*(9), 1075–1092.

MedlinePlus. (2018). *Clinical trials.* https://medlineplus.gov/clinicaltrials.html

MedReps.com. (2022, May 9). *How medical sales reps can influence prescriber behavior.* https://www.medreps.com/medical-sales-careers/how-medical-sales-reps-can-influence-prescriber-behavior

Meyer, R. (2014, September 8). Everything we know about Facebook's secret mood-manipulation experiment. *The Atlantic.* https://www.theatlantic.com/technology/archive/2014/06/everything-we-know-about-facebooks-secret-mood-manipulation-experiment/373648/

Mitchell, A., & Korenstein, D. (2020, December 4). Drug companies' payments and gifts affect physicians' prescribing. It's time to turn off the spigot. *STAT.* https://www.statnews.com/2020/12/04/drug-companies-payments-gifts-affect-physician-prescribing/

Moreno, R. (2006). Does the modality principle hold for different media? A test of the method-affects-learning hypothesis. *Journal of Computer Assisted Learning, 22*(3), 149–158.

National Commission for the Protection of Human Subjects of Biomedical and Behavioral Research. (1979). *The Belmont report: Ethical principles and guidelines for the protection of human subjects of research.* U.S. Department of Health and Human Services. https://www.hhs.gov/ohrp/regulations-and-policy/belmont-report/read-the-belmont-report/index.html

National Quality Forum. (2005). *Implementing a national voluntary consensus standard for informed consent: A user's guide for healthcare professionals.* Washington, DC: National Quality Forum. https://www.quality-forum.org/Publications/2005/09/Implementing_a_National_Voluntary_Consensus_Standard_for_Informed_Consent__A_User_s_Guide_for_Healthcare_Professionals.aspx

Nature. (2020). Henrietta Lacks: Science must right a historical wrong. *Nature, 585*, 7.

Occa, A., & Morgan, S. E. (2019). Animations about clinical trial participation for cancer patients and survivors. *Journal of Health Communication, 24*(10), 749–760.

Parekh, N., & Shrank, W. H. (2018). Dangers and opportunities of direct-to-consumer advertising. *Journal of General Internal Medicine, 33*(5), 586–587.

Peng, W., Occa, A., McFarlane, S. J., & Morgan, S. E. (2019). A content analysis of the discussions about clinical trials on a cancer-dedicated online forum. *Journal of Health Communication, 24*(12), 912–922.

PEW. (2013, November 11). *Persuading the prescribers: Pharmaceutical industry marketing and its influence on physicians and patients.* https://www.pewtrusts.org/en/research-and-analysis/fact-sheets/2013/11/11/persuading-the-prescribers-pharmaceutical-industry-marketing-and-its-influence-on-physicians-and-patients

Public Health Service. (2005). *Public Health Service (PHS) policies on research misconduct – 42 CFR Part 93 – June 2005.* https://ori.hhs.gov/public-health-service-phs-policies-research-misconduct-%E2%80%93-42-cfr-part-93-%E2%80%93-june-2005

Schwartz, L. M., & Woloshin, S. (2019). Medical marketing in the United States, 1997–2016. *JAMA, 321*(1), 80–96.

Shmerling, R. H. (2022, March 3). How direct-to-consumer ads hook us. *Harvard Health Ad Watch.* https://www.health.harvard.edu/blog/harvard-health-ad-watch-what-you-should-know-about-direct-to-consumer-ads-2019092017848

Shuster, E. (1997). Fifty years later: The significance of the Nuremberg Code. *The New England Journal of Medicine, 337*(2), 1436–1440.

Silverman, E. (2013). Everything you need to know about the Sunshine Act. *BMJ, 347*, 1–2.

Skloot, R. (2010). *The immortal life of Henrietta Lacks.* Crown.

Spitzberg, B. H., & Cupach, W. R. (1984). *Interpersonal communication competence.* Sage.

van Diemen, J., Verdonk, P., Chieffo, A., Regar, E., Mauri, F., Kunadian, V., Sharma, G., Mehran, R., & Appelman, Y. (2021). The importance of achieving sex- and gender-based equity in clinical trials: A call to action. *European Heart Journal, 42*(31), 2290–2294.

Ventola, C. L. (2011). Direct-to-consumer pharmaceutical advertising: Therapeutic or toxic? *Pharmacy and Therapeutics, 36*(10), 669–684.

Verma, I. M. (2014). Editorial expression of concern and correction. *PNAS, 111*(29), 10779.

Wakefield, A. J., Murch, S. H., Anthony, A., Linnell, J., Casson, D. M., Malik, M., Berelowitz, M., Dhillon, A. P., Thomson, M. A., Harvey, P., Valentine, A., Davies, S. E., & Walker-Smith, J. A. (1998). Ileal-lymphoid-nodular hyperplasia, non-specific colitis, and pervasive developmental disorder in children. *The Lancet, 351*(9103), 637–641.

Wauters, A., & Van Hoyweghen, I. (2016). Global trends on fears and concerns of genetic discrimination: A systematic literature review. *Journal of Human Genetics, 61*, 275–282.

In-class Activities

1. Divide the class into two groups and assign them to argue for or against whether the Facebook study was ethical or not according to the principles of respect for autonomy, nonmaleficence, beneficence, and justice.
2. Visit the FDA's website on prescription drug advertising: https://www.fda.gov/drugs/information-consumers-and-patients-drugs/prescription-drug-advertising. Compare and contrast the examples they provide of correct and incorrect product claim, reminder, and help-seeking ads. Have students share examples of drug advertising they've seen, and see whether they think the ads follow FDA guidelines.

Discussion Questions

1. In the 2001 edition of their book *Principles of Biomedical Ethics*, Beauchamp and Childress present the case of a 69-year-old man who was diagnosed with inoperable, incurable prostate cancer. His doctor, who had been treating him for many years, was faced with breaking the news; however, he was torn. The cancer was early stage and slow growing. He knew that the patient was neurotic and had previously suffered severe depressive episodes when he faced other serious health problems in the past. The patient had only recently recovered from severe depression and a suicide attempt following the death of his wife, who died from cancer. And he was actually looking very forward to

a trip to Australia that had opened up to him. When the physician met with his patient to deliver the diagnosis, the patient asked, "Am I okay? I don't have cancer, do I?" The doctor replied, "You're as good as you were ten years ago." Was the doctor's decision to withhold the bad news ethical? Consider the ethical principles and rules presented in the text to guide discussion.

2. During the COVID-19 pandemic, numerous health policies came under public debate, such as stay-at-home orders, mandatory mask wearing, and vaccine requirements. How do the tensions around these policies demonstrate the dilemmas in the ethical principles of respect for autonomy, nonmaleficence, beneficence, and justice?

3. Imagine you have been tasked with implementing a CBPR program in your home-town with the goal of increasing clinical trial participation. How would you involve community members in your CBPR program? How would you ensure the three communication strategies that McFarlane et al. (2022) identified were enacted?

Unit V

Societal-Level Health Communication Concerns

The Phone That Won't Stop Ringing

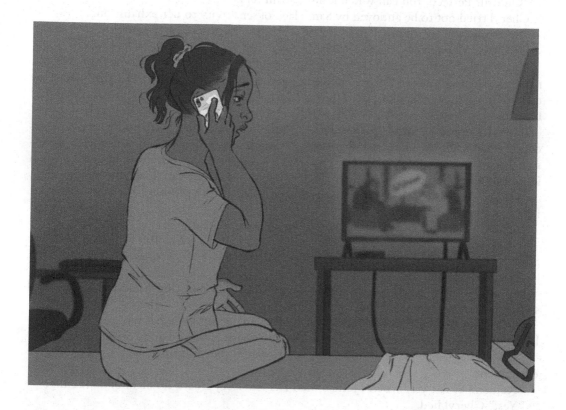

Cheryl had just finished a grueling 10-hour shift and was transitioning to being on call. As she opened the door to her hospital's on-call room, she was startled by the sound of the television blaring. Whoever had been in there last was not kind enough to turn it off. As she reached for the remote, something in the commentary caught her attention. She turned around to see a talk show host on the screen interviewing a leading expert in breast cancer research. Cheryl became engrossed in the report.

"Proving all the ways in which environmental contaminants can increase the risk of breast cancer is very difficult," the expert explained. "But when you look at the last three decades of research all together, there appears to be a very clear link." She went on to tell the host that the important take-away was that pollutants in both the air and water could be major contributors to breast cancer risk.

This was not entirely new information to Cheryl. She was familiar with the American Cancer Society's argument for the theoretical connection between environmental

DOI: 10.4324/9781003214458-28

pollutants and breast cancer. But the timing was fortuitous as Cheryl had just recently learned that breast cancer rates in her hometown were increasing at a suspiciously higher rate than nearby towns in the region. Could environmental factors be at play in her town? Before she could take herself too far down that rabbit hole, her phone rang.

"Hi, Sam," Cheryl said as she turned the television off.

"Have you seen the latest episode?" Sam shouted, clearly excited about something.

Cheryl didn't have to ask what show they were talking about. Sam, who was now twenty and in their second year of college, had been obsessively watching *Queer Eye*.

"No, Sam. I've been working all day and now I'm on call. But I'll call you as soon as I watch it."

"On call? Perfect! You can watch it now," Sam replied.

Cheryl tried not to be annoyed by Sam's lack of sensitivity to her exhaustion.

"Seriously? I'm wiped out, Sam. Can't it wait till tomorrow? What is it with you and this show?" Cheryl asked.

There was a short pause on the phone, then Sam answered. "I don't know. I guess it just makes me feel seen to see these empowered, gay, wonderfully unique individuals from the queer community embracing who they are in front of the entire world. It makes me feel like I'm not alone."

Cheryl dropped her head. She should have known better. She understood where Sam was coming from. It's the same way she felt growing up seeing Black women in major professional roles—especially doctors. She even had a Miranda Bailey poster on her wall in high school. It made her feel seen, and it made her decision to chase her dreams seem realistic.

"Okay. I promise that I'll put it on right now. But I can't promise that I'll stay awake. Deal?" Cheryl bargained.

"DEAL!" Sam shouted and promptly hung up the phone.

Cheryl reached for the remote so she could try to find the show. But to her surprise, her phone rang again. This time it was her Uncle Michael.

"Hey, Uncle Michael," Cheryl answered.

"What's good, Cheryl? You're not going to believe the meeting I had today," Michael stated in a frustrated tone.

Cheryl was thrilled that her uncle didn't expect an answer to "what was good." Between her shift and the television report, she really didn't have anything good to share.

"What happened?" Cheryl replied, trying to hide her exhaustion and channel some excitement.

"Remember last year when I joined the FDA Advisory Board for alcohol marketing?"

"Yes," Cheryl lied.

"Well, here I thought I'd be helping shepherd this FDA into a new era of alcohol marketing regulations consistent with the clear science showing the harms of alcohol on humans. But no. Because do you know who else was at the meeting? Is at *every* meeting?"

Uncle Michael had paused. Cheryl was hoping it was for dramatic effect, but it quickly became clear that he expected an answer this time.

"Kermit the Frog?" Cheryl joked.

"Ha! I wish. I would welcome that green guy with open arms. But no. I am stuck with the most vocal industry representatives, all from major alcohol corporations. At every meeting. And do you know what they care about?"

"Money?" Cheryl quickly responded, assuming a guess was again expected from her.

"You're darn tootin' money. And it doesn't matter at what cost to health. I do not understand why they're allowed to be part of these discussions. This is supposed to be an impartial advisory board. How in the world is an industry representative—who just cares about the bottom line—impartial?"

"Only in a capitalist society, I guess." Cheryl really hoped that her answer didn't get her uncle going. Fortunately, she heard him start talking to someone else in the room.

"Oh hey, Cheryl. I'm sorry. I have to run. But I'll call you tonight and tell you everything!"

"Sounds good, Uncle Michael. Bye."

Cheryl pocketed her phone and flopped onto the small bed. She felt bad to be letting Sam down by not watching the Fab Five on *Queer Eye*, but she knew there was no way she could stay awake for an episode. She closed her eyes, her brain still processing the television report and the challenges of alcohol marketing regulations. Just as she was falling asleep, her phone rang again.

"Hello?" Cheryl mumbled, without looking at who was calling.

"Cheryl." It was Sally. "I have bad news."

Cheryl sat up, knowing this was about Savannah. She had been in the hospital for the last few weeks after finally contracting COVID-19. Cheryl listened as Sally told her that Savannah had succumbed to the disease.

"She passed a few minutes ago," Sally said quietly. "I wanted to call you first. One of the last things she said is how proud she is of you."

"Oh, Mom." Cheryl broke down and sobbed.

Notes

You can read more about the composition of FDA advisory committees here: https://www.fda.gov/drugs/information-consumers-and-patients-drugs/advisory-committees-critical-fdas-product-review-process

The U.S. Department of Health and Human Services periodically generates a *Report on Carcinogens*, which provides a list of substances "known or reasonably anticipated" to cause cancer. In the ninth edition of the report, published May 15, 2000, alcohol was added to the list: https://www.federalregister.gov/documents/2001/05/30/01-13485/national-toxicology-program-ntp-availability-of-the-report-on-carcinogens-ninth-edition. In the 15th edition of the report, published December 21, 2021, evidence of the carcinogenicity of alcohol is reviewed further: https://ntp.niehs.nih.gov/ntp/roc/content/profiles/alcoholicbeverageconsumption.pdf

Even with the availability of the vaccine, deaths from COVID-19 continue to haunt families. The CDC track cases, deaths, hospitalizations, and vaccinations here: https://covid.cdc.gov/covid-data-tracker/#datatracker-home

12 Health Communication in the Media

Think of a health topic, any topic. Did you think about eating tasty food? About talking to a healthcare provider? About safety protocols at work? Maybe you thought about starting that exercise routine you've been putting off? No matter what you thought about, there's been an episode covering the topic on *Grey's Anatomy*, it's been the subject of discussion on a sub-Reddit, and some journalist somewhere has written on it. The pervasive coverage of health across media platforms isn't surprising because people are mortal creatures who care about issues surrounding life and death. But media platforms do more than just convey neutral content about health topics. How they cover topics has the potential to shape the perceptions and behaviors of audiences.

Media content has the potential to influence people's knowledge about health; understanding of healthcare systems, practices, and approaches; attitudes toward diseases and preventive behaviors; and beliefs about what causes diseases and how to cure them. It also can influence which health topics people think are the most pressing at any given time. Sometimes, media can be used as a tool to help people live healthier lives. But other times, media can be used as a way to manipulate or confuse viewers. Whether for good or evil, there's no denying the effect of media on the health-related perceptions and behaviors of audiences.

In this chapter, we'll highlight the key ways that media can influence health. We'll start by reviewing research showing media's relationship to health perceptions and behaviors, including the role of celebrities and parasocial relationships and the power of advertising. Following that, we'll explore two communication strategies for promoting good health: public health communication campaigns and entertainment-education. To accompany this comprehensive review, we've included two theory tables for your learning enjoyment.

Media and Health

Media messages are important because research shows that they influence audience perceptions and behaviors. In recent decades, communication researchers have been especially focused on behaviors that pose the greatest risk to viewers' health. These include alcohol use, smoking (and in recent years, vaping), violence, risky sex, and seeing unrealistic body images in television, film, and advertising. In particular, classic media theories have been especially essential to building scholarly understanding of the extent to which media can influence not only viewer perceptions about health but also viewer behavior. Let's look at some examples of how.

Regarding perceptions, numerous media theories (see Table 12.1), including **cultivation theory** (Gerbner et al., 1986) and **agenda setting** (McCombs & Shaw, 1972), outline explanations for how media can affect how audiences see the world. This is especially true regarding the media's obsession with unrealistic beauty ideals. For women, this typically

DOI: 10.4324/9781003214458-29

comes in the form of celebrating thin, white women as the ultimate beauty standard (Redmond, 2003). For men, this typically comes in the form of a hyper-muscular body type (Jung, 2011). The question is whether these biased depictions of femininity and masculinity are influencing the perceptions of consumers. Qian Huang and colleagues (2021) sought to answer this question through a meta-analysis of 127 internationally diverse studies representing the United States, United Kingdom, Australia, Belgium, Canada, Germany, France, Netherlands, Israel, and Fiji. They found that "more appearance-related media exposure was significantly associated with negative body-image outcomes" (p. 14). Interestingly, the researchers did not find a difference in the effect between men and women. However, they did note that "media contents without obtrusively commercial purposes, such as television programs and music videos, may produce greater effects on negative body outcomes than commercial contents, such as television advertisements" (Huang et al., 2021, p. 42).

Regarding behavior, **social cognitive theory** (Bandura, 1986; see Table 12.1), as well as its predecessor, **social learning theory** (Bandura, 1969), is one of the most cited theories for examining media influence on audience behavior. The theory posits that people will often "model" the behaviors they witness, particularly if those behaviors are positively rewarded in some way. A large body of research supporting the influence of media use on behavioral modeling targets cigarette smoking. As one example, in a longitudinal study of more than 2,500 adolescents living in Vermont or New Hampshire, Madeline Dalton and colleagues (2003) found that adolescents with the highest amount of exposure to smoking in movies were 2.71 times more likely to smoke than adolescents with the lowest exposure. They concluded that "viewing smoking in movies strongly predicts whether or not adolescents initiate smoking, and the effect increases significantly with greater exposure" (Dalton et al., 2003, p. 284). Such findings are what led to a 2007 decision by the Motion Picture Association of American (MPAA) to include smoking and tobacco imagery as a factor in their ratings (MPAA, 2018). And just in case you weren't convinced that smoking deserves to be listed as a warning at the start of films, a study by James Sargent and colleagues (2012) estimated that if the MPAA were to give an "R" rating to movies with smoking, the number of teen smokers would be reduced by 18%, preventing up to 1 million deaths from smoking. That's a lot of lives being put at risk by exposure to media content.

Media has a clear ability to influence viewer perceptions and behaviors regarding health. So far, our examples have centered on general media consumption, such as movies and

Table 12.1 Theoretical Frameworks in Mediated Health Communication

Theory/Model	Brief Summary	Citation
Agenda Setting	Media priorities shape audience priorities in that the media don't tell audiences what to think, but through their coverage of certain topics, they do tell audiences what to think about.	McCombs and Shaw (1972)
Cultivation Theory	Exposure to media shapes how audiences perceive the world.	Gerbner et al. (1986)
Social Cognitive Theory	Individual perceptions and behaviors are a product of individual experiences, observing the actions of others, and environmental factors.	Bandura (1986)
Social Learning Theory	People learn new behaviors by observing others' behavior. Behaviors that are rewarded are more likely to be repeated. Self-efficacy, or a person's belief that they're capable of engaging in a particular behavior, is a central construct.	Bandura (1969)

Note. See *Supplemental Online Theory Table* for additional theories/models.

television shows. But celebrity stories in the media can also influence people's health. The next section will explore this idea further.

Celebrity Health Narratives

What is it about watching someone on the screen save the world, fall in love, shoot the game-winning shot, or talk at their audience for hours that makes people feel such a strong connection to them? Viewers are unlikely to ever meet the celebrities they love most, yet if the celebrities asked them to, their fans might be willing to follow them off a cliff. Okay, hopefully no one idolizes any celebrity *that* much. But it turns out that the most beloved celebrities can influence perceptions and behaviors. Long before the term "influencers" entered our media vocabulary, celebrities, including actors, athletes, musicians, politicians, and the wealthy, were leveraged for their ability to persuade audiences, including around the topic of health.

Sometimes celebrities are compensated for their endorsement of health-related products, such as being paid for commercial advertising. But other times, celebrities share their health opinions and experiences for the simple reason of seeking human connection during often difficult or challenging times. These moments are referred to as **health events**, and they can include everything from planned press conferences to leaks in the press. Research has found that the more viewers identify or connect with a particular celebrity, the more likely they're to be affected by the celebrity's health event (Kresovich & Noar, 2020). Research has also found that a health event often expands into a larger celebrity **health narrative**, where celebrities must navigate the public–private communication tension of publicly sharing their private health journeys (see Beck et al., 2015).

One of the most widely discussed examples of a health event that turned into a health narrative involves legendary basketball player Earvin "Magic" Johnson and his 1991 press announcement that he was HIV-positive. Immediately following the announcement, the Centers for Disease Control and Prevention (CDC) reported a rise in calls to their National AIDS Hotline that lasted months (Rogers, 2002). This rise was echoed in local city hotlines across the United States (e.g., Cohn et al., 1992). In addition, researchers found that Mr. Johnson's biggest fans developed greater concerns about sexual responsibility (Brown & Basil, 1995). Keep in mind, this influence was found pre-social media. Magic Johnson's health event was an intentional effort to raise awareness for HIV/AIDS prevention (Iyer, 1991), and he took on the mantle of becoming a public health spokesperson for HIV/AIDS prevention. However, even when celebrity health events don't lead to taking on official spokesperson roles, they can still have similar outcomes.

For example, in 2013, actor, director, and humanitarian Angelina Jolie announced that she had tested positive for the $BRCA_1$ gene mutation, putting her at high risk for developing breast cancer. As a result, she underwent an elective double mastectomy, a procedure that greatly reduces the risk of developing breast cancer (National Cancer Institute, 2020). In an op-ed in *The New York Times*, Jolie (2013) wrote that she was sharing her decision in the hope "that other women can benefit from [her] experience" and that she wanted

> to encourage every woman, especially if you have a family history of breast or ovarian cancer, to seek out the information and medical experts who can help you through this aspect of your life, and to make your own informed choices.
>
> (n.p.)

Jolie's op-ed is a prime example of a celebrity recognizing that her decision could influence the decisions of countless other women. Yet, unlike Magic Johnson, she stopped short of dedicating herself as a spokesperson for the cause.

Still, the impact of her health event on audiences was so strong that in a cover story, *Time* magazine labeled the aftermath of her op-ed as the "Angelina Effect" (Park, 2013), with researchers finding similar audience outcomes to Magic Johnson's health event. Within a week of the publication of Jolie's op-ed, the National Cancer Institute (NCI) reported a 795-fold increase in the number of online visitors to their fact sheet page, *Preventative Mastectomy* (Juthe et al., 2015). Similarly, in a longitudinal analysis from 1997 to 2016, Alexander Liede and colleagues (2018) reported finding a statistically significant increase in genetic testing for the $BRCA_1$ gene mutation and in risk-reducing mastectomies among women 18 and older *after* Jolie's health event. Although most studies center on U.S. audiences, these effects were not exclusive to Americans. D. Gareth Evans and colleagues (2014) analyzed 21 family history clinics and regional genetics centers in the United Kingdom and found that both referral rates and requests for BRCA testing almost doubled following Jolie's op-ed.

The health events of Magic Johnson and Angelina Jolie, both of which grew into larger health narratives, are just two examples of the potential power of celebrity health narratives to influence audiences. But why do health narratives have such a powerful influence on audience health perceptions and behaviors? One explanation is that it occurs due to a strong bond the audience feels with the celebrity or a character played by the celebrity. This bond is called a parasocial relationship.

Parasocial Relationships

Parasocial relationships are the one-sided interactions between viewers and media personalities leading to a connection that extends beyond the moments of watching the show (Liebers & Schram, 2019). Parasocial relationships can be connections built with fictional characters or with the celebrities themselves. For example, we will forever argue that there was a great loss to the scientific community when Spock decided not to attend the Vulcan Science Academy (even though he did pretty well as a member of Starfleet). Parasocial connections can have both positive and negative outcomes on people's health. Let's start with two positive examples.

Following the suicide of beloved actor Robin Williams, Cynthia Hoffner and Elizabeth Cohen (2018) were interested in how his death influenced the mental health help-seeking behaviors of people with a strong parasocial connection to him. To explore this question, the researchers surveyed 350 U.S. adults about their feelings toward Robin Williams, media exposure to coverage of his death, perceptions of depression, and willingness to seek mental health treatment. They found that adults with stronger parasocial connections to Williams had a greater willingness to seek treatment for depression and more frequent outreach to others experiencing depression or suicidal thoughts.

In another example, Nathan Walter and colleagues (2022) were interested in how celebrity parasocial relationships affected perceived susceptibility to COVID-19 and engaging in COVID-19 protective behaviors. Following analyses of a two-part survey among U.S. adults, the researchers concluded that having a parasocial relationship with "a celebrity who tested positive for COVID-19 can increase perceived susceptibility to the virus, in turn, positively affecting intent to engage in protective behaviors" (Walter et al., 2022, p. 609). They further argued that celebrities serve as important agents of public health education in that "celebrities, particularly those who were diagnosed with the virus, are well-positioned to increase awareness and join the effort to prevent not only the spread of the current pandemic but other enduring health threats as well" (Walter et al., 2022, p. 615).

Now that we've presented two positive examples of how parasocial relationships can influence audience health, let's look at one example from the other side of the coin. Keren

Eyal and Tali Téeni-Harari (2013) were concerned that media exposure might negatively affect adolescent body image. In a survey of 391 seventh and eighth graders in Israel, the researchers asked participants to report their favorite same-sex television character and complete a series of questions measuring their parasocial interaction with that character. Through their analysis, the researchers found that stronger parasocial relationships were "positively associated with greater social comparison with the favorite character, which was, in turn, associated with an enlarged discrepancy between the actual and ideal body shape; this discrepancy was negatively associated with body image" (Eyal & Téeni-Harari, 2013, p. 137). Thus, the strong parasocial tie made teenagers feel worse about their bodies.

In sum, the media, including celebrities and the characters they play, can influence the health perceptions and behaviors of audiences. Depending on the context, these influences can promote health in a positive or negative way. Health communication scholars seek to understand these influences to better understand individual health perceptions and behaviors and how to design interventions to overcome negative influences.

Media Influences on Health

Media influences audience health in a variety of ways. Cultivation theory shows how the media can influence perceptions of health. Social learning theory shows how the media can influence behaviors. Celebrity health events and health narratives also influence perceptions and behaviors. The concept of parasocial relationships is one explanation for why celebrities, and the characters they play, can be so influential for audiences.

Advertising

For decades, the power of advertising over audiences has fascinated media researchers—including health communication scholars. Corporate advertising for health-related products inherently navigates two tensions: making money and promoting healthy living. Sometimes these two goals can align, but when they don't, corporations will, for economic survival reasons, pick making money, which often comes at the expense of public health. Just ask anyone who needs to purchase insulin or an EpiPen. The need to prioritize making money wouldn't matter so much except for the mountain of evidence showing that advertising has a strong impact on consumers' health perceptions and behaviors. To demonstrate, we'll examine the literature on alcohol and tobacco advertising to show the implications of those messages on public health.

Regarding alcohol, there have been numerous studies on the influence of alcohol advertisements. In a review of such studies, Anders Hansen and Barrie Gunter (2013) begin by showing that early studies in the 1980s and 1990s concluded that exposure to alcohol advertising was associated with increased alcohol consumption. However, they go on to show how more recent studies suggested the relationship wasn't that direct. More specifically, they conclude that "What is also apparent is that if alcohol advertising does ultimately influence consumption, this process is more likely to be indirect than direct, operating via brand awareness and liking, or even via internalized cognitions about alcohol and its consumption" (p. 301). The recognition of contingent persuasive message effects has led to an era of more focused study on the features of alcohol messages that specifically result in more persuasive outcomes. For instance, a recent study found that young adult consumers hold a greater intention to drink when younger-looking models are featured (Alhabash et al., 2021).

The history of tobacco advertising is one of the most documented areas at the intersection of marketing and health. Reasons for this stem from the decades of tobacco industry coverup regarding the known consequences of tobacco use (Bero, 2003), the billions of dollars in advertising spent annually by the tobacco industry (Federal Trade Commission, 2021), and the evidence that the advertising by the tobacco industry worked to create generations of addicted tobacco users (e.g., Pierce et al., 1998). In addition, the tobacco industry is one of the few industries to face substantial legal consequences for their advertising practices. In the landmark 1998 tobacco *Master Settlement Agreement,* the deception of the tobacco industry and the irreversible damage their marketing caused for users—especially among minority populations (Public Health Law Center & American Lung Association California, 2021)—led to a lawsuit filed against the industry by 46 states, five U.S. territories, and the District of Columbia. The end agreement required the industry to annually, and indefinitely, pay the settling states billions of dollars, as well as imposing substantial restrictions on advertising, including forbidding advertiser to target youth in their marking (Public Health Law Center, n.d.).

Given the known power of advertising on consumer perceptions and behavior, most governments have some form of monitoring over commercial advertising. In the United States, most regulations on advertising stem from one of two federal agencies: the Federal Trade Commission (FTC) and the Food and Drug Administration (FDA). As is laid out in a 1971 memorandum of understanding, the FTC is the primary regulator of the truth or falsity of claims made in product advertisements, except ads for prescription drugs. The FDA is the primary regulator of prescription drug advertising (see Chapter 11), as well as regulating the content of product labels (FTC, 1971). This means that if a beer company wants to run an advertisement during the Super Bowl, the content of the commercial falls under the jurisdiction of the FTC. However, if you were to buy that beer at a store, the content you see on the label of the bottle falls under the jurisdiction of the FDA. Both regulatory agencies not only provide guidelines for what advertisers *can't* say, such as banning cigarette ads from claiming smoking has positive health effects (which is a lie and thus banned by both the FTC and FDA), but can also require advertisers to include specific content, such the FDA (2011) regulation for cigarette packages and advertisements to contain at least one of nine warning statements (e.g., WARNING: Cigarettes are addictive; WARNING: Cigarettes cause cancer; WARNING: Cigarettes cause strokes and heart disease).

The regulatory oversight, although successful in reducing public health consequences stemming from misleading and manipulative advertising, has not slowed industries from advertising their products on a mass scale to consumers. Advertisers continue to find novel and persuasive approaches to marketing their products. For instance, prior to the FDA's tightened regulations on the advertising of vaping products, vape companies featured celebrity endorsements in their Instagram marketing, which was shown to significantly increase positive perceptions of vaping (Phua et al., 2018).

Public Health Communication Campaigns

The prevalence of advertisements can make it feel like all media messages are created for the purpose of making money. But that isn't always the case. In fact, there's an entire subset of research focused on using the media as a tool to promote positive health behaviors regardless of whether anyone makes money on the changed behavior. Enter public health communication campaigns. **Public health communication campaigns** are

> purposive attempts to inform or influence behaviors in large audiences within a specified time period using an organized set of communication activities and featuring an

array of mediated messages in multiple channels generally to produce noncommercial benefits to individuals and society.

(Rice & Atkin, 2013, p. 3)

Through this definition, you can discern the multiple aspects that make up a public health communication campaign.

First, public health communication campaigns are *purposeful*, or intentional. They're not messages that just happen to inform or influence a large audience. Instead, they require dedicated resources, detailed planning, and specific end goals to achieve changes in specific audiences. Second, they're *time bound*. Public health communication campaigns don't run indefinitely but are planned for dissemination during a specific period of time. Third, public health communication campaigns use an *organized set of communication activities*. The term "organized" refers to approaches being grounded in evidence, building on knowledge of what has worked in the past, and having theoretical foundations that provide logical guidelines for persuasive efforts. Finally, and most notably, public health communication campaigns *do not produce a commercial benefit*. Although there may be economic benefits, such as reduced waste of resources to treat preventable diseases, nobody's pockets are being lined.

Because public health communication campaigns are noncommercial, they're somewhat different from advertising campaigns. **Advertising campaigns** promote commercial goods and services that range from the substantial to superficial, whereas public health communication campaigns promote one central, ego-involved, and supremely important topic: people's health (Elliott, 1987). For example, an advertising campaign might market an easily obtainable product that you want (maybe a delicious slice of pizza), whereas a public health communication campaign might advocate for you to avoid risky health behaviors that are often enjoyable ("Put that pizza down!"). Similarly, a public health communication campaign might also advocate for adopting behaviors that involve a short-term sacrifice, such as checking your heart rate or running for 30 minutes, for the sake of long-term benefits that are not necessarily guaranteed, such as a reduced risk of cardiovascular disease.

Although researchers don't expect public health communication campaigns to have the same effects as advertising campaigns (predominantly due to the lack of resources relative to those typically invested in an advertising campaign), research shows that these campaigns have evolved over time in terms of design sophistication and outcome expectations to be quite effective at changing perceptions and behaviors (Rice & Atkin, 2013). Indeed, effective public health communication campaigns can result in *small to moderate* effects among *large to very large* groups of people. Although "small to moderate" may not sound impressive, these effects are very important when you consider entire populations. For instance, a 1% improvement in the health of the U.S. population means more than 3 million people would see improvement in their health. But not every public health threat is appropriate for a public health communication campaign.

Daniel Catalán-Matamoros (2011) suggests that public health communication campaigns are most appropriate when the following conditions apply:

- Wide exposure is desired
- The timeframe is urgent
- Public discussion is likely to facilitate change
- Awareness is a main goal
- Media authorities (e.g., journalists, editors, producers, stations) are on your side
- Other program components support change
- Long-term release of information is feasible
- A generous budget exists

- The behavioral change is simple
- The agenda includes public relations to increase wide-ranging exposure

Additionally, Noar (2006) concluded that health communication campaign success is more likely when campaign designers adhere to the following guidelines:

- Conduct formative research
- Use theory as a foundation for the campaign
- Segment the audience (split it up based on relevant characteristics)
- Use a targeted message design focus (design messages based on the relevant targeting characteristics)
- Place messages in strategic communication channels
- Conduct a process evaluation
- Use a sensitive outcome evaluation that will generate causal arguments about the campaign's influence on attitudes and behaviors

With such complexity involved in developing a successful campaign, understanding how and why campaigns work is essential. Most campaign scholars study the campaign process in three distinct phases: formative evaluation, process evaluation, and summative evaluation. The following sections will take you through the processes and goals of each phase.

Phases of Public Health Communication Campaign Implementation

Public health communication campaigns are implemented through three distinct evaluation phases:

- Formative evaluation (design stage)
- Process evaluation (implementation stage)
- Summative evaluation (outcome evaluation stage)

Design and Formative Evaluation

Formative evaluation, often called the design phase, is the stage of the campaign process when all the decisions are made before the public ever sees any content related to the campaign. The following paragraphs will highlight five key areas of formative evaluation: goal identification, theoretical foundations, audience targeting, channel selection, and message design. In this phase, it's also important to determine an evaluation plan. However, because the plan isn't needed until the last phase, we'll discuss evaluation plans in a later section. Across the five areas we're discussing now, campaign designers should keep in mind the role of culture in every aspect of their planning. Campaigns that don't recognize the cultural nuances of their audiences' health behavior goals, preferred communication channels, and language are unlikely to be successful. For instance, Natalie Tindall and Jennifer Vardeman-Winter (2011) conducted a closer examination of the United States' Heart Truth campaign (colloquially known as the Red Dress campaign), which was intended to be inclusive of all women for heart disease prevention. In their interviews with Black, Latina, and Asian American women, the researchers discovered that the campaign might have treated women too much as a monolith, with women of color not connecting with, or changing their behavior in response to, the campaign messages.

Another example is a qualitative case study examining health insurance literacy, a study that was designed to be able to provide key lessons for public health education and campaigns. Elizabeth Sayers and her colleagues (2021) analyzed focus group discussions from members of marginalized Haitian Creole, Mandarin, Native American, and Vietnamese communities. In their analysis, the authors identified the following five important lessons for public health education and campaigns regarding cultural sensitivity in messaging: (a) use culture-centered materials to build empathy and trust, (b) ensure appropriate and salient translations of materials into local languages, (c) use community-specific channels to disseminate messages and materials, (d) incorporate interpersonal communication opportunities for community members, and (e) leverage organizational partners to build networks and increase the overall reach of messages and materials. As you read the following sections, keep in mind the cultural aspects that could be different for different audiences.

Goal Identification

Like any project, the first step in campaign design is to decide what you're actually trying to accomplish. Determining your public health communication campaign *goal* is the most important step of campaign design because it sets the stage for everything to come. Drawing on the work of Gael O'Sullivan and colleagues (2003), Kami Silk and colleagues (2022) think of this stage as a "conceptual analysis" where campaign designers approach the situation "to understand the behavioral aspects of the health problem and to determine which actions should be performed by which people in order to improve health outcomes" (p. 336). In other words, focused campaign goals should tell you *what* you're hoping to change in *whom*. What you change might be a behavior, such as improving the number of vegetable servings someone eats per day. But it could also be an intention to perform a behavior or perceptions surrounding how people think about the behavior (e.g., improve attitudes toward the idea of eating vegetables).

When deciding who your audience will be, you have two choices. The recipient of your message might be the person who is going to directly benefit from the changed behavior, such as the person you'd like to eat more servings of vegetables. But it could also be people around that person who have an influence on what the person does. For example, if you were trying to increase the number of vegetable servings a child eats, you might try to target parents, who purchase the foods kept at home, or school boards, who determine which foods are available in schools. Before you can do anything else in your campaign, you must determine a focused, clear "what" and "who." Moving forward, every decision comes back to what makes the most sense for your attitude/intention/behavior and audience.

Target Audience

Once you know broadly whose behavior (or attitude or intention) you're trying to change, it's important to target that audience as specifically as possible. For example, if you're trying to reduce vaping among teens, you might be interested in lowering the national vaping rate, but you also might be interested in lowering the vaping rate in regions with the highest rate of use or among certain at-risk populations with the highest rate of use. Michael Slater (1996) presents a thorough discussion of various characteristics along which audiences can be *segmented*, including psychographics, demographics, geographics, and other relevant theoretical constructs and variables. Since Slater's review, changes in technology have only made it easier to segment audiences based on these characteristics by using data from people's online information (including information about behavior) as a means to reach and target individuals (Evans et al., 2019). Moreso, social media platforms typically include tools that allow messages to target a variety of audience characteristics, such as age, race, gender, education, employment, hobbies, interests, search history, and many more. The ability to use these tools has substantially improved researchers' ability to reach their intended audience. For instance, in a thirdhand smoke awareness campaign guided by McGuire's communication-persuasion model (see Table 12.2), Rachael Record and colleagues (2023) used Facebook's advertising algorithm to target California adults who were either most at risk of exposure to thirdhand tobacco smoke themselves or who had children or pets who would be at risk. They reached 1.89 million users in only four months (and for only $10,500, which means they paid less than a penny per person).

Theoretical Foundations

When designing campaigns, there are a lot of moving parts to consider. The best way to guide the decision-making process is to draw upon communication theory to inform choices and strategies. Some of these theories are presented in Table 12.2. To date, there is no overarching theory of campaigns. Instead, campaign designers employ theory at various stages in the process to guide all aspects of the formative evaluation stage. Some theories provide guidance for creating messages. For instance, the *extended parallel process model* (Witte, 1992) provides a foundation for creating messages that seek to scare audiences into behavior change. Other theories provide guidance for audience targeting. For example, through the lens of the *transtheoretical model*, also known as the stages of change model (Prochaska & Velicer, 1997), behavior change is understood as a series of stages that people go through. This model posits that in order to get people to the larger end goal of behavior change, you need to know where they are now (e.g., maybe they're not even aware they

Table 12.2 Theoretical Frameworks in Health Communication Campaigns

Theory/Model	Brief Summary	Citation
Extended Parallel Process Model	Fear appeals trigger relationships between perceived threat and efficacy. When an individual perceives their efficacy to be greater than the threat, they will work to control and prevent the threat. When an individual perceives the threat to be greater than their efficacy, they will work to control the fear instead of the threat.	Witte (1992)
McGuire's Communication-Persuasion Model	Campaign designers' evidence-based decisions about five key inputs (goal, source, message, channel, and receiver) will trigger 12 outputs (ranging from exposure to the communication to post-behavioral consolidating) as mediating steps in the persuasion process.	McGuire (2013)
Theory of Planned Behavior	Attitude, subjective norms, and behavioral control will predict behavioral intention, which in turn predicts actual behavior.	Ajzen (1985)
Transtheoretical Model	The transtheoretical model posits that health behavior change involves progress through five stages of change: precontemplation (not seriously considering behavior change), contemplation (actively considering behavior change), preparation (committed to behavior change), action (engaging in modified behavior), and maintenance (sustained enactment of newly developed behavior).	Prochaska and Velicer (1997)

Note. See *Supplemental Online Theory Table* for additional theories/models.

should change their behavior) and work to move them to the next step, as opposed to jumping straight to the end goal, which might be a few steps away.

Perhaps the most cited model for considering the comprehensive development of all the parts of the campaign process is **McGuire's communication-persuasion model**, or input-output matrix (see McGuire, 2013). This model provides a framework for what goes into and what comes out of a campaign. The inputs are the communication factors: source, message, channel, receiver (audience), and destination (campaign goal). The outputs are the steps to persuasion, ranging from tuning in and attending to the communication to changing behavior and even encouraging others to do so (e.g., an evangelical former smoker). You might think of McGuire's Matrix like a recipe for a campaign, where you get to change the ingredients based on your goals. Just as following a recipe is much more likely to get you an edible cake, using theory to guide campaign design is much more likely to lead to positive outcomes.

Channel Selection

Where you decide to post your campaign messages can make or break a great campaign plan, for what's the point of having a great campaign if no one you intended to see the messages ever does? Campaign designers will achieve greater effects when they find the means for getting persuasive messages to their target audience, as opposed to disseminating messages among larger audiences who aren't as likely to be persuaded. For example, commercial messages targeting women's heart health should be broadcast on the channels that report the highest numbers of women viewers. The key to this endeavor is closely examining where and when your segmented audience consumes media.

Today, with advances in technology, campaigns can also be improved by finding ways to interact with audience members through the use of the internet, especially social media. Instead of traditional 30-second public service announcements on TV, campaigns can now include opportunities for audiences to visit a website, interact in a discussion forum, or complete activities, such as through an online learning module. Similarly, on social media, audiences can like, share, or comment on the campaign messages. For example, Rachel Powell and colleagues (2022) launched a campaign seeking to prevent unintended pregnancy among women living in Puerto Rico. Guided by the theory of planned behavior (see Table 12.2), the campaign launched during the 2016–2017 Zika virus outbreak when concerns were rising over adverse Zika-related pregnancy and birth outcomes. As one element of their campaign strategy, the researchers launched an interactive Facebook page that allowed for two-way communication between their team and the target audience. In addition, Facebook users who visited the campaign page could invite others to join the conversation through tagging and sharing. The authors concluded that the campaign successfully raised awareness of available services, such as access to contraceptives, with the Facebook page having the largest audience reach.

Message Design

At last. We're finally at the place we bet you were expecting us to start: designing the campaign messages. Most people are surprised at how much work goes into designing a campaign before ever considering what you're going to say in your campaign messages. But until you know who your audience is, what you're trying to ask of your audience, and where you're going to reach your audience, you cannot know with any assurance what you should say to them. Effective public health communication campaign messages will include clear **calls to action**, or statements telling their audience exactly what you want (or don't want) them to do, such as "Don't do drugs!" "Eat your veggies!" or "Schedule a medical visit today!" Most importantly, messages should be designed to culturally resonate with the identified target audience.

For instance, Stephanie Chao and Samuel So (2011) carefully detailed the design decisions that went into creating messages for the Jade Ribbon Campaign that was designed to increase awareness of Hepatitis B among Asians and Pacific Islanders. In their account, they demonstrate the need to understand current cultural practices and integrate feedback from the target audience. For example, they used an image of a traditional awareness ribbon, but they modified it slightly to appear as the Chinese character for "people," symbolizing "the united voices of those fighting hepatitis B and liver cancer worldwide" (Chao & So, 2011, p. 48). Such design considerations let them develop a campaign that was not only successful but also meaningful. Once you have your messages designed, it's time to pretest them with your target audience.

Indeed, one of the things campaign planners tend to forget is that just because they think something will be well received by a target audience doesn't mean it will be. You won't know for sure unless you double-check with your target audience. In public health communication campaigns, this happens by pretesting messages. **Pretesting** allows campaign designers to gather feedback on their messages and make changes before the campaign launches. Whereas quantitative methods, such as surveys and experiments, are often most effective for evaluating whether a campaign is likely to influence behavior in the target audience, qualitative methods, such as interviews and focus groups, are often most effective for identifying which aspects of messages are resonating with audiences and which are falling flat. Silk and colleagues (2022) note that gathering feedback from pretesting is especially helpful in assessing "whether the audience regards the content and style as informative, believable, motivating, convincing, useful, on-target, and enjoyable rather than too preachy, disturbing, confusing, irritating, or dull" (p. 337). Although all feedback doesn't have to result in changes to the messages, reasonable and sound suggestions should be taken into account before finalizing the messages. And ideally, if resources are available, the revised messages will be pretested again before going into final production.

Implementation and Process Evaluation

You have designed a campaign grounded in theory, with clear goals for a specific audience that will see your persuasively designed messages in pre-planned channels. Now you just need to sit back and wait for the pre-determined campaign end date to see if the campaign worked—or maybe it's not time to sit back just yet. After campaign design, the implementation work, or the process evaluation phase, begins. The process evaluation stage is the most straightforward phase of the campaign stages in that it seeks to answer one simple question: Is everything going according to plan? **Process evaluation** monitors exposure and attention to campaign messages while the campaign is running. This information is useful for determining the success of campaign management and identifying any unexpected obstacles to campaign effectiveness. For print-based campaigns, such as billboard ads, this could mean driving by the billboard to make sure the advertisement was actually installed and that it hasn't been vandalized. For print newspaper advertisements, this could mean opening each issue of the newspaper to make sure the advertisement actually appears on the page. For online messages, such as YouTube videos or Facebook posts, this could mean setting a daily or weekly schedule to make sure that the platform hasn't taken down the messages or that the links aren't broken. For online messages, you may also have to hide any extremely negative or irrelevant comments. What's important during the process evaluation phase is that the campaign designers be able to confidently report that the messages were in fact disseminated to their target audience as planned.

Campaign Effects and Summative Evaluation

Congratulations! You designed and launched your campaign and made sure it went according to plan. You're now in the **summative evaluation**, or outcome evaluation, phase. This phase seeks to answer the question: Did your campaign achieve the goal that you set at the beginning of the formative design stage? To answer this question, you need to have determined an **evaluation plan** prior to the start of the campaign. The reason an evaluation plan needed to be decided before now is because outcome evaluation procedures often run alongside campaign design and implementation activities. We'll demonstrate what we mean as we discuss the most common experimental designs for evaluating a campaign's effectiveness.

At this point in your life, you've probably heard the expression "correlation is not causation." This expression refers to the fact that just because two things appear together doesn't mean that one is causing the other to occur. For instance, ice cream sales go up around the same time of the year that burglaries increase. This association does not mean that ice cream sales are causing more burglaries or vice versa (even though successful burglars may think they deserve an ice cream cone as a reward for their heist). The causal factor explaining increases in ice cream sales and burglaries is the time of year: People tend to eat more ice cream in the summer, and people also tend to leave the windows of their homes open in the summer, making it more likely for their homes to be burgled.

Teasing out causation from correlation is relevant to campaign designers because from the beginning, the goal has been to cause some sort of change in a particular belief or behavior. So how do campaign designers establish that their campaign actually caused a change in behavior and that the effect wasn't just correlational coincidence? Thomas Valente and Patchareeya Kwan (2013) give a detailed overview of the research methods used to determine the effects of a campaign. For the most part, these methods include cross-sectional or longitudinal field experiments that allow for causal arguments about the relationship between campaign exposure and attitude or behavior change. We'll briefly review two types of experimental designs often used by campaign designers to evaluate the effectiveness of their campaigns. For additional reading, we encourage you to check out Ronald Rice and Charles Atkin's (2013) book on the subject.

Pretest/Posttest Control Group Design

One of the most traditional, straightforward experimental designs is that of the pretest/posttest control group design. First, data is collected before the campaign is launched (pretest). Second, data is collected after the campaign ends (posttest). In addition, data is collected not only from members of the target audience who saw the campaign messages but also from members of the target audience who did *not* see the campaign messages (the control group). These two groups should be as similar as possible in every way *except* campaign exposure to rule out other potential explanations for any campaign effects. Campaign designers then analyze the data to see whether there was a statistically significant pre-post change in the outcome variable for the target group but not for the control group. If so, the campaign is deemed effective. Let's look at an example.

Sara LaBelle and colleagues (2020) worked with students in an undergraduate strategic communication course to develop a public health communication campaign called

Rethink. Guided by the theory of planned behavior, the *Rethink* campaign targeted college students and had a goal of decreasing misuse of prescription stimulants, such as Adderall, Ritalin, and Concerta. The campaign was run on one campus, which served as the experimental group. Another campus similar to the experimental campus was selected as the control group. Communication students on both campuses were recruited to complete a pretest survey before the implementation of the campaign. Two weeks after the campaign was implemented at the experimental campus, the same students on both campuses completed a posttest survey. In examining posttest scores between the experimental and control groups, the researchers found that although students exposed to the *Rethink* campaign held significantly lower attitudes toward the misuse of prescription stimulants, the "behavioral elements" were not different between the two groups (LaBelle et al., 2020, p. 22). Similarly, differences in perceived social norms regarding the misuse of prescription stimulants did not vary as expected by the researchers. The authors concluded that although the campaign did not effectively change behavior, it did promote changes in attitudes, which is an important predictor of behavior change. In other words, it was a step in the right direction.

Pretest/Posttest Non-Control Group Design

Sometimes identifying a control group isn't feasible for campaign designers. There can be numerous reasons for this. For instance, researchers who design a nationwide campaign for COVID-19 prevention that targets all U.S. adults might not be able to find a reasonable comparison nation. Other times, resources might not be available to gather data from a control group. In these circumstances, campaign planners might rely on simply finding a statistical difference between pre- and post-campaign measures among members of the target audience. Although they might have lower confidence in their results (because something other than the campaign messages could have influenced the target audience), they can still provide provisional support that the campaign worked. Let's look at an example that includes some of your favorite textbook authors—us!

Guided by the theory of planned behavior, Record and colleagues (2017) developed a campaign called *Let's Clear the Air* to improve compliance with a smoke-free college campus policy. Specifically, their goal was to reduce the number of undergraduate students smoking on a campus where smoking was no longer allowed. Survey data was collected from students three weeks before campaign implementation and three weeks after. To determine campaign effectiveness, the researchers compared pretest survey responses to posttest responses, finding a significant decrease in the self-reported number of cigarettes that individuals estimated smoking on campus. Although the researchers concluded that the campaign effectively achieved its goal, they also noted that the inclusion of a control group would have strengthened their claim of campaign effectiveness.

In sum, public health communication campaigns are an essential tool for promoting health and well-being. Unlike marketing and advertising campaigns, these efforts don't produce financial benefits for the creators and are often operating with minimal resources. Yet, the last few decades have clearly shown that public health communication campaigns, when theoretically driven and carefully designed for a specific target audience, can effectively improve public health (see Noar, 2006).

Entertainment-Education

In addition to public health communication campaigns, another strategy that health researchers and advocates use to leverage the persuasive power of the media is through entertainment-education, or edutainment. **Entertainment-education** is "the process of purposely designing and implementing a media message both to entertain and educate, in order to increase audience members' knowledge about an educational issue, create favorable attitudes, and change overt behavior" (Singhal & Rogers, 1999, p. 9). Most often, entertainment-education occurs when health professionals work with writers and producers to create original storylines for well-known programs and characters. Let's look at this through a study on a crime drama called *Numb3rs* to demonstrate the complexities and characteristics of entertainment-education.

Using a case study approach, Lauren Movius and colleagues (2007) analyzed an episode of *Numb3rs*. For the episode, show creators had collaborated with the Norman Lear Center (NLC), a center that pairs "TV writers with information experts and other resources to develop health storylines" (p. 6), to develop a story about black-market organ trade in the United States. Of course, there actually is no market for illegally harvested organs in the United States, but NLC experts worked to include some accurate information on legitimate organ donation in the imaginary tale. Although the fictional organ-harvesting plot drove the drama behind the episode, writers also included facts and statistics concerning the number of people waiting for organs in the United States in various scenes. Furthermore, the episode included a subplot in which a main character was convinced by others to become an organ donor himself. A follow-up survey conducted by the NLC found that viewers of this episode were more likely than viewers of other dramas featuring storylines about organ donation to think about the importance of organ donation, sign up to become an organ donor, and encourage others to become donors (Movius et al., 2007). It seems, then, that presenting medically reliable information through fictional narratives can produce prosocial effects.

But why are entertainment-education approaches influential? One explanation is that they work through the process of **narrative transportation**, or the extent to which individuals are pulled into the experience, imagery, and emotions of a narrative (Green et al., 2004). Think back to the last TV episode or movie you watched that absolutely consumed you—the one where you were so engrossed in the storyline that you barely noticed anything else going on around you. This experience you had is what media researchers call transportation. For example, Sheila Murphy and colleagues (2011) surveyed 167 regular viewers of the show *Desperate Housewives* about a lymphoma storyline that was aired as part of the series. The researchers found that transportation experiences were the strongest predictors of viewer knowledge, attitudes, and behaviors. They argue that the findings suggest that "transported viewers are likely to devote more of their cognitive resources and pay closer attention to the unfolding drama" and that "transportation into a narrative may reduce counterarguing and, as a consequence, increase the likelihood that viewers will process the information conveyed in a less critical manner" (pp. 423–424).

Entertainment-education is a complex field that must balance the capitalist drive to make money through entertaining audiences with the social responsibility to positively influence audiences' health perceptions and behavior. To aid the entertainment industry in walking this fine line, various communication-based resources are available to the public free of charge for crafting positive public health content that is still entertaining. One of the largest is the CDC's *Resources for Writers*, housed on their *Gateway to Health Communication* resource page (CDC, 2020). There, entertainers can connect with the CDC's consulting resources for assistance with writing scripts. In addition, the NLC, which is housed at the University of California, Los Angeles, "is a nonpartisan research and public policy center that studies the social, political, economic and cultural impact of entertainment on the world" (Norman Lear Center, n.d., para. 1). The NLC conducts media-based research projects and hosts educational events on a variety of leading media topics, including entertainment-education.

Entertainment-education continues to be a flourishing area of research within the media and health communication disciplines. If you're looking for additional information about entertainment-education, we encourage you to read Arvind Singhal and Everett Roger's (1999) book *Entertainment-Education: A Communication Strategy for Social Change*. With thousands of television channels and hundreds of streaming services at everyone's fingertips, the potential for entertainment-education feels endless.

Entertainment-Education

Entertainment-education is the process of purposely designing and implementing a media message both to entertain and educate in order to increase audience members' knowledge about an educational issue, create favorable attitudes, and change overt behavior. It occurs when health professionals work with writers and producers to create original storylines for well-known programs and characters. Research indicates that accurate information needs to be portrayed in ways that engage audiences so that they connect with characters, stories, and fictional environments.

Conclusion

It's clear that media and health intersect in numerous ways. Through these intersections, there's great potential for the media to influence audience perceptions and behaviors. Some sources of influence, such as celebrities, might not be intentionally seeking to affect audience health, but they do so through their status and parasocial connections. Other influences, such as advertising and public health communication campaigns, do intentionally seek to leverage the power of media to affect audience health. Whether from traditional media, celebrity narratives, or campaigns, these influences can either make it hard to choose the healthy option or help people live healthier lives. Media technology will continue to evolve, leading to changes in how audiences use and engage with media. It's essential that health communication scholars examine how these social and individual changes will influence audience health. We hope that having read this chapter, you are now more aware of the ways that media can influence your perceptions and behaviors and will, therefore, be better equipped to seek out the positive influences and avoid the negative ones.

References

Ajzen, I. (1985). From intentions to actions: A theory of planned behavior. In J. Kuhl & J. Beckmann (Eds.), *Action-control: From cognition to behavior* (pp. 11–39). Springer.

Alhabash, S., Mundel, J., Deng, T., McAlister, A., Quilliam, E. T., Richards, J. I., & Lynch, K. (2021). Social media alcohol advertising among underage minors: Effects of models' age. *International Journal of Advertising, 40*(4), 552–581.

Bandura, A. (1969). Social-learning theory of identificatory processes. In D. A. Goslin (Ed.), *Handbook of socialization theory and research* (pp. 213–262). Rand McNally.

Bandura, A. (1986). *Social foundations of thought and action: A social cognitive theory*. Prentice-Hall.

Beck, C. S., Chapman, S. M. A., Simmons, N., Tenzek, K. E., & Ruhl, S. M. (2015). *Celebrity health narratives and the public health*. McFarland & Company.

Bero, L. (2003). Implications of the tobacco industry documents for public health and policy. *Annual Review of Public Health, 24*(1), 267–288.

Brown, W. J., & Basil, M. D. (1995). Media celebrities and public health: Responses to "Magic" Johnson's HIV disclosure and its impact on AIDS risk and high-risk behaviors. *Health Communication, 7*(4), 345–370.

Catalán-Matamoros, D. (2011). The role of mass media communication in public health. In K. Smigorski (Eds.), *Health management: Different approaches and solutions* (pp. 399–414). InTech.

Centers for Disease Control and Prevention. (2020, August 4). *Gateway to health communication: Resources for writers.* https://www.cdc.gov/healthcommunication/toolstemplates/entertainmented/index.html

Chao, S., & So, S. (2011). The Jade Ribbon Campaign: A systematic, evidence-based public awareness campaign to improve Asian and Pacific Islander health. *Journal of Communication in Healthcare, 4*(1), 46–55.

Cohn, D. L., Miller, L. A., Yamaguchi, K. J., & Douglas, J. M. (1992). Denver's increase in HIV counseling after Magic Johnson's HIV disclosure. *American Journal of Public Health, 82*(12), 1692.

Dalton, M. A., Sargent, J. D., Beach, M. L., Titus-Ernstoff, L., Gibson, J. J., Ahrens, M. B., Tickle, J. J., & Heatherton, T. F. (2003). Effect of viewing smoking in movies on adolescent smoking initiation: A cohort study. *The Lancet, 362*(9380), 281–285.

Elliott, B. J. (1987). *Effective mass communication campaigns: A source book of guidelines: Conception, design, development, implementation, control and assessment of mass media social marketing campaigns.* Transportation Research Board of the National Academies: Victoria, Australia.

Evans, D. G. R., Barwell, J., Eccles, D. M., Collins, A., Izatt, L., Jacobs, C., Donaldson, A., Brady, A. F., Cuthbert, A., Harrison, R., Thomas, S., Howell, A., Miedzybrodzka, Z., & Murray, A. (2014). The Angelina Jolie effect: How high celebrity profile can have a major impact on provision of cancer related services. *Breast Cancer Research, 16*(5), 1–6.

Evans, D. W., Thomas, C. N., Favatas, D., Smyser, J., & Briggs, J. (2019). Digital segmentation of priority populations in public health. *Health Education & Behavior, 46*(2S), 81–89.

Eyal, K., & Te'eni-Harari, T. (2013). Explaining the relationship between media exposure and early adolescents' body image perceptions. *Journal of Media Psychology, 25*(3), 129–141.

Federal Trade Commission. (1971, May). *Memorandum of understanding between the Federal Trade Commission and the Food and Drug Administration.* https://www.ftc.gov/policy/cooperation-agreements/memorandum-understanding-between-federal-trade-commission-food-drug

Federal Trade Commission. (2021). *Federal trade commission cigarette report for 2020.* https://www.ftc.gov/system/files/documents/reports/federal-trade-commission-cigarette-report-2020-smokeless-tobacco-report-2020/p114508fy20cigarettereport.pdf

Food and Drug Administration. (2011, June 22). *Required warnings for cigarette packages and advertisements.* https://www.federalregister.gov/documents/2011/06/22/2011-15337/required-warnings-for-cigarette-packages-and-advertisements

Gerbner, G., Gross, L., Morgan, M., & Signorielli, N. (1986). Living with television: The dynamics of the cultivation process. In J. Bryant & D. Zillman (Eds.), *Perspectives on media effects* (pp. 17–40). Lawrence Erlbaum Associations.

Green, M. C., Brock, T. C., & Kaufman, G. F. (2004). Understanding media enjoyment: The role of transportation into narrative worlds. *Communication Theory, 14*(4), 311–327.

Hansen, A., & Gunter, B. (2013). Alcohol, advertising, media, and consumption among children, teenagers, and young adults. *Communication Yearbook, 36*, 277–315.

Hoffner, C. A., & Cohen, E. L. (2018). Mental health-related outcomes of Robin Williams' death: The role of parasocial relations and media exposure in stigma, help-seeking, and outreach. *Health Communication, 33*(12), 1573–1582.

Huang, Q., Peng, W., & Ahn, S. (2021). When media become the mirror: A meta-analysis on media and body image. *Media Psychology, 24*(4), 437–489.

Iyer, P. (1991, November 18). *Health it can happen to anybody. Even Magic Johnson.* http://content.time.com/time/subscriber/article/0,33009,974293,00.html

Jolie, A. (2013, May 14). My medical choice. *The New York Times.* https://www.nytimes.com/2013/05/14/opinion/my-medical-choice.html

Jung, J. (2011). Advertising images of men: Body size and muscularity of men depicted in *Men's Health* magazine. *Journal of Global Fashion Marketing, 2*(4), 181–187.

Juthe, R. H., Zaharchuk, A., & Wang, C. (2015). Celebrity disclosures and information seeking: The case of Angelina Jolie. *Genetics in Medicine, 17*(7), 545–553.

Kresovich, A., & Noar, S. M. (2020). The power of celebrity health events: Meta-analysis of the relationship between audience involvement and behavioral intentions. *Journal of Health Communication, 25*(6), 501–513.

LaBelle, S., Ball, H., Weber, K., White, A., & Hendry, A. (2020). The Rethink campaign to reduce the normalization of prescription stimulant misuse on college campuses. *Communication Quarterly, 68*(1), 1–28.

Liebers, N., & Schramm, H. (2019). Parasocial interactions and relationships with media characters – An inventory of 60 years of research. *Communication Research Trends, 38*(2), 4–31.

Liede, A., Cai, M., Crouter, T. F., Niepel, D., Callaghan, F., & Evans, D. G. (2018). Risk-reducing mastectomy rates in the US: A closer examination of the Angelina Jolie effect. *Breast Cancer Research and Treatment, 171*(2), 435–442.

McCombs, M. E., & Shaw, D. L. (1972). The agenda-setting function of mass media. *Public Opinion Quarterly, 36*(2), 176–187.

McGuire, W. J. (2013). McGuire's classic input-output framework for constructing persuasive messages. In R. E. Rice & C. K. Atkin (Eds.), *Public communication campaigns* (4th ed., pp. 133–146). Sage.

Motion Picture Association of American. (2018). *G is for golden: The MPAA film ratings at 50.* https://www.motionpictures.org/wp-content/uploads/2018/11/G-is-for-Golden.pdf

Movius, L., Cody, M., Huang, G., Berkowitz, M., & Morgan, S. (2007). Motivating television viewers to become organ donors. *Cases in Public Health Communication and Marketing, 1*, 1–20.

Murphy, S. T., Frank, L. B., Moran, M. B., & Patnoe-Woodley, P. (2011). Involved, transported, or emotional? Exploring the determinants of change in knowledge, attitudes, and behavior in entertainment-education. *Journal of Communication, 61*(3), 407–431.

National Cancer Institute. (2020, November 19). *How can a person who has inherited a harmful BRCA1 or BRCA2 gene variant reduce their risk of cancer?* BRCA gene mutations: Cancer risk and genetic testing. https://www.cancer.gov/about-cancer/causes-prevention/genetics/brca-fact-sheet#how-can-a-person-who-has-inherited-a-harmful-brca1-or-brca2-gene-variant-reduce-their-risk-of-cancer

Noar, S. M. (2006). A 10-year retrospective of research in health mass media campaigns: Where do we go from here? *Journal of Health Communication, 11*(1), 21–42.

Norman Lear Center. (n.d.). *The Lear Center: For the study of entertainment, media & society.* https://learcenter.org/about/

O'Sullivan, G. A., Yonkler, J. A., Morgan, W., & Merritt, A. P. (2003). *A field guide to designing a health communication strategy.* Johns Hopkins Bloomberg School of Public Health/Center for Communication Programs. https://pdf.usaid.gov/pdf_docs/Pnacu553.pdf

Park, A. (2013, May 27). The Angelina effect. *Time.* https://time.com/3450368/the-angelina-effect/

Phua, J., Lin, J.-S., & Lim, D. J. (2018). Understanding consumer engagement with celebrity-endorsed E-Cigarette advertising on Instagram. *Computers in Human Behavior, 84*, 93–102.

Pierce, J. P., Choi, W. S., Gilpin, E. A., Farkas, A. J., & Berry, C. C. (1998). Tobacco industry promotion of cigarettes and adolescent smoking. *JAMA, 279*(7), 511–515.

Powell, R., Rosenthal, J., August, E. M., Frey, M., Garcia, L., Sidibe, T., Mendoza, Z., Romero, L., & Lathrop, E. (2022). Ante La Duda, Pregunta: A social marketing campaign to improve contraceptive access during a public health emergency. *Health Communication, 37*(2), 177–184.

Prochaska, J. O., & Velicer, W. F. (1997). The transtheoretical model of health behavior. *American Journal of Health Promotion, 12*(1), 38–48.

Public Health Law Center. (n.d.). *Commercial tobacco control: Countering the tobacco epidemic, Master Settlement agreement.* https://www.publichealthlawcenter.org/topics/commercial-tobacco-control/master-settlement-agreement

Public Health Law Center & American Lung Association California. (2021, June). *Endgame policy platform – Version 1.* https://www.trdrp.org/about/endgame-policy-platform-version-1.pdf

Record, R. A., Greiner, L. H., Wipfli, H., Strickland, J., Owens, J., Pugel, J., & Matt, G. E. (2023). Evaluation of a social media campaign designed to increase awareness of thirdhand smoke among California adults. *Health Communication, 38*(3), 437–446.

Record, R. A., Helme, D., Savage, M. W., & Harrington, N. G. (2017). Let's clear the air: A campaign that effectively increased compliance with a university's tobacco-free policy. *Journal of Applied Communication Research, 45*(1), 79–95.

Redmond, S. (2003). Thin white women in advertising: Deathly corporeality. *Journal of Consumer Culture, 3*(2), 170–190.

Rice, R. E., & Atkin, C. K. (2013). *Public communication campaigns.* Sage.

Rogers, E. M. (2002). Intermedia processes and powerful media effects. In J. Bryant, D. Zillmann, & M. B. Oliver (Eds.), *Media effects: Advances in theory and research* (2nd ed., pp. 209–224). Routledge.

Sargent, J. D., Tanski, S., & Stoolmiller, M. (2012). Influence of motion picture rating on adolescent response to movie smoking. *Pediatrics, 130*(2), 228–236.

Sayers, E. L. P., Bouskill, K. E., Concannon, T. W., & Martin, L. T. (2021). Creating culture-centered health and health insurance literacy resources: Lessons learned from Haitian Creole, Mandarin, Native American, and Vietnamese communities. *Journal of Communication in Healthcare, 14*(4), 312–323.

Silk, K., Smith, T. L., Salmon, C. T., Thomas, B. D. H., & Poorisat, T. (2022). Public health communication campaigns. In T. L. Thompson & N. G. Harrington (Eds.), *The Routledge handbook of health communication* (3rd ed., pp. 335–352). Routledge.

Singhal, A., & Rogers, E. M. (1999). *Entertainment-education: A communication strategy for social change.* Routledge.

Slater, M. (1996). Theory and method in health audience segmentation. *Journal of Health Communication, 1*(3), 267–283.

Tindall, N. J., & Vardeman-Winter, J. (2011). Complications in segmenting campaign publics: Women of color explain their problems, involvement, and constraints in reading heart disease communication. *Howard Journal of Communications, 22*(3), 280–301.

Valente, T. W., & Kwan, P. P. (2013). Evaluating communication campaigns. In R. E. Rice & C. K. Atkin (Eds.), *Public communication campaigns* (4th ed., pp. 83–98). Sage.

Walter, N., Cohen, J., Nabi, R. L., & Saucier, C. J. (2022). Making it real: The role of parasocial relationships in enhancing perceived susceptibility and COVID-19 protective behavior. *Media Psychology, 25*(4), 601–618.

Witte, K. (1992). Putting the fear back into fear appeals: The extended parallel process model. *Communication Monographs, 59*(4), 330–349.

In-class Activities

1. Have the students keep a health communication media journal for one day, making a list of every health communication mediated message they encounter. They should come to the next class period prepared to share their journal. In small groups, have the students compare and contrast the messages they saw. Were they promoting healthy or unhealthy behaviors? What behaviors did they cover? Where did students tend to see the messages? Have each group compile a summary report to share with the class.

2. Break the class into small groups. Give each group a public health problem relevant to their state, city, or campus. Problems could be smoking, exercise, alcohol, bullying, cancer screening, COVID-19 prevention, etc. Task the students with developing a public health communication campaign to improve their public health problem. Each group should consider the five key areas of formative evaluation (goal identification, theoretical foundations, audience targeting, channel selection, and message design) and outline an evaluation plan.

Discussion Questions

1. Think about your favorite public health communication campaign. After reading this chapter, critically analyze the campaign. What was it about? What features were employed? What made it your favorite campaign? How could it have been improved?

2. What health-related issue do you perceive as the most in need of awareness? If you were tasked with creating a public health communication campaign to increase awareness of this issue, what would your campaign plans be? Why would your strategy be effective?

3. Think about a time you experienced an especially effective example of entertainment-education. What features of your example (e.g., messages, characters, drama) made it so effective? How could those features influence future entertainment-education efforts?

A Blast from the Past

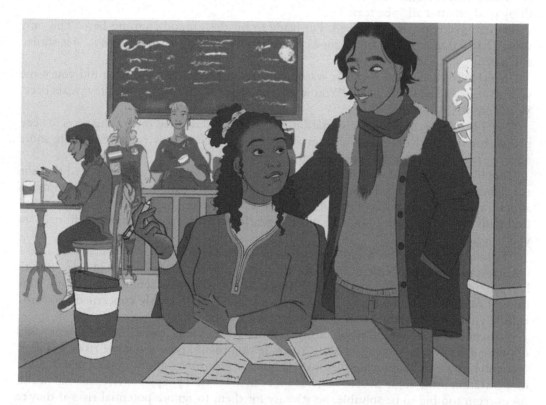

Several years passed. Cheryl had been treating her own patients for a while now. Given her continuing interest in environmental health, she was constantly on the lookout for information she could share with her patients. As part of her searching, she'd recently found a report that shook her to her core. A team of researchers had confirmed that the water in her hometown had been contaminated with cancer-causing pesticides from nearby agricultural farms. Moreover, the suspiciously high rates of breast cancer were officially linked to the water contamination. Her grandmother was by all accounts among the first victims. And of course, the Black women in her town were experiencing disproportionately high rates of breast cancer. This alarming news made her redouble her efforts to share the risks of environmental contaminations with all of her patients. Despite her best attempts, though, the vast majority of them didn't appear overly concerned. No matter how much she emphasized the risks, she couldn't seem to convince them of the importance of monitoring environmental exposures around their homes and in their communities.

DOI: 10.4324/9781003214458-30

Cheryl was reflecting on this very predicament at her local coffee shop early one morning before work when a young man with hazel green eyes approached her table.

"Mind if I sit?" came a familiar voice.

"Nathian!" Cheryl exclaimed. "Oh, my gosh! Yes, please sit."

"Thanks," Nathian replied as he sat down.

"What are you doing here?" Cheryl asked, so happy to see her old friend from college.

"I just moved here about a week ago," Nathian shared. "I'm starting a tenure-track position at the University."

"Wow, that's fantastic! So that means you finished your PhD?"

"Sure did," Nathian replied. "Back in May."

"That's wonderful," Cheryl said. "Dr. Juarez, professor. I guess that communication thing paid off after all," she teased.

Nathian grinned. "It did indeed. I'm ready to hit the ground running here. The only thing I had left to do was to find a good coffee shop. I think this one might be it." He smiled at Cheryl.

Cheryl felt her cheeks get a little warm and start to blush. "So, uh, what did you write your dissertation on?" she asked. "You were doing patient advocacy work a few years back. Was it on that?"

"No. I liked that, but for my dissertation, I really wanted to focus on finding ways to keep people healthy. So I developed a program to train clinicians how to communicate more effectively with their patients about environmental health risks."

"Stop!" Cheryl gasped, and Nathian jumped a little, but Cheryl was so excited that she continued on. "That's what I've been trying to do with my patients! I've learned so much about how indoor and outdoor pollutants affect health. I keep sharing all the information I find with my patients, but I just can't seem to get them to prioritize prevention efforts. Can you help me?"

"Tell me how you've been approaching them," Nathian asked.

Cheryl explained to Nathian the research she'd found and how she would share it with her patients during office visits, giving them handouts and even sending emails if a new finding came out. But somehow her patients just didn't seem overly concerned about the risks of environmental toxins for developing cancer.

Nathian was nodding the whole time. "I think you're up against some self-efficacy and response efficacy issues," he told her. "You're letting them know about the risks, but then you gotta let them know what they can do about it. Can they afford bottled water? Or a new filtration unit? Some people can, but a lot can't. To most people, environmental health issues seem too big to be solvable. So it's easy for them to ignore potential risks if they're feeling overwhelmed."

Cheryl was nodding along, following his explanation. Somehow, though, this perspective made her feel more defeated.

"So, what do we do? Just tell patients nothing and let them go on with their lives not attempting to prevent the risks?" Cheryl asked, trying not to show her frustration.

"No, of course not. It sounds like you're just giving them a lot of good information. But I think you also need to give people hope. You can acknowledge the barriers they face by admitting that prevention could mean some additional cost or require extra time and effort, but emphasize that those investments will be worth a healthier future for them and their family. Maybe you can partner with nonprofit organizations to help people find financial support or other resources to address some of the barriers. But to your credit, often simply raising awareness is a huge win."

"I can assure you, it doesn't feel like a huge win in the moment," Cheryl replied.

"Probably not. But for all you know, your patients thought about the information you gave them on their way home. Maybe they talked to someone else about it or bought a water filter system after all. If people aren't aware, they certainly can't be expected to do anything. So you're probably helping in ways you can't see," Nathian said with a smile.

"Thanks, Nathe," Cheryl said, unintentionally using the nickname she used to call him. "You have made me feel better—and given me some ideas for how I can better broach the topic with my patients."

"Happy to help, Cher," Nathian replied. "So, how is everyone else? How's Sam doing?"

"Just great. They're twenty-two now and, unlike my patients, totally caught up in environmental issues. And they're obsessed with Greta Thunberg. I mean intensely obsessed," Cheryl shared.

"Really? Well, Greta's a pretty great role model," Nathian replied.

"Yup. Sam actually organizes walkouts and protests at their college to coincide with the ones Greta schedules. They probably don't realize it, but everyone's really proud of them. Sam cares so much that they very well could be the one to stop this impending global disaster," Cheryl said, feeling proud of her younger sibling.

Nathian glanced at his phone. "Listen, I really wish I had more time, but I gotta go to a faculty orientation. I'd would love to catch up more, though. Maybe we could grab dinner this weekend?" Nathian asked.

"That would be nice," Cheryl smiled. "And I might also pick your brain about that communication PhD. I'm starting to think I need some of that advanced training myself to better serve my patients."

"Sounds great. I'll text you."

"I'll keep my eyes open," Cheryl smiled through warm cheeks.

13 Environmental Health Communication

Where are you right now? Look around. Does the space look clean? If you take a deep breath, does the air feel fresh? Is there clean water available to drink? Do you currently feel safe? These questions, although simple, are important because they relate to your health. And for each of them, everyone deserves to live in a place where they can answer yes. But sadly, that isn't the case for many people around the world whose environments are not clean or safe. This chapter seeks to highlight how communication plays a role in understanding and promoting healthy environments.

In this chapter, we'll review the growing body of communication literature centered on the interaction between health and the environment, or **environmental health risks**. Our review will include a discussion of science communication, an area of research that addresses the challenge of communicating complex science related to environmental health risks through both media coverage and healthcare provider communication. In addition, we'll highlight health impacts across three pressing environmental health topics: climate change, pollution (air and soil), and survival resources (food and water). Finally, we'll conclude with a review of how social media plays a role in environmental health communication practices. One thing we hope you take away from this chapter is an understanding of the many underdiscussed ways in which people can be exposed to environmental health risks. And we hope this chapter will prompt you to start discussing these issues with your family, friends, and elected officials (if you haven't already!). We'll begin by demonstrating the link between the environment and human health.

The Environment and Human Health

When you read the word "environment," you probably think of outdoor spaces. Historically, that is how the term was used. But in more recent years, the term has expanded to also include indoor spaces. In a thorough discussion of how people define and understand the term environment, John Barry (2007) explains that most definitions describe an **environment** as the circumstances or conditions by which a person is surrounded. Barry sees this as an overly simplistic approach to environments, which he argues are complex interactions of natural and social experiences (we'll come back to this shortly). Considering that the average American spends 87% of their time indoors (Klepeis et al., 2021), it makes sense that environmental considerations include both outdoor and indoor spaces. More to the point of this chapter, given how much time people spend indoors, clean and safe indoor environments are just as essential to protecting health as outdoor environments. Let's see how.

In her book *The Healthy Indoor Environment: How to Assess Occupants' Wellbeing in Buildings*, Philomena Bluyssen (2009) makes the case that for indoor environments to comprehensively benefit and promote health, the design, construction, and use of indoor space need to consider all five human senses. We're talking about everything from lighting and

DOI: 10.4324/9781003214458-31

temperature control to air quality and noise control. Bluyssen goes on to say that the construction of indoor environments is important to human health because "External stress factors can influence all three control systems of the human body and can result in both mental and physical effects" (Bluyssen, 2009, p. 9). (The three control systems Bluyssen references are the nervous system, immune system, and endocrine system.) These built environment factors are so influential that the label **sick building syndrome (SBS)** has been used to discuss the group of physical and psychological health problems caused by the quality of indoor environments. In a review of the literature, Yousef Al Horr and colleagues (2016) presented evidence documenting how "Uncomfortable temperature and humidity, chemical and biological pollution, physical condition, and psychosocial status are some of the factors identified as root causes of SBS" (p. 5). Further, they note that symptoms of SBS include "irritation of the eyes, nose, and throat, headache, cough, wheezing, cognitive disturbances, depression, light sensitivity, gastrointestinal distress and other flu like symptoms" (Al Horr et al., 2016, p. 5). They then show how these outcomes can result in an increased absence from work, reduced work productivity, and increased hospitalizations, particularly among women. And what about outdoor environments?

Like indoor environments, how outdoor spaces are designed, built, and used can influence human health. For example, James Sallis and colleagues (2009) were interested in how outdoor environments "help adults meet health-enhancing physical activity guidelines" (p. 485). To explore this question, they surveyed more than 11,000 adults living in cities across 11 countries (Belgium, Brazil, Canada, Colombia, China [Hong Kong], Japan, Lithuania, New Zealand, Norway, Sweden, and the United States). They found that individuals were 47% more likely to exercise if they lived in neighborhoods with sidewalks, 32% more likely if they had a transit stop in the neighborhood, 29% more likely if there were shops nearby, 21% more likely if there were bicycle facilities, and 16% more likely if a low-cost recreational facility was nearby. This is one example of research demonstrating how the design of outdoor environments can influence human health. Such findings have led to increased considerations of environmental health risks when designing new commercial, residential, or public outdoor spaces. One important outdoor consideration is green spaces.

According to the U.S. Environmental Protection Agency (EPA; n.d.), **green spaces** are open spaces of land that are partly or completely covered with grass, trees, shrubs, or other vegetation. They can include parks, community gardens, or cemeteries. The presence of green spaces in communities can benefit public health by providing a venue for increased physical activity and improved mental health and psychological well-being (see Lee & Maheswaran, 2011). Such spaces also can improve physical health. For example, a systematic review of 12 studies "found evidence of a reduction of the risk of CVD [cardiovascular disease] mortality in areas with higher residential greenness" (Gascon et al., 2016, p. 63). In other words, including green spaces in community planning can help save lives.

Regardless of the size or location of the environment, within each environment there exists a socio-ecosystem. This is the complexity that Barry (2007) was referencing in his argument for understanding environments. Understanding the impact of environments should include recognizing how people interact with the systems of environments and the policies affecting environments. Through this lens, you can see how and why environmental health risks can be different in geographically similar regions and for different groups of people. For example, this lens allows you to see how and why predominantly low-income Black residents of Flint, Michigan were exposed to lead contamination in their home water supply for years when residents of nearby towns were not (much more on this to come later in the chapter).

An equitable approach to environmental health risks argues that all people deserve to live in safe and healthy environments. To that end, the Centers for Disease Control and Prevention (CDC) launched the National Center for Environmental Health (NCEH;

2021) with the mission to "promote a healthy environment and prevent premature death, avoidable illness and disability caused by non-infectious, non-occupational environmental and related factors" (para. 1). Under their purview, the NCEH lists numerous relevant topics at the intersection of the environment and health. Topics include pest control (e.g., ticks, mosquitos), food safety (e.g., foodborne illnesses, preparation), climate change, water, natural disasters, environmentally triggered conditions (e.g., asthma), and toxic pollutants (e.g., carbon monoxide, mold, lead). Recognizing the numerous ways in which environments—indoors and outdoors—affect health is important to ensuring that all communities are designed as healthy spaces to live and grow.

The evidence of the strong relationship between the environment and health is indisputable—just ask anyone who lived in Flint, Michigan over the last 20 years. Yet, promoting healthy environments, especially through regulation, has proved challenging. This may come as a surprise to our readers who are members of the most vocal generation of environmental activists in modern history, but environmental communication research is still a new and growing field of study. A major part of the field includes a focus on science communication.

Science Communication and Environmental Health

It's easy to point the finger at social media as the primary cause of the conspiracy theories plaguing the world. Although social media is certainly a contributing factor, particularly because of the speed at which messages can spread, misinformation and resistance to scientific progress have been dark clouds over the scientific community for centuries (just ask Galileo, who was imprisoned under house arrest for daring to promote the idea that the earth revolved around the sun). There are numerous reasons that misinformation continues to afflict the scientific community. One reason, and the one most applicable to environmental health, stems from the challenge of communicating complex scientific ideas to audiences that do not have the same scientific training as researchers.

Science communication is a growing area of study that approaches science translation (making science understandable to the general public) and dissemination (sharing scientific findings with the general public) as an evidence-based endeavor. In other words, as science. The science of **science communication** is "an empirical approach to defining and understanding audiences, designing messages, mapping communication landscapes, and—more important—evaluating the effectiveness of communication efforts" (Hall Jamieson et al., 2017, p. 1). The approach "relies on evidence that is transparent and reliable, theory driven, and generalizable" (Hall Jamieson et al., 2017, p. 1). Environmental health science communication acknowledges that there is some degree of environmental health literacy required in order to fully understand how the environment affects health and how to reduce environmental health risks. Further, how science communication approaches message senders and receivers is key to successfully communicating complex science.

Dan Kahan (2017) explains that science communication considers the general public not as illiterate and unable to process the more challenging nuances of science but as an audience experiencing information overload and mixed messages from a variety of interpersonal and mediated sources. In addition, he notes that science communication considers scientists not as persons too smart to effectively and clearly communicate with lay audiences but as messengers of complex topics whose messages go through various social, cultural, and political filters. You can think of science communication as the messaging bridge between the public and scientists. What's important about this bridge is that when miscommunication occurs, science communicators don't blame either audience. Instead, they blame the construction of the bridge by assuming that the message wasn't crafted appropriately.

Communicating Complex Science

Science communication is an empirical approach to defining and understanding audiences, designing messages, mapping communication landscapes, and evaluating the effectiveness of communication efforts. Science communication relies on evidence that is transparent and reliable, theory-driven, and generalizable. In science communication, it's important to recognize that (a) the general public experiences information overload and mixed messages from a variety of interpersonal and mediated sources and (b) scientists are messengers of complex topics whose messages go through various social, cultural, and political filters.

There are countless examples of the need for science communication to overcome science hesitation and misinformation. Often, tensions between scientific findings and misinformation about those findings are encased in contentious political rhetoric. We'd like to briefly demonstrate with climate science, a prime example of such a tension (Björnberg et al., 2017). You might be surprised to learn just how long scientists have known about the threat of climate change.

In 1824, French scientist Joseph Fourier calculated a discrepancy in the earth's temperature, arguing that something in the atmosphere must be trapping heat because the earth was hotter than it should be. More than 30 years later, scientist (and women's rights activist) Eunice Foote found the source of the discrepancy: carbon dioxide and water vapor trapping heat. Over the next 100 years, a handful of scientists would further document the concerns and risks of an overheating planet, with Canadian physicist Gilbert Plass officially formulating the carbon dioxide theory of climate change in 1956 (Shaftel et al., 2023). In an analysis of documents from the major fossil fuel giant ExxonMobil, a team of investigative journalists showed that in 1977 Exxon scientists warned their executives that "there is general scientific agreement that the most likely manner in which mankind is influencing the global climate is through carbon dioxide release from the burning of fossil fuels" (Banerjee et al., 2015, para. 2). Despite the clear and compelling science predicting the catastrophic effects of climate change, only recently have the leaders of the world come together to address the global climate change crisis—and they're not doing a very good job of it.

For decades, there was widespread denial of climate change, and pockets of deniers remain quite vocal to this day. There are numerous reasons that climate change denial has been so pervasive, including politics, profit, human psychology, and, of course, communication challenges. We'll focus on four of the challenges here. First, there has been the obvious challenge of processing such complex science messaging. This is evidenced through questions such as, "If the world is getting warmer, why is it so cold?" Second, disinformation campaigns from corporate interests, such as the fossil fuel industry, have worked to persuade the public that corporations are not to blame for the crisis (Farrell, 2016)—despite their own research scientists confirming that fossil fuel is the primary contributor to climate change (Banerjee et al., 2015; Supran et al., 2023). Third, and similarly, corporate donations to political parties, particularly from the fossil fuel industry, have resulted in polarized political rhetoric surrounding climate change (Dunlap et al., 2016). Finally, Gabrielle Wong-Parodi and Irina Feygina (2020) argue that climate change denial also stems from biased reasoning, "whereby the desire to avoid acknowledging the reality of climate change is achieved through biased cognitive strategies which result in dismissal or doubt regarding the scientific consensus around climate change" (p. 61). Biased reasoning includes a desire to protect the current status quo, intertwined identity perspectives with political affiliations, social normative pressures, and difficulty in recognizing personal contributions to the problem. But why is all this important? Because climate change denial did not occur because there was weak climate science or compelling scientific counterarguments. It occurred because science communication could not effectively keep up with the substantial mis- and disinformation efforts, and changing closed human minds is incredibly difficult (Harrington, 2020).

In order to effectively engage in science communication, it's important to know why audiences are struggling to support an issue. In a review of environmental communication research, Amy Chadwick (2022) argues that there are three primary barriers hindering public action against environmental health threats. First, *individual political ideology*, particularly in the United States, is a powerful heuristic. The politicization of topics can make people feel like if they don't support their political party's argument, then they're going against their larger personal beliefs. For example, Republican voters who recognize the risks of climate change may find themselves in a bind because their party, on the whole, has historically rejected climate change (Dunlap et al., 2016). They often have to choose between voting for the Republican candidate and respecting their understanding of the desperate need for climate change mitigation. Second, people engage in *internal risk and benefit analyses* to determine whether something is worth preventing, and that analysis can get complicated. For example, purchasing a new air filtration system to prevent exposure to toxic particles in the air, such as lead or nicotine, may seem too expensive to mitigate a risk you cannot confirm you're experiencing without expensive testing or seeing it with your own eyes. Third, *social support* is essential to coping with health-related threats. For environmental risks where awareness or perceived risk might be low, however, requesting and receiving social support might be unlikely. For example, even though radon exposure is a real threat in several areas in the United States, homeowners might receive some quizzical glances from their neighbors if they installed a mitigation system for their home. Therefore, they might avoid attempting to prevent exposure because they don't think others will support their efforts.

Knowing barriers to processing information is only half of the battle. Having a credible source for the information you share is also important. The following paragraphs will review the role of media and healthcare providers in engaging in environmental science communication.

Role of the Media in Environmental Science Communication

As is true of most topics, how the media report and cover environmental health issues affects how audiences perceive and respond to environmental risks (see Chapter 12). Communication researchers can evaluate media coverage of topics through a research method called content analysis. **Content analysis** allows researchers to evaluate the extent to which content is discussed (such as the coverage of topics and representation of groups), as well as the ways in which it is discussed (such as the framing of controversial issues). The following sections will further reveal how the media have historically shaped environmental health conversations and the implications for promoting effective science communication moving forward.

Coverage and Representation

Just because something can negatively influence human health doesn't mean that it's receiving media attention. Instead, because media industries are themselves corporations that need to prioritize the bottom line in order to make money and stay in business, they typically give priority to stories that they believe will attract audiences. In addition, the extent to which media coverage addresses how groups are affected differently by various environmental health threats is also at the discretion of media industries. Communication research has served an important role in shedding light on coverage priorities and gaps. These priorities and gaps matter because they can influence audience perceptions of environmental health threats. We'll demonstrate with an example.

Alyssa Mayeda and colleagues (2019) conducted a content analysis of eight major newspapers in four western U.S. states "to examine how health-related water issues are reported, what health risks are emphasized, and the overall volume of news coverage noting the health implications of water issues" (p. 927). All 326 of the stories they analyzed were published during a drought that occurred between January 2012 and December 2014. The analysis coded for the water-related health risks of contamination, illness and disease, weather-related incidents, lack of water and dehydration, respiratory-related illness, recreational activities and accidents, and general health. The authors concluded that their findings revealed "limited representations of health-related water issues in the news both in terms of quantity of coverage and manner of framing" (p. 938). They also concluded that newspaper coverage may not accurately reflect "the nature of health impacts associated with water, which often are long-term" (p. 926). Through this example, we hope you can see how *not* covering the *long-term* implications of water issues could be limiting public awareness of the crisis. Such gaps in media coverage can leave the public vulnerable to important—and often preventable—environmental health risks.

In addition to identifying priorities and gaps in coverage, content analyses also reveal how much attention different aspects of particular topics receive. For example, Susan Mello (2015) was concerned that U.S. media reporting of environmental health risks to fetuses and newborns was minimal and varied arbitrarily by chemical type. Given the importance of this information for new and expecting parents, she analyzed more than 2,500 popular media texts, including magazines and websites, published from September 2012 to February 2013, looking for stories that addressed environmental health threats around pregnancy and childbirth. She found that the most discussed topics were food additives, cigarette smoke, pesticides, and mercury. The least discussed topics were flame retardants, polychlorinated biphenyls (a cancer-causing chemical compound formerly used in industrial and consumer products), drinking water quality, and arsenic. Most importantly, she found the level of coverage did not reflect the priority levels of the EPA. For instance, the EPA did not list food additives as being of high concern, yet that topic received the most media coverage. Likewise, the four topics that received the least coverage were all on the EPA's list of high concerns. This coverage discrepancy could send mixed messages to parents about what factors do and do not pose the greatest environmental health risks.

There's growing pressure for more accurate media representation around topics of environmental health. This pressure stems from the growing movement of environmental justice. **Environmental justice** is the principle that all people in all communities are entitled to equal protection under environmental and public health laws and regulations (Bullard, 2004) and the recognition that systemic structures result in different communities, mostly marginalized and underserved communities of color, disproportionately experiencing negative environmental impacts (see Bullard, 1994). Media coverage of environmental issues has been an essential tool in combating environmental injustices. For example, Jordan Neil and colleagues (2018) investigated political discourse surrounding *fracking*, or the extraction of underground natural gas and oil through a process that releases toxic and carcinogenic (cancer-causing) air pollutants and contributes to climate change. Through a content analysis of national media in the United Kingdom (UK), the researchers investigated the "interplay between multiple political stakeholders and how this interplay influences political discourse and policy through message strategy and information subsidy utilization" (p. 184). Their analysis found that anti-fracking advocacy groups in the UK were more successful than corporations at influencing media content in terms of message frames and tone, resulting in increased public awareness of and support for this globally contentious issue. The Neil et al. study serves as an example of the media's ability to advance environmental concerns. The next study we review shows how the media can reveal environmental injustices.

Analyses of media coverage in the aftermath of Hurricane Katrina in 2005 revealed numerous concerns around environmental injustices. One such example is a rhetorical analysis by Samuel Sommers and colleagues (2006), who presented three ways in which Black citizens were more negatively portrayed in the press than their white counterparts. First, the researchers revealed differences in language use that cast biased portrayals. For example, the authors noted that a Black man would be described as "looting," whereas a white couple, engaged in comparable behavior, would be described as "finding food" (p. 2). Second, they showed how in the aftermath of the hurricane, many story angles heavily focused on violence among survivors, who were predominantly people of color. The authors added that the largest problem with this practice was the possibility of deterring rescue efforts and aid. Finally, they explored what they called "new media" reporting, which included "weblogs, listservs, on-line bulletin boards, and mass e-mails" (p. 9). (You'll recall from Chapter 5 that this is now called citizen journalism.) The analysis drew the conclusion that these accounts from citizen journalists were beyond simple accusations of violence in that they were "not content to portray the survivors of Katrina as common criminals, but rather go further, focusing on bodily function and barbaric behavior" (p. 11). Research analyses such as this one by Sommers et al. are important because they hold such media accountable for how they represent groups experiencing environmental health risks, which is essential for increasing awareness of ongoing environmental injustices.

Framing

Framing is the concept that there are different ways to present, or frame, information for any given topic. More specifically, to **frame** information is to select "aspects of a perceived reality and make them more salient in a communicating text, in such a way as to promote a particular problem definition, causal interpretation, moral evaluation, and/or treatment recommendation" (Entman, 1993, p. 52). A very clear example of framing can be seen with political news coverage, where a right-leaning outlet (e.g., Fox News) will highlight different aspects of a story than a left-leaning outlet (e.g., MSNBC). How media choose to frame a story is important because framing theory says that how information is framed influences how audiences perceive the topic (Chong & Druckman, 2007). Table 13.1 presents framing theory along with two other theories that have been used to guide environmental communication research.

Content analyses that consider framing shed light on how important environmental health topics are being discussed, identifying gaps for awareness and potential informational needs. For example, a study by Aoife De Brún and colleagues (2016) analyzed how newspapers in Ireland and the UK covered the 2008 Irish dioxin crisis. Dioxin is a highly toxic compound that's a byproduct of certain manufacturing processes. The crisis was caused when animal feed was contaminated with the toxin and then fed to livestock. This resulted in a global recall of all Irish pork products and the slaughter of 100,000 pigs. The cause of the contamination was traced back to the use of an oil not meant for animal feed by a food recycling plant and a lapse in government inspection of that plant in 2008. De Brún et al. wanted to know how newspapers framed the crisis and whether there was a difference between Irish and UK coverage.

Table 13.1 Theoretical Frameworks in Environmental Communication

Theory/Model	Brief Summary	Citation
Construal-level Theory	Adopting a distal versus proximal perspective changes the way people make behavioral plans, resolve value conflicts, negotiate with others, and cope with self-control problems. The choices people make for psychologically distant situations are guided by their general attitudes, core values, and ideologies, which increase in influence as the distance shrinks.	Trope and Liberman (2010)
Deficit Model of Public Attitudes	Skepticism toward scientific explanations, particularly regarding climate change, stems from a lack of public understanding or knowledge.	See Sturgis and Allum (2004)
Framing Theory	Audiences will be influenced by the selection of aspects of a perceived reality used to promote a particular problem definition, causal interpretation, moral evaluation, and/or treatment recommendation.	Entman (1993)

Note. See *Supplemental Online Theory Table* for additional theories/models.

The researchers reviewed 15 months of newspapers, from right before the crisis to just after, and identified 141 articles for analysis. Their content analysis showed that the most common frame, appearing in 38 of the stories, was the adverse economic impact on the agribusiness industry. This was followed by blaming the feed supplier for the crisis (found in 37 of the stories) and health implications (reported in 30 of the stories, with 19 of the 30 emphasizing how there was *no risk to health* from the contamination). Regarding framing, De Brún et al. (2016) found differences between Irish and UK newspaper coverage in that "Irish media emphasized the impact of the crisis on Irish agribusiness and the wider economy, whereas UK media were more likely to portray the issue as relevant to public health" (p. 1240). They explain that "Comparing countries may reveal different media concerns and political motivations and could therefore indicate different understandings of the same issue" (p. 1240).

Framing analyses have also demonstrated how frames can perpetuate environmental injustices and be slow to draw attention to environmental crises, particularly when such injustices and crises impact marginalized and underserved communities. We'll demonstrate this through the media reporting surrounding the Flint water crisis in Flint, Michigan, where residents were exposed to lead contamination in their home water supply. Michael Carey and Jim Lichtenwalter (2020) were interested in how national media reporting used language to frame stories about the crisis. Through content analysis, the researchers examined 135 articles from *The New York Times* and *The Wall Street Journal*. Their analysis concluded that the articles typically described Flint residents, who were predominantly low-income people of color, by using *urban pathology language*, which is language that frames communities in terms of their problems. The authors argue that this frame leads readers to see those communities entirely in terms of their problems, suggesting a lack of agency among residents and reducing broader environmental justice concerns. Carey and Lichtenwalter (2020) point to the work by Jennifer Johnson and her team (2018) as demonstrating possible alternative frames that the media could have considered using, such as highlighting voices of the community working to promote positive change in their community.

Thus far, we've presented the media as a major source of environmental health information, and we've considered their role in calling attention to or minimizing environmental concerns. In addition, we've shown how communication research can be used to hold media reporting accountable. Another important source of information on the environment and its influence on health is healthcare providers. We turn our attention to them next.

Role of the Healthcare Provider in Environmental Science Communication

Although the vast majority of environmental communication research focuses on the media, there's a growing body of interdisciplinary literature focused on the communicative role of healthcare providers in reducing environmental health risks. The slow growth of research in this area may be rooted in the lack of environmental health training during medical school, which is minimal at best (Pelletier, 2016). But surveys of medical students show that many of them recognize the inadequacy of their training and the need for an increased focus on environmental health risks (e.g., Gehle et al., 2011). Leading medical organizations, including the National Medical Association, American Medical Association, and American Academy of Pediatrics, have endorsed a position statement calling for discussions of environmental health to be part of routine primary care and for an increase in training and education for clinicians (National Environmental Education Foundation, n.d.). We think this change in practice cannot come soon enough.

Beyond the lack of training on environmental health risks, there's also a lack of training on how to communicate with patients about those health risks. In a survey of pediatricians in Georgia, Nikki Kilpatrick and colleagues (2002) found that more than half of the surveyed pediatricians reported having a patient who was seriously affected by an environmental exposure. Their analyses revealed that pediatricians showed "A high level of interest in children's environmental health, a high level of belief in the impact of environmental exposures on their patients' health, and a high level of interest in learning more about the field" (p. 826). However, analyses also found that "Pediatricians reported very little prior training in taking environmental histories and low self-efficacy regarding taking these histories, discussing environmental exposures with parents, and locating diagnosis and treatment resources related to environmental exposures" (p. 826). The authors suggest that their findings demonstrate both the need and interest in more resources to help pediatricians talk with patients about environmental health risks.

Given the importance of provider communication with patients about environmental health risks, efforts are being made to improve educational resources during medical school. For example, Benjamin Kligler and colleagues (2021) tested the efficacy of a six-week interactive module for first-year medical students at Hackensack Meridian School of Medicine. During the students' second year of medical school, the researchers conducted a follow-up survey with them, finding a significant increase in students' perceived preparedness to discuss environmental health issues with their patients. The authors concluded that although students of this generation are already highly concerned about environmental health risks, their study results show that "a relatively brief six-week environmental health module combining didactic and experiential elements can significantly increase medical students' self-reported sense of preparedness to discuss environmental health issues, including climate change, with their patients" (p. 5). But what about communication training for providers after they leave medical school?

There are two main ways that practicing providers who have already completed medical school receive additional education and training. The first is through continuing education credits, often called **continuing medical education credits (CME)**. As you might recall from Chapter 3, continuing education activities are designed to help providers keep their knowledge current, as well as acquiring new knowledge and skills, including about communication. Nearly all 50 U.S. states have CME regulations (CECentral, 2023). Often healthcare employers require CMEs that focus on communication skills training. Such training has been shown to effectively improve clinician confidence in communicating with patients about environmental health risks. For example, Brandon Walling and colleagues (2021) found that pediatricians who completed CME training on environmental risks for breast cancer reported adopting recommended communication strategies for discussing the risks with their patients.

The second way to provide practicing clinicians with additional education and training is through publishing updated resources in medical journals. For example, research is showing new harms of tobacco exposure, such as through thirdhand smoke residue, which is the toxic tobacco residue left behind in environments after the smoking stops. To help providers navigate the new evidence, Ware Kuschner and colleagues (2011) published informational materials targeting practicing clinicians in the *International Journal of General Medicine* to better prepare them to talk with patients about thirdhand smoke exposure risks. The objective of their publication was to help providers prepare for and answer possible questions from patients.

Healthcare providers are vital not only for educating patients about environmental health risks but also for identifying patterns of emerging health threats within communities at large. Due to their training, providers are uniquely qualified to serve as community watchdogs for environmental health risks. And there is arguably no better example of such importance than Dr. Mona Hanna-Attisha, a physician working at Hurley Children's Hospital in Flint, Michigan. Dr. Hanna-Attisha discovered the lead water crisis through her observations of the symptoms of lead poisoning in her pediatric patients (Abbasi, 2021). Although it's not the responsibility solely of providers to keep people safe from environmental health risks, they are an important piece of the prevention puzzle.

Trending Topics in Environmental Health Communication

Thus far, we've reviewed the complexities of communication science and considered the role of the media and healthcare providers in communicating about environmental health risks. The following paragraphs will highlight three of the most pressing environmental health issues currently facing the planet: climate change, pollution, and water resources. Within each of these topics, we'll explore specific impacts on health, environmental justice concerns, and communication challenges. Around the world, all three of these challenges are felt at their most extreme in low-income and underdeveloped countries. We'll demonstrate how communities experience each of these environmental health challenges differently through a closer examination of disparities within the United States.

Climate Change

The CDC (2022) has compiled substantial evidence on the negative health effects due to climate change. Figure 13.1 depicts how the evidence points to four categories of climate change that are causing weather events that produce eight substantial impacts on human health—many of which ExxonMobil research scientists predicted back in 1978 would happen (Banerjee et al., 2015). These broad and substantial impacts are putting everyone on the planet at increased health risk. However, some communities and regions are experiencing these threats more profoundly than others.

The EPA (2021) released a report warning that individuals who have low income or are racial minorities are the most likely to experience the consequences of climate change. More specifically, low-income, Hispanic/Latino, and Black/African American individuals are more likely to currently live in areas with the highest increases in climate change-induced

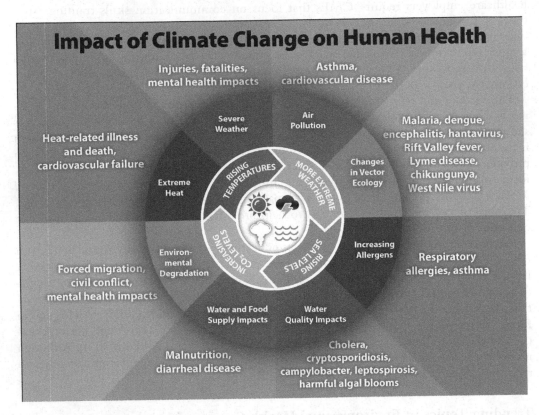

Figure 13.1 CDC's Impact of Climate Change on Human Health.
Source: CDC (2022).

childhood asthma and labor-hour losses for weather-exposed workers. In addition, low-income and Hispanic/Latino individuals are more likely to live in areas with the highest increases in traffic delays associated with high-tide flooding; low-income and Black/African American individuals are more likely to live in areas with the highest increases in mortality rates from climate-driven changes in extreme temperatures; and low-income individuals are more likely to live in areas with the highest percentage of land lost to inundation. As the planet continues to warm, the risk levels increase further.

There are numerous communication challenges surrounding climate change education and mitigation. As previously noted, climate change is particularly challenging following decades of denial, lobbying, and political rhetoric (Banerjee et al., 2015; Dunlap et al., 2016; Farrell, 2016; Wong-Parodi & Feygina, 2020). But now that the negative effects of climate change are impossible to ignore, people are more willing to listen to the science and support mitigation. Although climate change can feel like too big of a problem to solve with individual behavior change, research shows that there is hope—or rather, that hope might be the key. Chadwick (2015) has shown that messages that appeal to hope increase attention to messages about climate change and interest in climate change mitigation. In addition to research on messaging, health agencies and climate change advocates are ready to meet the public with information, resources, and tools to help them become involved in mitigation efforts. In the United States, the CDC (2019) is overseeing much of the national communication plan, which targets 11 priority health actions for mitigating the health consequences

Table 13.2 CDC Priority Health Actions for Climate Change

1. Serve as a credible source of information on the health consequences of climate change for the U.S. population and globally.
2. Track data on environmental conditions, disease risks, and disease occurrence related to climate change.
3. Expand capacity for modeling and forecasting health effects that may be climate-related.
4. Enhance the science base to better understand the relationship between climate change and health outcomes.
5. Identify locations and population groups at greatest risk for specific health threats, such as heat waves.
6. Communicate the health-related aspects of climate change, including risks and ways to reduce them, to the public, decision makers, and healthcare providers.
7. Develop partnerships with other government agencies, the private sector, nongovernmental organizations, universities, and international organizations to more effectively address U.S. and global health aspects of climate change.
8. Provide leadership to state and local governments, community leaders, healthcare professionals, nongovernmental organizations, the faith-based communities, the private sector and the public, domestically and internationally, regarding health protection from climate change effects.
9. Develop and implement preparedness and response plans for health threats such as heat waves, severe weather events, and infectious diseases.
10. Provide technical advice and support to state and local health departments, the private sector, and others in implementing national and global preparedness measures related to the health effects of climate change.
11. Promote workforce development by helping to ensure the training of a new generation of competent, experienced public health staff to respond to the health threats posed by climate change.

Note. From CDC (2019).

of climate change—all of which are grounded in communication strategies. The actions are presented in Table 13.2.

Pollution: Air and Soil

It should come as no surprise that human health is affected by the quality of the air people breathe into their lungs and the chemicals that seep into the ground. **Pollution**, or the introduction of harmful materials into the environment, comes in many forms. The most notable forms are air and soil pollutants. Exposure to air and soil pollution is of such concern that substantially reducing the number of deaths and illnesses from hazardous chemicals in air, water, and soil is a sustainability goal for the United Nations (see U.N. Sustainable Development Goals in Chapter 1).

Air pollution—both indoors and outdoors—can cause a variety of adverse health effects, including increased risk of respiratory infections, heart disease, chronic obstructive pulmonary disease, and lung cancer (World Health Organization [WHO], 2019, 2021). The most common sources of air pollution are inefficient modes of transportation, inefficient combustion of household fuels, coal-fired power plants, agriculture, and waste burning (WHO, 2019). For indoor environments, this list expands to include tobacco smoke, radon, carbon monoxide, and mold (Seguel et al., 2017). Each year, the WHO (2021) estimates that 3.8 million people die prematurely from illnesses attributable to the household air pollution caused by the inefficient use of solid fuels and kerosene for cooking. Similarly, airborne metals, such as mercury, cadmium, and lead, have been found to increase the risk of postmenopausal breast cancer among women in the United States (White et al., 2019). Like air pollution, soil pollution can cause adverse health outcomes through inhalation, ingestion, or skin absorption of the toxicants in soil or from soil transfers to dust, air, water, or food. Depending on the contamination, negative health effects vary widely from cancer (e.g., arsenic) and organ necrosis (e.g., copper) to increased risks for childhood development disorders (e.g., lead) and neurological disorders (e.g., manganese).

The CDC (n.d.) maintains an *Environmental Justice Dashboard* that tracks how environmental exposures, including pollution, vary for different groups and communities. As of 2022, data show that 11.9 million people in the United States are living with unhealthy air quality and that air pollution disproportionately affects racial and ethnic minorities. Similarly, communities with low incomes have disproportionate exposure to environmental hazards because of proximity to a superfund site (a place where hazardous waste has been dumped into the ground) and are more likely to have older homes that may have asbestos or lead paint and pipes.

The communication challenges surrounding pollution often stem from the feeling that pollution, whether in the air or the soil, is either not an imminent threat (e.g., "I wouldn't develop cancer for at least 20 years") or is unavoidable (e.g., "I can't afford to move elsewhere"). Research suggests that these challenges can be overcome with communication efforts that seek to increase pollution awareness and exposure prevention by highlighting personal risks and self-efficacy (Yang & Huang, 2019) and finding creative ways to visualize the impacts of pollution (Kuchinskaya, 2018). For example, when communicating the health risks surrounding poor air quality, A. Susana Ramírez and colleagues (2019) call for a greater focus on the translation of the complex science using noncomplex terminology and a clear emphasis on risks and prevention behaviors.

Water: Access and Quality

When it comes to environmental communication surrounding water, the two key areas of concern are access and quality. A joint report from the WHO and UNICEF (2021) shows that 2 billion people around the world continue to lack access to safe drinking water at home, with 800 million of those individuals having less than basic home access (i.e., drinking water from an improved source; designated collection time from a central source that is not more than 30 minutes for a round trip, including lining up and waiting). Notably, universal access to safe drinking water, adequate sanitation, and hygiene has the potential to reduce the global disease burden by 10% (WHO, 2012). That would mean improving the health of more than 800 million people! However, the world is not on track to meet the Sustainable Development Goal of universal access to safely managed water by 2030, with only 16 countries on track (WHO & UNICEF, 2021).

A joint report by Dig Deep, a human rights nonprofit working to ensure that every American has clean, running water, and the US Water Alliance (2019) states that approximately 2 million Americans live without running water and basic indoor plumbing, with many more living with sanitation barriers. Concerningly, quality tests of private wells (which the U.S. Geological survey [2019] reports are relied upon by 15% of the population) found that 23% were contaminated with toxicants such as arsenic, nitrates, and *E. coli*. Access to water is of greatest challenge to rural, Native American, and low-income populations. More specifically, Native American families are 19 times more likely than white households to not have indoor plumbing. Similarly, African American and Latinx households are almost twice as likely as white households to lack indoor plumbing.

Communication challenges surrounding water are broad. As previously noted, one challenge is the under-reporting of water-related health risks in the media (Mayeda et al., 2019).

Other communication challenges include competing interests in managing limited water supplies, such as between agricultural industries and environmental groups (Hundemer & Monroe, 2021). Because these challenges cannot be easily resolved, it's important for communication efforts to continue to raise public awareness of water-related health issues. To that end, the WHO lists March 22 as **World Water Day**, a day for celebrating water, raising awareness of people living without access to safe water, and taking action to tackle the global water crisis (World Water Day, 2023). In addition, as new strategies for water security emerge, communication research is needed to prepare the public for such changes. For instance, recycled wastewater is seen as one strategy for adding to the potable water supply. But, as you can image, the general public tends to have a lot of hesitancy around its consumption. (And we're not so sure we disagree with that hesitancy.) In an experimental test of affective (emotional) response to recycled wastewater among Australian adults, Tameika Greenaway and Kelly Fielding (2020) found that messages emphasizing positive aspects of recycled water (e.g., the water is purified, people can't tell the difference) as opposed to negative aspects (e.g., emphasis on wastewater treatment plants) elicited more positive affective responses and higher acceptance of use. As the world continues to face extreme threats of water insecurity, such messaging strategies will be essential to promoting solutions and reducing uncertainty.

Trending Topics in Environmental Health Communication

Trending topic areas of environmental health communication research include climate change, pollution (air and soil), and water (access and quality). For all three areas, environmental health threats are experienced at a greater rate for underserved and minority communities. Communication efforts are needed to counter misinformation, raise awareness, and promote hope.

Social Media and Environmental Communication

This chapter has presented information about a lot of complex environmental problems. It can be easy to feel like these problems are too big for one person to make a difference. But we believe no problem is too big for any one person—let alone collections of dedicated people—to tackle and potentially solve. One tool that's made it substantially easier for people to get involved and try to make a difference is social media. Social media allows people to readily advocate for increased awareness of environmental health risks among both the public and policymakers. It's also used by individuals, groups, and activists working to promote equitable environmental health solutions and correct environmental injustices. The efficacy of social media is especially evident in online climate change activism.

It's hard not to think about climate change advocacy on social media without thinking about the passionate leader and activist Greta Thunberg. In 2018, Ms. Thunberg began protesting for climate justice by sitting in front of the Swedish parliament and refusing to go to school, documenting these actions on Twitter and Instagram (Jung et al., 2020). Less than a year later, her efforts had gone viral, and since January 2023, it's estimated that she's mobilized more than 18 million strikers at 166 thousand strike events across 233 countries in the name of climate change (Fridays for Future, 2023). Her extensively documented activism, predominantly on social media platforms, has been so powerful that a team of researchers labeled her success the "Greta Thunberg Effect," showing that U.S. adults who were more familiar with her held higher intentions of taking collective action to reduce global warming (Sabherwal et al., 2021). Shelley Boulianne and colleagues (2020) argue that the social media support, particularly on Twitter, surrounding Ms. Thunberg's climate change movement has been successful, in part, due to its ability to connect protests around world, strengthening the magnitude of the outcry, and to facilitate a global discussion. Although climate change activism on social media gets a substantial portion of research attention, it's by no means the only environmental health issue being promoted.

For example, the crisis of water scarcity has started to gain particular urgency in hotter desert climates, such as in Arizona. Government and advocacy groups are beginning to push water conservation agendas in an attempt to mitigate the present threat. To investigate the impact of an Arizona-based water conservation campaign called *Water—Use It Wisely*, Anne-Lise Boyer and colleagues (2021) content analyzed 3,500 tweets and 15,204 Twitter profile descriptions. They found that the water conservation discussions in Arizona made their way into global discussions. They concluded that the ability for water professionals and activists to publicly interact on the controversial challenges of water management served as a key tool for potentially persuading broader audiences to support such efforts. Across social media platforms, hashtags also serve as a central tool for promoting environmental health activism.

The use of hashtags on social media platforms is a communicative strategy to aggregate publicly available posts on a particular topic. Like following accounts and handles, users can follow hashtags as a way to stay apprised of ongoing conversations around a particular topic. In recent years, hashtags have served an important role in environmental activism. For instance, the use of English hashtags surrounding the 2019 fires that burned in the Brazilian Amazon, which included #PrayForAmazon, #ActForTheAmazon, and #AmazonFire, was found to successfully raise awareness of the crisis, including by promoting likes and retweets online and being a key factor in framing the environmental issue as a global concern (Skill et al., 2021). Similarly, Ladislav Pilař and colleagues (2020) content analyzed more than 38,000 Instagram posts using the hashtags #sustainability and #food from November 2017 to December 2018. They found that hashtags facilitated community discussions centered, predominantly, on healthy sustainable living, including discussions of ecological sustainability and supporting community development and local charities. Such means of aggregated communication create global conversations that promote and encourage #EnvironmentalActivism.

Social Media for Environmental Communication Advocacy

Social media has been a key tool for improving public awareness and putting pressure on decision makers to support environmental health protections. Social media is used by individuals, groups, and activists working to promote equitable environmental health solutions and correct environmental injustices. The use of hashtags in social media posts has been important for creating global dialogues about environmental health risks.

Conclusion

The **National Institute of Environmental Health Sciences (NIEHS)** is the branch of the National Institutes of Health charged with researching the vast ways in which the environment can affect human health. Underlying their many initiatives to improve understanding of environmental health impacts is a core belief in **community-based participatory**

research (**CBPR**; see Chapter 11), or the research method of working with and for communities to use research in a way that addresses their priorities and needs. CBPR is a key approach not only to the early identification of environmental health risks within particular communities but also for achieving environmental justice. For instance, Mohan Dutta and colleagues (2013) reported on the successes of a CBPR project showing how making room for community voices and ideas can provide meaningful solutions to structurally imposed challenges to food security. And what does NIEHS list as the core ingredient for all their CBPR efforts? If you thought communication, you would be right.

Communication efforts are central to the ability to raise awareness and reduce environmental health risks. Environmental health risks occur in both outdoor and indoor environments. Although they can be hard to see and they may feel bigger than any one individual can solve, they are not lost causes. Continued communication research, particularly on media and healthcare provider communication, is needed to educate the members of public on the various environmental health threats to which they could be exposed. In addition, environmental health problems persist globally, and global efforts are needed to craft equitable solutions to protect everyone. Although social media can't solve these problems, it continues to be an important tool for addressing these large, challenging, and important environmental issues.

References

Abbasi, J. (2021). Lead, mistrust, and trauma—Whistleblowing pediatrician discusses the legacy of Flint's water crisis. *JAMA, 325*(21), 2136–2139.

Al Horr, Y., Arif, M., Katafygiotou, M., Mazroei, A., Kaushik, A., & Elsarrag, E. (2016). Impact of indoor environmental quality on occupant well-being and comfort: A review of the literature. *International Journal of Sustainable Built Environment, 5*(1), 1–11.

Banerjee, N., Song, L., & Hasemyer, D. (2015, September 16). Exxon's own research confirmed fossil fuel's role in global warming decades ago. *Inside Climate News.* https://insideclimatenews.org/news/16092015/exxons-own-research-confirmed-fossil-fuels-role-in-global-warming/

Barry, J. (2007). *Environment and social theory.* Routledge.

Björnberg, K. E., Karlsson, M., Gilek, M., & Hansson, S. O. (2017). Climate and environmental science denial: A review of the scientific literature published in 1990–2015. *Journal of Cleaner Production, 167,* 229–241.

Bluyssen, P. (2009). *The indoor environment handbook: How to make buildings healthy and comfortable.* Earthscan.

Boulianne, S., Lalancette, M., & Ilkiw, D. (2020). "School strike 4 climate": Social media and the international youth protest on climate change. *Media and Communication, 8*(2), 208–218.

Boyer, A.-L., Vaudor, L., Le Lay, Y.-F., & Marty, P. (2021). Building consensus? The production of a water conservation discourse through twitter: The water use it wisely campaign in Arizona. *Environmental Communication, 15*(3), 285–300.

Bullard, R. D. (1994). The legacy of American apartheid and environmental racism. *Journal of Civil Rights and Economic Development, 9*(2), 445–474.

Bullard, R. D. (2004). *Environment and morality: Confronting environmental racism in the United States.* New York: United Nations Research Institute for Social Development.

Carey, M. C., & Lichtenwalter, J. (2020). "Flint can't get in the hearing": The language of urban pathology in coverage of an American public health crisis. *Journal of Communication Inquiry, 44*(1), 26–47.

CECentral. (2023). *State CME licensure requirements.* https://www.cecentral.com/licensure/cme/

Centers for Disease Control and Prevention. (2019, September 9). *CDC policy on climate change and public health.* https://www.cdc.gov/climateandhealth/pubs/Climate_Change_Policy.pdf

Centers for Disease Control and Prevention. (2022, November 29). *Climate and health.* https://www.cdc.gov/climateandhealth/default.htm

Centers for Disease Control and Prevention. (n.d.). *Environmental justice dashboard.* https://ephtracking.cdc.gov/Applications/ejdashboard/

Chadwick, A. E. (2015). Toward a theory of persuasive hope: Effects of cognitive appraisals, hope appeals, and hope in the context of climate change. *Health Communication, 30*(6), 598–611.

Chadwick, A. E. (2022). Communicating about the environment and health. In T. Thompson & N. G. Harrington (Eds.), *Handbook of health communication* (4th ed., pp. 489–503). Routledge.

Chong, D., & Druckman, J. N. (2007). Framing theory. *Annual Review of Political Science, 10*(1), 103–126.

De Brún, A., Shan, L., Regan, Á., McConnon, Á., & Wall, P. (2016). Exploring coverage of the 2008 Irish dioxin crisis in the Irish and UK newsprint media. *Health Communication, 31*(10), 1235–1241.

Dig Deep, & US Water Alliance. (2019). *Closing the water access gap in the United States.* http://uswateralliance.org/sites/uswateralliance.org/files/publications/Closing%20the%20Water%20Access%20Gap%20in%20the%20United%20States_DIGITAL.pdf

Dunlap, R. E., McCright, A. M., & Yarosh, J. H. (2016). The political divide on climate change: Partisan polarization widens in the US. *Environment: Science and Policy for Sustainable Development, 58*(5), 4–23.

Dutta, M. J., Anaele, A., & Jones, C. (2013). Voices of hunger: Addressing health disparities through the culture-centered approach. *Journal of Communication, 63*(1), 159–180.

Entman, R. M. (1993). Framing: Towards clarification of a fractured paradigm. *Journal of Communication, 43*(4), 51–58.

Farrell, J. (2016). Corporate funding and ideological polarization about climate change. *Proceedings of the National Academy of Sciences, 113*(1), 92–97.

Fridays for Future. (2023, January 14). *Strike statistics.* https://fridaysforfuture.org/what-we-do/strike-statistics/

Gascon, M., Triguero-Mas, M., Martínez, D., Dadvand, P., Rojas-Rueda, D., Plasència, A., & Nieuwenhuijsen, M. J. (2016). Residential green spaces and mortality: A systematic review. *Environment International, 86*, 60–67.

Gehle, K. S., Crawford, J. L., & Hatcher, M. T. (2011). Integrating environmental health into medical education. *American Journal of Preventive Medicine, 41*(4), S296–S301.

Greenaway, T., & Fielding, K. S. (2020). Positive affective framing of information reduces risk perceptions and increases acceptance of recycled water. *Environmental Communication, 14*(3), 391–402.

Hall Jamieson, K., Kahan, D., & Scheufele, D. A. (2017). *The Oxford handbook of the science of science communication.* Oxford University Press.

Harrington, N. G. (2020). On changing beliefs in the closed human mind. *Health Communication, 35*(14), 1715–1717.

Hundemer, S., & Monroe, M. C. (2021). A co-orientation analysis of producers' and environmentalists' mental models of water issues: Opportunities for improved communication and collaboration. *Environmental Communication, 15*(3), 320–338.

Johnson, J. E., & Key, K. (2018). Credit where credit is due: Race and recognition in responses to the drinking water crisis in Flint. *Progress in Community Health Partnerships: Research, Education, and Action, 12*(2), 215–221.

Jung, J., Petkanic, P., Nan, D., & Kim, J. H. (2020). When a girl awakened the world: A user and social message analysis of Greta Thunberg. *Sustainability, 12*, 2707, 1–17.

Kahan, D. (2017). On the sources of ordinary science knowledge and extraordinary science ignorance. In K. Hall Jamieson, D. Kahan, & D. A. Scheufele (Eds.), *The Oxford handbook of the science of science communication* (pp. 35–50). Oxford University Press.

Kilpatrick, N., Frumkin, H., Trowbridge, J., Escoffery, C., Geller, R., Rubin, L., Teague, G., & Nodvin, J. (2002). The environmental history in pediatric practice: A study of pediatricians' attitudes, beliefs, and practices. *Environmental Health Perspectives, 110*(8), 823–827.

Klepeis, N. E., Nelson, W. C., Ott, W. R., Robinson, J. P., Tsang, A. M., Switzer, P., Behar, J. V., Hern, S. C., & Engelmann, W. H. (2021). The national human activity pattern survey (NHAPS): A resource for assessing exposure to environmental pollutants. *Journal of Exposure Science & Environmental Epidemiology, 11*(3), 231–252.

Kligler, B., Pinto Zipp, G., Rocchetti, C., Secic, M., & Ihde, E. S. (2021). The impact of integrating environmental health into medical school curricula: A survey-based study. *BMC Medical Education, 21*(1), 1–6.

Kuchinskaya, O. (2018). Connecting the dots: Public engagement with environmental data. *Environmental Communication, 12*(4), 495–506.

Kuschner, W. G., Reddy, S., Mehrotra, N., & Paintal, H. S. (2011). Electronic cigarettes and thirdhand tobacco smoke: Two emerging health care challenges for the primary care provider. *International Journal of General Medicine, 4,* 115–120.

Lee, A. C., & Maheswaran, R. (2011). The health benefits of urban green spaces: A review of the evidence. *Journal of Public Health, 33*(2), 212–222.

Mayeda, A. M., Boyd, A. D., Paveglio, T. B., & Flint, C. G. (2019). Media representations of water issues as health risks. *Environmental Communication, 13*(7), 926–942.

Mello, S. (2015). Media coverage of toxic risks: A content analysis of pediatric environmental health information available to new and expecting mothers. *Health Communication, 30*(12), 1245–1255.

National Center for Environmental Health. (2021, April 22). *About NCEH.* https://www.cdc.gov/nceh/default.htm.

National Environmental Education Foundation. (n.d.). *Health professionals and environmental health education position statement.* https://www.neefusa.org/node/4395

Neil, J., Schweickart, T., Zhang, T., Lukito, J., Kim, J. Y., Golan, G., & Kiousis, S. (2018). The dash for gas: Examining third-level agenda-building and fracking in the United Kingdom. *Journalism Studies, 19*(2), 182–208.

Pelletier, S. G. (2016, September 27). *Experts see growing importance of adding environmental health content to medical school curricula.* AAMC News. https://www.aamc.org/news-insights/experts-see-growing-importance-adding-environmental-health-content-medical-school-curricula

Pilař, L., Kvasničková Stanislavská, L., Prokop, M., & Jaaskelainen, P. (2020). Food in the context of sustainability-Instagram social network analysis. In *Proceedings of the Agrarian Perspectives XXIX: Trends and Challenges of Agrarian Sector* (pp. 272–279). Czech University of Life Sciences Prague.

Ramírez, A. S., Ramondt, S., Van Bogart, K., & Perez-Zuniga, R. (2019). Public awareness of air pollution and health threats: Challenges and opportunities for communication strategies to improve environmental health literacy. *Journal of Health Communication, 24*(1), 75–83.

Sabherwal, A., Ballew, M. T., van Der Linden, S., Gustafson, A., Goldberg, M. H., Maibach, E. W., Kitcher, J. E., Swim, J. K., Rosenthal, S. A., & Leiserowitz, A. (2021). The Greta Thunberg effect: Familiarity with Greta Thunberg predicts intentions to engage in climate activism in the United States. *Journal of Applied Social Psychology, 51*(4), 321–333.

Sallis, J. F., Bowles, H. R., Bauman, A., Ainsworth, B. E., Bull, F. C., Craig, C. L., Sjöström, De Bourdeaudhuij, I., Lefevre, J., Matsudo, V. Matsudo, S., Dphil, D. J. M., Gomez, L. F., Inoue, S., Murase, N., Volbekiene, V., McLean, G., Carr, H., Heggebo, L. K., Tomten, H., & Bergman, P. (2009). Neighborhood environments and physical activity among adults in 11 countries. *American Journal of Preventive Medicine, 36*(6), 484–490.

Seguel, J. M., Merrill, R., Seguel, D., & Campagna, A. C. (2017). Indoor air quality. *American Journal of Lifestyle Medicine, 11*(4), 284–295.

Shaftel, H., Callery, S., Jackson, R., & Bailey, D. (2023, January 12). Climate change: How do we know? *Earth Science Communications Team at NASA's Jet Propulsion Laboratory, California Institute of Technology.* https://climate.nasa.gov/evidence/

Skill, K., Passero, S., & Francisco, M. (2021). Assembling Amazon fires through English hashtags: Materializing environmental activism within Twitter networks. *Computer Supported Cooperative Work (CSCW), 30*(5), 715–732.

Sommers, S. R., Apfelbaum, E. P., Dukes, K. N., Toosi, N., & Wang, E. J. (2006). Race and media coverage of Hurricane Katrina: Analysis, implications, and future research questions. *Analyses of Social Issues and Public Policy, 6*(1), 39–55.

Sturgis, P., & Allum, N. (2004). Science in society: Re-evaluating the deficit model of public attitudes. *Public Understanding of Science, 13*(1), 55–74.

Supran, G., Rahmstorf, S., & Oreskes, N. (2023). Assessing ExxonMobil's global warming projections. *Science, 379*(6628), 1–9.

Trope, Y., & Liberman, N. (2010). Construal-level theory of psychological distance. *Psychological Review, 117*(2), 440–463.

U.S. Environmental Protection Agency. (n.d.). *What is open space/green space?* https://www3.epa.gov/region1/eco/uep/openspace.html

U.S. Environmental Protection Agency. (2021, September). *Climate change and social vulnerability in the United States: A focus on six impacts.* https://www.epa.gov/system/files/documents/2021-09/climate-vulnerability_september-2021_508.pdf

U.S. Geological Survey. (2019). *Domestic (private) supply wells.* https://www.usgs.gov/mission-areas/water-resources/science/domestic-private-supply-wells#:~:text=More%20than%2043%20million%20people,their%20source%20of%20drinking%20water

Walling, B. M., Totzkay, D., Silk, K. J., Boumis, J. K., Thomas, B., & Smith, S. (2021). Evaluating the feasibility of continuing medical education for disseminating emerging science on the breast cancer and environment connection. *Journal of Health Communication, 26*(6), 391–401.

White, A. J., O'Brien, K. M., Niehoff, N. M., Carroll, R., & Sandler, D. P. (2019). Metallic air pollutants and breast cancer risk in a nationwide cohort study. *Epidemiology (Cambridge, MA), 30*(1), 20–28.

Wong-Parodi, G., & Feygina, I. (2020). Understanding and countering the motivated roots of climate change denial. *Current Opinion in Environmental Sustainability, 42*, 60–64.

World Health Organization. (2012). *Global costs and benefits of drinking-water supply and sanitation interventions to reach the MDG target and universal coverage.* https://apps.who.int/iris/bitstream/handle/10665/75140/WHO_HSE_WSH_12.01_eng.pdf?sequence=1&isAllowed=y

World Health Organization. (2019, November 15). *Health consequences of air pollution on populations.* https://www.who.int/news/item/15-11-2019-what-are-health-consequences-of-air-pollution-on-populations#:~:text=Exposure%20to%20high%20levels%20of,people%20who%20are%20already%20ill"

World Health Organization. (2021, September 22). *Household air pollution and health.* https://www.who.int/news-room/fact-sheets/detail/household-air-pollution-and-health

World Health Organization, & United Nations Children's Fund. (2021). *Progress on household drinking water, sanitation and hygiene 2000–2020: Five years into the SDGs.* https://washdata.org/sites/default/files/2021-07/jmp-2021-wash-households.pdf

World Water Day. (2023). *World water day 2023: Accelerating change.* https://www.worldwaterday.org/

Yang, J. Z., & Huang, J. (2019). Seeking for your own sake: Chinese citizens' motivations for information seeking about air pollution. *Environmental Communication, 13*(5), 603–616.

In-class Activities

1. Climate change remains a universal public health threat. Break the class into small groups. Within their groups, have the students consider Chadwick's (2022) three barriers to public action against environmental health threats (individual political ideology, internal risk and benefit analysis, and social support). Ask them to discuss which barrier they think is most applicable to climate change hesitation in their community and write a message designed to overcome that barrier. Have the groups share the messages they create with the class.

2. Break the class into small groups. Have each group identify an environmental health scenario relevant to their community. For their scenario, have the students serve as the lead campaign planners for increasing awareness of their environmental health threat. Students should prepare the following information:
   a. What is the environmental health impact and whom does it most impact?
   b. Now that you have identified who is most at risk, what will your message be to persuade this audience to take action against this health threat, and why do you think this message will be effective? (Be sure to include a specific action you want your audience to take!)
   c. What will your campaign messages look like, and where will you disseminate them? Be prepared to defend your answers.
   d. What hashtag do you think would go viral for this campaign?

Discussion Questions

1. Thinking back on your life, what environmental health risks have you encountered? (Think outdoor and indoor.) How did talking with other people help you prepare, navigate, or remediate the situation? Did you take action against the health risks? What ultimately happened?

2. Climate change is a clear example of a controversial environmental health risk. What other environmental health risks do you think spark controversial discussion, and how would you recommend persuading people to protect their health?

3. Think about the social media platforms you use most. Which environmental health issues do you see most often on each platform? How are these issues being framed? Do you think the approaches are effectively promoting awareness of the environmental health risk? How so?

Sam's Big March

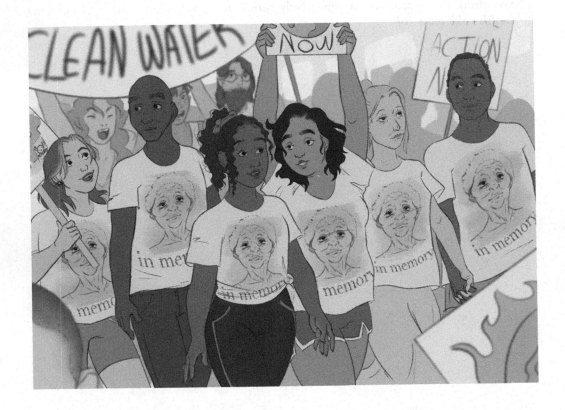

This was Cheryl's first trip home in many years. And she wasn't even through the front door before Sam threw their arms around her and pulled her into the house.

"I'm so happy you're here!" Sam beamed. "The march is gonna be so great! Look at the shirts I had made!"

Sam stepped back to show off the shirt they were wearing, which had a big picture of Helen's face on the front.

"Grams would be so touched, Sam," Cheryl said softly. "Thank you for bringing attention to her story."

"How could I not?" Sam stated. "All the evidence points to the water in this town being the cause of her cancer. We can't let anyone else go unaware of the risk."

Despite the research report about the water contamination in her town coming out over a year ago, local officials were slow to respond to the crisis. Cheryl's family had switched

DOI: 10.4324/9781003214458-32

to bottled water, but she was constantly worried about their health after what happened to her grandmother.

"Okay, T-minus two days. How can I help?" Cheryl asked.

"To the planning room!" Sam shouted. They turned and marched into the dining room, which was covered in signs.

Two days later, Sam's event was up and running. Although the state government had not declared the water contamination an official crisis, Sam was convinced that it was, and they were adamant that people be made aware of the dire state of things. Given all their thoughtful research, detailed planning, and careful communication, it was no surprise that the event drew thousands of people, including national media, leading public health experts, and environmental activists, as well as the entire Montgomery family and all of their neighbors and local friends. It seemed as if the only person who wasn't there was Greta Thunberg. Sam had actually invited her. It turned out she was already booked elsewhere, but she sent a kind letter wishing Sam good luck. The huge turnout made it clear to Cheryl that this was why Sam had worked so hard to prepare for today: They'd hoped the event would draw national attention and wanted to be ready to effectively communicate the details of the water contamination crisis in a way that would move people to see it for the crisis it was. And oh, did they. Sam was a natural leader.

As the event went on, Cheryl found herself moved by the numerous conversations with old friends and strangers alike. Sadly, almost every one of them had a similar story to her family's, with at least one relative affected by cancer like Helen had been. Cheryl had seen evidence of the water risks years ago in media reports and research articles, but she hadn't thought about how many people might not have access to the same information she did or be able to understand its implications. Sam's event was helping to rectify that. Cheryl's favorite part of the day was Sam's concluding speech. After the large group walked about two miles around their town center, Sam took to the stage to share about Helen.

"Helen was not my blood. But she was my Grams." Sam's delivery was powerful and eloquent. "She helped raise me to believe that we do have the power to call for change. And that's why we're here," Sam roared. "To demand change!" The crowd cheered so loud Cheryl could feel it.

After the event, the family went home to share a meal and celebrate Sam's success—which did end up making national headlines. Over dinner, Sam decided to ask a question that had been on their mind.

"Do you think Aunt Savannah would have supported the march, Mom?" Sam asked.

The table was quiet as all eyes turned to Sally. She'd had a hard time talking about Savannah ever since her death. Sally sometimes wished they'd tried a little harder with the COVID vaccine, but she had to admit that nothing would have worked. Savannah had been too swept up in all the conspiracies promoted in the media.

"I think she would have, yes," Sally said. "She loved you very much, Sam. And even if she still doubted climate change, she never doubted you."

Everyone smiled at that thought. They all sat quietly for a moment. Cheryl decided to break the silence to share some happy news.

"Everyone, I actually have an announcement. Today was a really powerful day for me, and I thank you for that, Sam. Although I'm happy with my work at the hospital, I've always felt disconnected from it, wanting to do something more. I've been accepted into a communication PhD program that specializes in community-based research. For years I've dreamed about opening a community-based breast cancer clinic in Grams' honor. And that's what I'm going to do. I've accepted the offer from the program, and in four years I intend to open *The Helen Montgomery Community Clinic for Breast Cancer Awareness and Prevention* right here in town."

The whole family broke into spontaneous applause. Cheryl had never felt so clear about what she wanted to do with her skills, passion, and life.

Note

Upset about environmental injustices and inaction? Environmental journalist Jane Marsh provides six ways to raise awareness about environmental issues here: https://environment.co/6-ways-to-raise-awareness-about-environmental-issues/

14 Public Health Crises

A decade ago, the phrase "public health crisis" carried little meaning to most people. But now, following the COVID-19 pandemic, most people are aware of not only the phrase but also its relevance and importance. By definition, a crisis is unpredictable. Even if you know a crisis might be looming, such as if you live in a region that experiences annual hurricanes, the specific details surrounding how individuals and communities will be affected by and move through the events of the crisis are unknown. One thing you can count on is that public health crises require increased levels of communication.

In this chapter, we'll review the characteristics of a public health crisis. From there, we'll consider common communication theories used to understand and navigate responses to public health crises, with a specific focus on the crisis and emergency risk communication (CERC) model and chaos theory. In addition, we'll examine the influence of leadership during times of crisis and share information on the concept of swarm intelligence as a way to understand effective crisis leadership. Finally, we'll examine how the media have shaped modern crisis experiences and how stakeholders prepare for potential known crises. Although it may not be possible to prevent all crises, preparing for them can save lives.

Public Health Crises and Crisis Communication

Within the discipline of communication, the field of risk and crisis communication houses the scholarly research on public health crises. This research is conducted at the intersection of public relations, organizational communication, and health communication. A **crisis** is defined as "a specific, unexpected, and non-routine event or series of events that create high levels of uncertainty and threat or perceived threat to an organization's high priority goals" (Seeger et al., 1998, p. 233). A **public health crisis** builds on this definition, with the added specification that the event or series of events is in some way affecting the health of people. Such events typically are separated into three categories: **infectious diseases** (e.g., outbreak, pandemic), **natural disasters** (e.g., earthquake, wildfire), and **human-caused disaster** (e.g., food contamination, oil spill). Public health crises are often studied as occurring in distinct stages, where crisis is viewed as beginning at some point pre-event, moving into some triggering event during the crisis, and ending post-crisis (see Reynolds & Seeger, 2005; Seeger et al., 1998). Risk and crisis communication includes the study of unique communication challenges that stem from unexpected, fast-moving events in which there is often a great deal of uncertainty and threat (Reynolds & Seeger, 2005).

More specifically, **crisis communication** is driven by the goal of preventing or lessening the negative outcomes of a crisis event, especially its effects on public health, while simultaneously protecting the interests of the organization at the heart of the crisis (Coombs, 2012). In a public health crisis, those organizations could be a corporation responsible for putting the public at risk (e.g., a food chain that had an *E. coli* outbreak) or a government

DOI: 10.4324/9781003214458-33

agency managing the response to a crisis that doesn't have a clear responsible party (e.g., the Federal Emergency Management Agency [FEMA] overseeing the response to a hurricane that they obviously didn't cause). Although protecting the interests of the responsible organization might seem counter to public health interests, research has shown that public perception of the crisis response, including the credibility of the communicating organization, is important for maintaining confidence in the public health system (Ballard-Reisch et al., 2007).

Definitions of Crisis Communication

A crisis is a specific, unexpected, and non-routine event or series of events that creates high levels of uncertainty and threat or perceived threat to an organization's high-priority goals.

A public health crisis is a crisis event that affects the health of people at local, regional, national, or global levels.

Crisis communication is driven by the goal of preventing or lessening the negative outcomes of crisis events as they affect public health.

Communication during a crisis can come in the form of warnings of pending threats, evacuation notifications, situational updates, and public asks. A **public ask**, sometimes referred to as a *call to action*, refers to the behaviors that the public is being asked to adopt, such as "wear a mask," "get vaccinated," or "evacuate." These communications serve numerous functions, including attempting to reduce uncertainty, contain harm, provide information, promote recovery, rationalize decisions, and, at times, apologize (Seeger et al., 2003). In other words, they can help keep people safe. Indeed, as the Centers for Disease Control and Prevention (CDC; 2018) states, "The right message at the right time from the right person can save lives" (para. 1). For students majoring in communication, this is probably not a surprising statement. But for non-communication majors, it might seem a bit grandiose. So we can all be on the same page, let's take a quick look at how communication can save lives during a public health crisis.

Imagine that the zombie apocalypse has finally arrived, and a hoard of zombies is approaching the town where you live. (We know, dramatic. But this is actually a common metaphor in crisis preparedness training.) Outside of seeing the zombies for yourself, how would you know the apocalypse was happening? Where a safe location is that's free of zombies? If you were bitten by a zombie, is there a treatment, or are you doomed? Should you fear someone who was bitten? Is it really your brains the zombies are after? Who's currently trying to rid the zombies from your town? (Unless the answer is Woody Harrelson, there's no hope for you. Sorry!) Communicating the answers to these questions efficiently and effectively could be the difference between life and death.

In the context of a crisis, what needs to be said by whom and to whom depends on numerous factors stemming from various aspects of the crisis. These aspects include the type of crisis event, the likelihood of a crisis occurring, the level of risk to public health, and the difficulty of the public ask for reducing the health threat. For instance, if a local grocery store determines that customers purchased contaminated food, the messaging would be localized to the specific community, it would ask the public to throw away the purchased food, and it would probably come from a local official. On the other hand, a large-scale event, such as an earthquake, will likely garner national attention, with messages about the event coming from local, state, and national sources, with messaging about where available resources can be found and when someone should request medical assistance. Such communications cannot be perfectly planned beforehand, but they can be anticipated. The people responsible for doing so are called crisis managers. **Crisis managers** include trained public health experts, elected leaders, heads of corporations, public relations experts, and trained crisis communicators. They are responsible for communicating with the public during crisis events.

Communication research examining public health crises is methodologically diverse. However, much of what is known about effective crisis communication in the context of protecting public health stems from case study analyses (Veil, 2011). In a **case study**, a single event is critically analyzed to identify communication-related themes that can be used to better understand similar events that might occur in the future. Through a case study analysis of the communication events before, during, and after a public health crisis, resources, tools, and "lessons learned" can be extracted. Let's look at an example of how a case study analysis can help prepare for the next public health crisis.

After a thorough review of crisis communication during the SARS, swine flu, H1N1, ZIKA, Ebola, and COVID-19 pandemics, Wouter Jong (2021) created the ACCP checklist, or the **Assessment tool for Crisis Communication during Pandemics**. This 30-item checklist covers five domains. First, *sense making* seeks to

> understand public needs, define communication goals, and enable practitioners to feel better prepared… It enables crisis communication professionals to quickly and proactively respond, based on insights into the volume of messages, underlying sentiments, important influencers, and the stance of stakeholders.
>
> (p. 966)

The next three domains are centered on particular groups: *public leadership*, *public health professionals and expert voices*, and *stakeholders*. These domains encompass an evaluation of the communications from the groups themselves, as well as communications about the groups, such as reports by media outlets. Finally, *instructions to the public* considers the extent to which communications contain balance in tone, reach diverse audiences, employ broad media channels, acknowledge lessons learned, and persuade audiences to follow the public ask. Jong concludes that "The checklist not only supports evaluators in assessing efforts within a team or country but also enables academics to make worldwide comparisons between affected countries" (p. 967). Although the specific details of the inevitable next pandemic are unknown, Jong's case study analysis of past pandemics demonstrates how researchers can use those experiences to develop tools that can assist experts in managing the next one.

Shari Veil (2011) noted that a public health crisis can emit warning signals long before it's officially declared a crisis event. Regardless of whether there are warning signals or not, the declaration of a crisis is important because it indicates that officials now have the power to access resources specifically designated to support crisis events. Until an event is officially declared a crisis, response resources are limited. Because crises can happen at the community, national, or global level, the responsibility for declaring an event a crisis will fall on different persons or agencies depending on the situation. Also depending on the situation, more than one agency or official may end up designating an event as a crisis. Let's consider an example.

You'll probably recall the Flint water crisis. This crisis happened at the local level in Genesee County, Michigan, and resulted from governmental mismanagement that exposed citizens to lead contamination in the water supply for years. Merrit Kennedy (2016), a writer for National Public Radio (NPR), noted that although the citizens of Flint reported complaints about their water in May 2014—less than a month after the city switched their water supply—it wasn't until December 2015 that the newly elected mayor of the city would declare a state of emergency. The City of Flint, Michigan website (2015) reported that "Declaring an emergency intends to help raise awareness of the issue that the water is still not safe to drink and activates the City's Emergency Support Plan in order to respond to the crisis" (para. 2). The website later reported that the emergency preparedness plan, which included providing immediate relief to citizens and rebuilding the city's water distribution infrastructure, officially request emergency resources from the governor of Michigan and the president of the United States (City of Flint, Michigan, 2016). Shortly after that, the governor declared a state of emergency in January 2016. Within two weeks of the state declaring the crisis, President Obama declared the event as a state of emergency, allowing for the deployment of FEMA resources to aid the citizens of Flint. Shortly after the federal declaration, the Environmental Protection Agency (EPA) ordered immediate protections for the citizens of Flint under the Emergency Order clause of the Safe Drinking Water Act. Federal resources were now able to be deployed alongside local and state resources. But during the 18-month period in which a crisis was not declared, the citizens of Flint, whose health was seriously at risk from the lead in their water supply, received minimal government resources and support.

As a public health crisis appears on the horizon, officials may feel overwhelmed by what they need to do and say. Fortunately, researchers have identified distinct patterns for the types of communication needed to most effectively reach and persuade the public. In particular, Matthew Seeger (2006) presented 10 guidelines for best practices in crisis communication. These guidelines are listed in Table 14.1. They provide "general standards rather than specific prescriptions about methods, channels, and messages. These best practices do not constitute a plan, but are the principles or processes that underlie an effective crisis communication plan and an effective crisis response" (p. 242). The focus on general standards and processes is what allows for adaptability during "inherently unpredictable, chaotic events" where public health is at risk (Seeger, 2006, p. 243). Two further guidelines, one focused on culture and the other on social media, have been added to this list. We'll discuss those shortly.

As previously noted, crisis communication research mostly consists of case studies on past crises and attempts to identify which communication responses were effective and which were ineffective. As part of this analysis, after a crisis is contained, crisis managers engage in what is called renewal discourse. **Renewal discourse** is a form of communication that

Table 14.1 Guidelines for Best Practices in Crisis Communication

1. Establish a policy program and process approach
2. Plan pre-event logistics
3. Partner with the public
4. Listen to the public's concerns and work to understand the audience
5. Communicate with honesty, candor, and openness
6. Collaborate and coordinate with credible sources
7. Meet the needs of the media, remaining accessible
8. Communicate with compassion, concern, and empathy
9. Accept uncertainty and ambiguity
10. Incorporate self-efficacy calls into messaging
11. Acknowledge and account for cultural differences and enact relevant narratives
12. Incorporate social media tools throughout the crisis communication plan

Note. The first 10 guidelines were provided by Seeger (2006), the 11th guideline was added by Sellnow and Vidoloff (2009), and the 12th was suggested by Veil et al. (2011).

strives to seek a balance between providing empathy and support for those affected by the crisis while simultaneously looking forward toward rebuilding in a manner that prevents similar crisis events. More specifically, renewal discourse has been characterized as follows (Seeger & Ulmer, 2002):

- Focusing on the future rather than trying to explain the past (note that case studies, by definition, focus on the past, but they do so to help in the future)
- Emphasizing rebuilding and reform to encourage growth
- Highlighting the positive opportunities rather than dwelling on the negative
- Being grounded in the values and vision of leadership and the ability to engender a shared vision

Through engaging in renewal discourse, communities have an opportunity to move forward while contributing to efforts to prevent or reduce the impact of unknown future threats to public health.

Cultural Considerations in Public Health Crises

One of the most important takeaways in understanding a crisis is recognizing that crises are not experienced equally by all the people affected. This means that in a public health crisis, some people experience greater health risks than others. This is so central to the understanding of crisis communication that Tim Sellnow and Kathleen Vidoloff (2009) proposed adding a guideline to Seeger's (2006) original 10 guidelines for effective crisis communication: *Acknowledge and account for cultural differences and enact relevant narratives* (see Table 14.1). This additional recommendation calls attention to the importance of reaching marginalized populations and working to understand how messages could be interpreted differently across cultural, ethnic, racial, and socioeconomic groups. Social determinants of health play a substantial role in how individuals experience a crisis. Let's clarify this with a hypothetical scenario.

Imagine for a moment that a crisis is pending that will require you to evacuate your city. Do you have someone out of state you could call right now and stay with? Do you have transportation to get to this person? Do you have funds to support these unexpected travel plans? If you happened to get injured along the way, do you have health insurance to cover any needed care? Often, when a crisis is reported, audiences are quick to judge the individuals who are "choosing" not to evacuate. But for many people, choosing not to evacuate doesn't feel like a choice at all because they have nowhere to go or no means to support getting there. Case studies examining how different groups of people experience crisis-related events consistently show that differences occur by social determinants of health, especially based on race and disability. Let's look at a few examples for each, starting with race.

Going back to the Flint water crisis, social justice advocates have repeatedly argued that the reason public officials attempted to sweep the issue under the rug was because the residents of the town are predominantly low-income minorities (Campbell et al., 2016). Similarly, in the aftermath of Hurricane Katrina, which devastated New Orleans in 2005, research quickly mounted showing crisis-associated disparities between Black and white residents. For instance, James Elliott and Jeremy Pais (2006) reported that if Black residents, especially low-income residents, were to evacuate at all, they were more likely to evacuate after the hurricane, rather than before as recommended. In addition, Black residents experienced significantly higher stress levels and were more likely to have lost their jobs post-crisis. In both of these examples, Black residents experienced greater health risks than their white counterparts.

Regarding disability, individuals with mobility limitations, such as needing a wheelchair, typically experience some of the greatest barriers to crisis evacuation (Elklit et al., 2018). But crisis disparities arise for people with other disabilities, as well. For example, the COVID-19 pandemic led to mask mandates that were essential to protecting public health. Wearing masks, however, created unique communication barriers for members of the deaf community who rely on reading lips. Although clear face masks, interpreters, and captioning apps were potential resources to support this community during the pandemic (McKee et al., 2020), these resources were not consistently available throughout the pandemic and certainly not required in public spaces, such as grocery stores, banks, and mass transportation. In both of these examples, having a disability resulted in needing to navigate additional challenges that able-bodied individuals did not.

What makes a crisis so difficult is the unexpected details surrounding what exactly will happen and to whom it will happen. Although researchers don't have the ability to see into the future (yet), they do know enough about how crises unfold to provide frameworks for preparing for a crisis event. Indeed, risk and crisis communication scholars have worked diligently to develop evidence-based models to aid with communication decision making during times of crisis.

Theoretical Frameworks for Crisis Communication

Impending public health crises can pose severe threats to life, infrastructure, and economic stability. Crisis managers must, therefore, seek to understand the complex needs, backgrounds, and cultures of audiences, determining the stressors they're experiencing. With this information, crisis managers are responsible for communicating messages that resonate with individuals, provide necessary information, and promote action to prevent negative post-crisis outcomes. Table 14.2 presents some of the most common theories and models for anticipating and examining communication during a public health crisis. Included in the table are the CERC model and chaos theory. The following sections will review each, including examples of their application.

Table 14.2 Theoretical Frameworks for Public Health Crises

Theory/Model	*Brief Summary*	*Citation*
Crisis and Emergency Risk Communication (CERC)	Assumes that crises will develop in largely predictable and systematic ways that can be examined in five distinct stages: precrisis, initial event, maintenance, resolution, and evaluation. Within each stage, the model suggests consideration of six core communication principles: be first, be right, be credible, express empathy, promote action, and be respectful.	Reynolds et al. (2002)
Chaos Theory	This theory attempts to explain the behavior of systems that do not unfold in a linearly predictable, conventional cause-and-effect manner over time. It emphasizes four interacting elements: bifurcation, fractals, attractors, and self-organization.	Murphy (1996)
Situational Crisis Communication Theory	To adequately protect an organization's reputation, management must adjust their communication to account for possible past crises about which relevant publics are aware.	Coombs and Holladay (2002)

Note. See *Supplemental Online Theory Table* for additional theories/models.

Crisis and Emergency Risk Communication

Developed in 2002 through a collaboration between the CDC and public health officials, the **crisis and emergency risk communication (CERC) model** seeks to address both the urgency of crisis communication and the need to explain risks and benefits to stakeholders and the public. Originally designed as a training program to educate and equip public health professionals for their expanding communication responsibilities in emergency situations, CERC provides communication strategies and recommendations for navigating a crisis (Reynolds et al., 2002). The CERC model "assumes that crises will develop in largely predictable and systematic ways: from risk, to eruption, to clean-up and recovery on into evaluation" (Reynolds & Seeger, 2005, p. 51). Following these assumptions, the model examines crisis events in five distinct stages. Within each stage, the CERC model suggests the consideration of six core communication principles. The following paragraphs will review each stage, present the six principles, and provide examples of case studies using the CERC model to evaluate the effectiveness of crisis communication for protecting public health.

The first stage is **precrisis**. At this stage, a crisis event is possible, but the date, time, and location of the potential event are mostly unknown. Communication during this stage predominantly includes risk, warning, and preparation messages. For example, in the state of California, the risk of an earthquake occurring is relatively high. However, experts don't know exactly when or where the next earthquake will happen. Messaging regarding earthquakes in California focuses on preparedness and awareness of how to respond in the event of an earthquake. Next is **initial event**. In this stage, the crisis event has officially occurred in some capacity. Communication in this stage centers on uncertainty reduction, self-efficacy, and reassurance. For example, if a large earthquake occurred, messaging would change to encouraging the enactment of crisis preparedness plans, such as going to emergency evacuation points. The third stage is **maintenance**, where communication echoes that of the second stage but is marked by a sense of informational certainty around the event. For instance, when a hurricane first hits, *initial event* communication will share what is known at the time about emergency resources and the extent of the damage. As time goes on, more information will come to light as additional resources and emergency plans become available. Communication about these resources and their availability, as well as any changes in resources, occurs in the *maintenance* stage. Next is **resolution**. In this stage, the risk to health and life is almost zero, and communication efforts now focus on reflection with the public about what exactly occurred, including how the crisis was resolved, discussions about its cause, and new understandings of risk. Finally, the last stage is **evaluation**. In this stage, communication shifts to renewal discourse with a focus on evaluation of the adequacy of the crisis response and lessons learned. The purpose of the evaluation stage is to honestly and accurately share what is perceived to have gone right and wrong during the crisis.

Across all five stages, the CERC model emphasizes six **communication principles** to be valued and upheld within each stage: be first, be right, be credible, express empathy, promote action, and be respectful (U.S. Department of Health and Human Services, 2018). *Be first* acknowledges the time sensitivity of a crisis, recognizing that communicating in a timely manner is crucial because the first source of information often becomes the preferred source. *Be right* recognizes that it's essential to provide accurate information. This includes being accurate about what is known, what isn't known, and what's being done to fill in the gaps. The third principle, *being credible*, means that honesty and truthfulness should not be compromised during crises. Similarly, *expressing empathy* is essential during a crisis because crises create harm, and addressing what people are feeling, including the challenges they face, builds trust and rapport. *Promoting action* refers to giving people meaningful things to do to calm anxiety, help restore order, and promote a sense of control. Finally, *being respectful* is essential during times of crisis when the public often feels the most vulnerable. When people feel disrespected, they're less likely to respond positively to messages.

The CERC model has been used by numerous crisis communication scholars to examine communication effectiveness during a crisis. In a systematic review of CERC-related research conducted prior to 2018, Ann Neville Miller and colleagues (2021) analyzed 400 articles reviewing, critiquing, or applying the CERC model. A little more than half of these studies examined a crisis or disaster in North America ($n = 202$). The authors coded the studies for the type of crisis/disaster they covered and found that almost half ($n = 167$) covered crises "in general." As far as studies that covered specific crises, the most common crisis by far was infectious disease ($n = 127$), with coverage 10 times that of the next closest crisis categories (droughts, weather events, and radiological or chemical incidents, all coming in at $n = 13$). Although it is clear that CERC is widely used within the academic discipline (400 articles in the 16 years since the model's inception is impressive), the authors conclude that their findings show that "although a robust body of research has cited and applied the CERC model in case studies, few projects have empirically tested CERC" (Miller et al., 2021, p. 19).

In more recent years, the CERC model has been especially helpful in understanding how social media has played a role in crisis communication efforts. For instance, Emily Kinsky and colleagues (2021) examined 13 FEMA-related Twitter accounts during four major hurricanes that hit the U.S. over a three-month period in 2017 (Harvey, Irma, Maria, and Nate). The researchers scraped 1,095 tweets, coding each for hurricane, content (word use, tagging, quoting, and information type), and user engagement (original tweets, retweets, and replies). Their findings showed that FEMA messaging predominantly occurred during the later CERC stages of maintenance, resolution, and evaluation. Importantly, the authors concluded that the FEMA messages clearly followed four of the six CERC communication principles, as we detail next.

First, "Credible sources were developed through the use of authority figures and consistent use of hashtags and tagging of authoritative organizations" (Kinsky et al., 2021, p. 8). Second, "Empathy was built using personal pronouns to create identification with stakeholders" (Kinsky et al., 2021, p. 8). Third, tweets were action-oriented in their promotion of self-efficacy and management procedures. Finally, FEMA's tweets demonstrated respect by providing "Links and visual elements (that) helped connect to various stakeholders" and "Providing facts and instructions for safety and health during storms...particularly when tweets place value on what is important to stakeholders, which could include pets and property as well as human lives" (Kinsky et al., 2021, p. 8). In addition, the authors found that despite the changing threats occurring between each hurricane, FEMA consistently paid attention to the specific community's needs. Although the authors didn't comment on whether FEMA followed the communication principles of being first and being right, Twitter, as a platform, did allow FEMA to be first, and there's no evidence that they shared information that wasn't right. So we are comfortable claiming that FEMA did consider all six principles.

The CERC model provides a clear framework of expected communication patterns before, during, and after a crisis event. This model has been a useful tool for crisis communication scholars working to identify the most and least effective approaches to crisis communication, as well as determining the extent to which agencies are following the tenets of the crisis model. Although the CERC model lays out five stages of a crisis along a linear path, sometimes things aren't always so linear. Indeed, crisis events can often create moments of chaos that can be challenging for crisis scholars to organize, examine, and evaluate. In those moments, other frameworks, such as chaos theory, can be useful for scholars seeking to learn from public health crises.

Chaos Theory

Chaos theory posits that a predictable pattern of organization can be detected within seemingly chaotic events. Priscilla Murphy (1996) explains that "Although it incorporates elements of chance, chaos is not random disorder. Rather, chaos theory attempts to understand the behavior of systems that do not unfold in a linearly predictable, conventional cause-and-effect manner over time" (p. 96). Curtis Liska and colleagues (2012) elaborate, stating that chaos theory "offers perspective for analyzing crisis communication and response strategies beyond traditional linear views of cause and effect during postcrisis situations" (p. 180). Specifically regarding crisis communication, chaos theory has been used as a metaphor to better understand the unexpected, dynamic, and complex events of natural disasters, terrorist attacks, and other public health crises.

The roots of chaos theory are grounded in theories of the physical universe articulated by scientists such as Galileo, Bacon, Descartes, and Newton (Murphy, 1996). Chaos theory emphasizes four interacting elements. First, *bifurcation* refers to the fundamental disruption of order, where radical change (e.g., a crisis) has resulted in sensemaking challenges for those experiencing the change. Due to the unexpected nature of the crisis, the bifurcation creates uncertainty in those experiencing the event (Seeger et al., 2003). Second, *fractals*, which are a unit of measurement for organizational patterns, are sources of information that exist in various pieces and from various sources. Fractals can be processed in a variety of different ways by different people, resulting in different crisis responses and perspectives (Liska et al., 2012). Third, *attractors* refer to "values, principles, and social assumptions that draw people together in pursuit of common goals" (Murphy, 1996, p. 183). Because a crisis has the potential to either tear communities apart or bring them together, attractors serve as opportunities to create meaning for people to unite around (Seeger, 2006). Finally, *self-organization* refers to a group's ability to adapt to the crisis event and implement positive changes for moving forward (Wheatley, 2007). According to chaos theory, these four interacting elements do not happen in a linear process but, instead, are dynamic and interdependent, wherein changes to one produce changes in the others throughout the ongoing crisis event (Liska et al., 2012).

Unlike CERC, which suggests that crisis managers can effectively move the public through five distinct stages of crisis communication, chaos theory recognizes that mass groups can respond in unpredictable, and sometimes irrational, ways that reduce the power of agencies to influence the public's behaviors (Murphy, 1996). Thus, CERC is most easily applied to a crisis where messaging can clearly signal each of the five stages, and chaos theory is uniquely situated to examine a crisis in which the current stage is hard to discern. For instance, historically, pandemics have been treated as public health crises, not fodder for political gain. Throughout the stages of pandemics, leaders would deliver credible, fact-based information to guide appropriate public response and quell fears. However, in the United States, the COVID-19 pandemic saw traditionally credible sources spreading misinformation and contradicting evidence from public health officials (Prasad, 2021). This resulted in competing narratives about how people should be responding during the pandemic, leaving the public less prepared and protected throughout the crisis (Mian & Khan, 2020). The resulting lack of consistent stakeholder and public response led to a repeating cycle of crisis stages, with a blurring of whether the pandemic was in the initial event, maintenance, or resolution stage. We don't need to tell you, dear reader, that chaos, defined in its traditional sense, is a reasonable adjective to describe what living through COVID-19 has felt like. Thus, it is not surprising that a theory that recognizes patterns from non-linear, chaotic events is helpful in analyzing the effective and ineffective communication moments during those events.

Through the lens of chaos theory, communication strategies should not seek to move through a general preparedness plan intended to reduce perceived threats and uncertainty. Instead, communication strategies should focus on in-the-moment responses to the bifurcations, fractals, and attractors currently at play as a means to produce self-organization. We'll demonstrate what we mean by this through our own analysis of communication messaging during the COVID-19 pandemic. Going back to the bifurcation of the COVID-19 pandemic in the United States, we can see how communication strategies began by following a general pandemic playbook: Communicate preventive behaviors with the public and make them feel empowered to perform said behaviors (e.g., practice social distancing, wear a mask, get vaccinated). But as previously noted, the public did not respond as expected to these messages, in large part due to the fractals of misinformation that flooded their media environments. The public's resistance to messaging halted planned communication and left public health experts largely surprised by the challenges in persuading the public to engage in simple, sensible prevention behaviors. Eventually, communication strategies shifted toward creating attractors for the public, such as messages that addressed saving lives, vaccine safety, and the hope of finally ending the pandemic. Through these attractor messages, self-organizing was able to move forward, albeit slowly, to increase vaccination rates and reduce the spread of infection.

Across the various crisis communication theories and models, including CERC and chaos theory, one factor consistently plays a role in making or breaking the effectiveness of crisis management. That factor is crisis leadership. Whoever is taking lead on communicating with the public bears an enormous responsibility, one that can decide the success or failure of a crisis response. It's easy to sit in the comfort of our homes and judge the decisions made by local, national, and global leaders. But most people will never truly know the complexities of the decisions that leaders have to make during a crisis.

Public Health Crisis Leadership

What does it mean to be a good leader? Ideally, good leaders are expected to have the problem-solving skills of MacGyver, the intelligence of Marie Curie, the charisma of Oprah Winfrey, the grace of Misty Copeland, the grit of John Lewis, the patience of Nelson Mandela, and the selflessness of Ghandi. Basically, good leaders are expected to be superheroes. But at their core, leaders are just your standard human in a position of power. What leaders choose to do in their leadership positions can elevate others to do their best, keep things at the status quo, or doom everyone. Leaders, therefore, are not defined by who they are but by what they choose to do and say in their positions of power.

Yuen Wu and colleagues (2021) define **crisis leadership** as "a process in which leaders act to prepare for the occurrence of unexpected crises, deal with the salient implications of crises, and grow from the disruptive experience of crises" (p. 3). In addition, the researchers argue that research on crisis leadership is different from research on crisis management in that crisis leadership includes a critical analysis of the effectiveness of the leader during the crisis, such as how a crisis influences leaders, how leaders exert influence over others during the crisis, and why some leaders are more effective than others in a crisis. Thus, crisis leadership is part of crisis management but more comprehensive in its examination of the role of the leader. This is important because how a leader chooses to respond can make or break the success of a crisis response, which in a public health crisis can mean life or death.

The literature is laden with examples of successful moments of leadership during a crisis, such as Massachusetts Governor Deval Patrick's coordination during the 2013 Boston marathon bombing (Marcus et al., 2014), New Zealand Prime Minister Jacinda Ardern's communication during the COVID-19 pandemic (McGuire et al., 2020), and former President Barak Obama's renewal discourse and planning following the 2014 Ebola outbreak (Schismenos et al., 2020). On the other side of the coin, researchers have also documented numerous examples of ineffective leadership during a crisis, such as the U.S. presidential mishandling of the COVID-19 pandemic (Schismenos et al., 2020), Senator Ted Cruz's absence from the 2021 severe winter weather crisis in Texas (Faktorovich, 2021), and most government officials' behavior during the Flint water crisis (Kennedy, 2016). But what is the major differentiator between effective and ineffective leaders? That is a question that's been explored by researchers from the Harvard National Preparedness Leadership Initiative.

Launched after the 9/11 terrorist attack, the **Harvard National Preparedness Leadership Initiative (NPLI)** is a joint program offered by Harvard's T.H. Chan School of Public Health and Center for Public Leadership (Marcus & Gergen, 2023). One of the many aspects of leadership studied by NPLI researchers is leadership behavior during crisis events, with the goal of identifying strategies and patterns that lead to effective crisis leadership. One of NPLI's findings suggests that a possible model for effective crisis leadership is one that typically applies to animal behavior: swarm intelligence. According to Leonard Marcus and colleagues (2014), **swarm intelligence** is a phenomenon in nature where no single individual is directly in charge, yet remarkable achievements are made. It's characterized by the principles of a unity of mission, a spirit of generosity, respect for others, removal of assigned credit/blame, and strong preexisting relationships.

For an example of the phenomenon of swarm intelligence, Marcus et al. (2014) point to the leadership following the 2013 Boston marathon bombing, in which two homemade pressure cooker bombs detonated 12 seconds and 210 yards apart near the finish line of the race, killing three people and injuring hundreds of others. In their analysis of leadership behavior in the aftermath of the event, they "discovered an extraordinary though unspoken (and unconscious) compliance to these principles among the Boston MBR [marathon bombings response] leaders" (p. 11). For example, no leader tried to steal the spotlight or grandstand. Instead, they demonstrated respect for each other's authority in their respective jurisdictions and forged "extraordinary cooperation…across organizational lines of authority" (p. 15). Marcus et al. caution that the full potential of a swarm intelligence leadership approach can be easily lost due to factors such as politics, rivalries, glory-seeking, lack of awareness, and failure to come together. However, the closer crisis management comes to a swarm intelligence approach, the more successful leaders will be in their crisis management.

Crisis Communication Leadership: Definition and Characteristics

Crisis leadership is a process in which leaders act to prepare for the occurrence of unexpected crises, deal with the salient implications of crises, and grow from the disruptive experience of crises. Research suggests that a swarm intelligence approach is the most effective leadership strategy during a crisis. This approach is characterized by the principles of a unity of mission, a spirit of generosity, respect for others, removal of assigned credit/blame, and strong preexisting relationships.

When lives are on the line, leaders can be a key factor in successful crisis management. But they're not the only factor. Beyond messages from individuals and organizations, communication research on public health crises has also found the message channel to be an essential factor in the effectiveness of crisis communication. Importantly, the substantial technological advancement over the last few decades has changed, and improved, the ways in which crisis managers can communicate with the general public during a crisis.

Media Facilitation of Crisis Communication

With its ability to reach mass audiences, the media has always been a key tool for crisis communicators. In fact, Larsåke Larsson (2010) went so far as to say that media "constitute the most important information path to citizens" (p. 716) during a crisis. This importance stems from the ability of media to efficiently communicate with large audiences quickly and simultaneously as the crisis unfolds. But media platforms are not just simply tools for communicating to the public. Rather, they are large corporate entities with their own vested interests and financial goals. Thus, crisis managers need to facilitate a working relationship with media entities in order to establish honest and open dialogues that will facilitate media access during times of crisis (Ulmer et al., 2007). But as is true of most relationships, establishing mutually beneficial exchanges is easier said than done.

During a crisis, crisis managers need media platforms in order to get information out to the public. And at the same time, media entities need crisis managers in order to report the details of stories that attract audiences. But just because they both need each other doesn't mean that they always work together cohesively. For example, Robert Littlefield and Andrea Quenette (2007) conducted a rhetorical analysis of 52 news stories published in *The New York Times* or *Times-Picayune of New Orleans* covering the government's response to the 2005 Hurricane Katrina crisis that devastated New Orleans. The researchers recognized that although the media initially served their primary function of providing the public with information on the crisis, by the end of the crisis the media had lost their objectivity and were pointing blame. Littlefield and Quenette argue that blaming is problematic because "the association of negative terms with those in authority may result in the premature placement of blame by the public and the effectiveness of those in authority may be compromised" (p. 43). The authors aren't saying that incompetent or malicious authorities shouldn't be held accountable. Rather, their argument is that evaluations of crisis response effectiveness should prioritize conclusions from crisis communication experts, not accounts from journalists who may be more focused on attracting readers than drawing sound conclusions about crisis response. Such tensions surrounding media reporting during a crisis contribute to the efforts of crisis managers to use media platforms outside of traditional channels.

Historically, television was the medium most relied on during times of crisis (Heath & O'Hair, 2009). However, more recent research suggests that social media is quickly becoming the leading medium for communicating with audiences during a crisis (Austin et al., 2012). Reasons for this include that the platforms deliver messages quickly, reach large numbers of people, can facilitate dialogue, and are already embedded into daily social and organizational communication habits. Social media has been identified as such an essential tool during times of crisis that Shari Veil and colleagues (2011) argued that guidelines for effective crisis communication should officially consider social media, coming to the following recommendation: *Incorporate social media tools throughout the crisis communication plan* (see Table 14.1). Further, in order to have preestablished credibility with the public before the onset of a crisis, Jeannette Sutton (2018) suggests that public health organizations should actively engage in social media posting through routine, daily communications on social media—especially in an era of bot-based misinformation efforts.

Over the last decade, research has closely examined the use of social media for crisis communication. Use, in this context, has two distinct meanings: (a) the role of social media in facilitating public awareness of a crisis and (b) the degree to which the public engages in their own crisis communication via social media. Let's take a brief look at each area of research.

Regarding the role of social media in facilitating public awareness of a crisis, most research has found social media to be the primary channel for crisis awareness, including during the global COVID-19 pandemic (Ehondor & Unakalamba, 2021), the Flint water crisis (Day et al., 2019), and the 2009 H1N1 influenza outbreak (Reynolds, 2010). For all of these crises, and many more, social media was found to be a primary source for learning about the ongoing crisis. Interestingly, but probably not surprising to avid social media users, crisis managers appear to be using social media platforms differently for different purposes. For instance, Jeanine Guidry and colleagues (2017) examined the Twitter and Instagram posts by the CDC, World Health Organization, and Doctors without Borders during the 2014 Ebola crisis. They found that public health organizations used the two platforms differently, noting that "posts on Instagram were significantly more likely than those on Twitter to feature risk perception variables, such as information about adverse or dreaded outcomes" (p. 483). They note this finding as one possible reason that user engagement was higher with Instagram posts than Twitter posts. This finding is important because which social media platform people are on could influence the crisis communication information they receive.

Regarding the degree to which the public engages in their own crisis communication via social media, research has revealed two patterns. First, members of the public have reported crisis stories on their social media accounts before mainstream media were able to pick them up. For example, the 2009 emergency plane landing in the Hudson River was first reported on Twitter by a nearby ferry passenger (Memmott, 2014). Second, the public uses social media as a means to communicate their own experiences and perspectives during a crisis. For instance, following the 2011 earthquake that hit off the coast of Japan, causing a tsunami that led to a radiation disaster, there was an immediate public outpouring of crisis-related user experiences on Twitter, including calls to action, expressions of emotions, and provision of information (Cho et al., 2013). In addition to information seeking and sharing, some researchers have found social media to be an essential tool for individuals affected by a crisis to simply reach out to and communicate with their own friends and family, such as was true during Hurricane Maria, which ravaged Puerto Rico in 2017 (Bui, 2019).

As discussed in earlier chapters, the digital divide produces gaps in access to communication technologies. These gaps are products of social determinants of health wherein individuals with a lower socioeconomic status have a harder time accessing and critically consuming media. Although social media has leveled the playing field slightly, mainstream media sources, such as newspapers and streaming services, still require fees to access. Crisis communicators are not responsible for solving the systemic problems and structural racism that underlie digital divide issues. They are, however, responsible for recognizing the reality of the digital divide and communicating equitably in order to reach all members of the at-risk public. For example, Ashleigh Day and colleagues (2019) found that during the Flint water crisis, social media use and content varied by race such that African Americans were the most likely to obtain current information about the crisis via Instagram. Because this group was also the most at risk during the crisis, public health efforts prioritizing crisis-related messaging on Instagram would have been an equitable communications strategy.

Preparing for the Unexpected

Crises almost always result in sadness and loss. But with all challenging life experiences, if you look hard enough, silver linings can be found. For crises, sometimes the events, moments, and missteps that were terrible—or maybe even made things worse—can lead to changes to reduce the risk of such events happening again or reducing loss if they do. For example, the 1999 Columbine school shooting that shook America to its core led to state (Seeger et al., 2001) and federal (Vossekuil et al., 2002) changes to school-based crisis response plans. Although the United States still has a long, long way to go in preventing school-based shootings, such communication crisis plans are important tools to have in place. The point is that with each crisis, people ideally learn from what went wrong so they can do better next time. Today, numerous public health program officials, event coordinators, and government agency leaders have created communication plans or invested resources to prepare for worst-case scenarios.

For example, public health programs such as Harvard's NPLI exist to prepare individuals and organizations for communicating during a crisis event. The NPLI conducts research and creates educational programs that prepare leaders for potential crisis challenges (Marcus & Gergen, 2023). The program provides online training delivered by NPLI staff and self-administered programs for leaders looking to sharpen their skills during times of crisis.

In addition to public health programs, crisis communication researchers also host and attend events to share, discuss, and learn about the latest research in crisis communication. Such events include the *International Crisis and Risk Communication (ICRC) Conference* held annually at the University of Central Florida (ICRC, n.d.). Finally, government-funded agencies are among the most notable entities providing crisis communication plans, education, and resources. For instance, the CDC (2020) hosts an online *Emergency Preparedness and Response* page with immediate resources for current crises and links for ongoing communication programs, such as CERC. Over the last 100 years and through many crises, public health programs, event coordinators, and government agencies have worked to create crisis preparedness plans. Although all of the people involved in these efforts hope to never need them, the plans remain available to enhance effective crisis response should they be necessary.

Preparing for a Crisis Situation

To prepare for a crisis, individuals should seek information from credible organizations, such as government and public health agencies. Following these organizations on social media now, before a crisis occurs, can, in the event of a crisis, help you receive crisis-related information right as it becomes available. If you're at risk of experiencing a crisis, such as living in a region with extreme weather events, you should review crisis preparedness resources from local and national government and public health agencies. Effective preparation can save lives.

Conclusion

Thanks to the COVID-19 pandemic, the general term "public health crisis" is now a household phrase—one that will elicit emotional reactions for generations to come. Although it's safe to say that no one wants to relive the pandemic years (we hope!), the experience should remind everyone of the importance of crisis preparedness. This chapter sought to provide a broader and deeper understanding of what a public health crisis is and what it entails.

Through research-based examinations of past crises and analysis of crisis communication, lessons learned can be gathered and used to better prepare for the next crisis. With 12 working guidelines for crisis communication, appropriate preparedness involves education on crisis communication processes, competent leadership, and effective use of media resources.

Although the details surrounding the next big crisis will always remain unknown, everyone can take comfort in knowing that preparing for the unknown isn't futile. For example, different groups of people have different resources and abilities to respond during a crisis, and considering those differences will be essential to the effectiveness of the crisis management plan. A crisis communication plan is not static. It will fluctuate and change as new research is published and as social communication patterns change. The best that government agencies, public health officials, and leaders can do is commit to creating, updating, and implementing crisis preparedness plans that include a comprehensive communication strategy. And should we ever find ourselves face-to-face with another public health crisis, let's remember the empowering words of author C. S. Lewis from his work *Voyage of the Dawn Treader*: "Hardships often prepare ordinary people for an extraordinary destiny." Here's to extraordinary.

References

Austin, L., Fisher Liu, B., & Jin, Y. (2012). How audiences seek out crisis information: Exploring the social-mediated crisis communication model. *Journal of Applied Communication Research, 40*(2), 188–207.

Ballard-Reisch, D., Clements-Nolle, K., Jenkins, T., Sacks, T., Pruitt, K., & Leathers, K. (2007). Applying the crisis and emergency risk communication (CERC) integrative model to bioterrorism preparedness: A case study. In M. W. Seeger, T. L. Sellnow, & R. R. Ulmer (Eds.), *Crisis communication and the public health* (pp. 203–219). Hampton.

Bui, L. (2019). Social media, rumors, and hurricane warning systems in Puerto Rico. In *Proceedings of the 52nd Hawaii International Conference on System Sciences*. https://scholarspace.manoa.hawaii.edu/bitstream/10125/59704/1/0264.pdf

Campbell, C., Greenberg, R., Mankikar, D., & Ross, R. D. (2016). A case study of environmental injustice: The failure in Flint. *International Journal of Environmental Research and Public Health, 13*(10), 1–11.

Centers for Disease Control & Prevention. (2018, January 23). *Crisis & Emergency Risk Communication (CERC)*. https://emergency.cdc.gov/cerc/index.asp.

Centers for Disease Control & Prevention. (2020, March 19). *Emergency preparedness and response*. https://emergency.cdc.gov/

Cho, S. E., Jung, K., & Park, H. W. (2013). Social media use during Japan's 2011 earthquake: How Twitter transforms the locus of crisis communication. *Media International Australia, 149*(1), 28–40.

City of Flint, Michigan. (2015, December 15). *Mayor Karen Weaver declares state of emergency*. https://www.cityofflint.com/mayor-karen-weaver-declares-state-of-emergency/

City of Flint, Michigan. (2016, January 14). *Genesee County Commissioners declare emergency*. https://www.cityofflint.com/genesee-county-commissioners-declare-emergency/

Coombs, W. T. (2012). *Ongoing crisis communication: Planning, managing, and responding* (3rd ed.). Sage.

Coombs, W. T., & Holladay, S. J. (2002). Helping crisis managers protect reputational assets: Initial tests of the situational crisis communication theory. *Management Communication Quarterly, 16*, 165–186.

Day, A. M., O'Shay-Wallace, S., Seeger, M. W., & McElmurry, S. P. (2019). Informational sources, social media use, and race in the Flint, Michigan, water crisis. *Communication Studies, 70*(3), 352–376.

Ehondor, B., & Unakalamba, C. (2021). Social media for crisis communication in the Coronavirus (COVID-19) outbreak: A study of NCDC. *Journal of Media Research, 14*(2), 45–69.

Elklit, A., Simonsen, L. D., & Todorovac, A. (2018). *No one left behind-The accessibility of medical and psychosocial services following disasters and other traumatic events: Experiences of physical disabled individuals, in Denmark*. Federal Office of Civil Protection and Disaster Assistance. http://eunad-info.eu/fileadmin/EUNAD-Downloads/Research/Denmark_Report_Physically.pdf

Elliott, J. R., & Pais, J. (2006). Race, class, and Hurricane Katrina: Social differences in human responses to disaster. *Social Science Research, 35*(2), 295–321.

Faktorovich, A. (2021). The blackout in Quanah, Texas. *Pennsylvania Literary Journal, 13*(1), 91–340.

Guidry, J. P. D., Jin, Y., Orr, C. A., Messner, M., & Meganck, S. (2017). Ebola on Instagram and Twitter: How health organizations address the health crisis in their social media engagement. *Public Relations Review, 43*(3), 477–486.

Heath, R. L., & O'Hair, H. D. (Eds.). (2009). *Handbook of risk and crisis communication*. Routledge.

International Crisis and Risk Communication Conference. (n.d.). *History*. https://communication.ucf.edu/icrcc/history/

Jong, W. (2021). Evaluating crisis communication. A 30-item checklist for assessing performance during COVID-19 and other pandemics. *Journal of Health Communication, 25*(12), 962–970.

Kennedy, M. (2016, April 20). Lead-laced water in Flint: A step-by-step look at the makings of a crisis. *NPR*. https://www.npr.org/sections/thetwo-way/2016/04/20/465545378/lead-laced-water-in-flint-a-step-by-step-look-at-the-makings-of-a-crisis

Kinsky, E. S., Chen, L., & Drumheller, K. (2021). Crisis and emergency risk communication: FEMA's Twitter use during the 2017 hurricane season. *Public Relations Review, 47*(4), 102094.

Larsson, L. (2010). Crisis and learning. In W. T. Coombs & S. J. Holladay (Eds.) *The handbook of crisis communication* (pp. 713–717). Wiley.

Liska, C., Petrun, E. L., Sellnow, T. L., & Seeger, M. W. (2012). Chaos theory, self-organization, and industrial accidents: Crisis communication in the Kingston coal ash spill. *Southern Communication Journal, 77*(3), 180–197.

Littlefield, R. S., & Quenette, A. M. (2007). Crisis leadership and Hurricane Katrina: The portrayal of authority by the media in natural disasters. *Journal of Applied Communication Research, 35*(1), 26–47.

Marcus, L. J., & Gergen, D. (2023). Co-director's welcome. *National preparedness leadership initiative*. https://npli.sph.harvard.edu/about/co-directors-welcome/

Marcus, L. J., McNulty, E., Dorn, B. S., & Goralnick, E. (2014). Crisis meta-leadership lessons from the Boston marathon bombings response: The ingenuity of swarm intelligence. *National Preparedness Leadership Initiative*. https://cdn1.sph.harvard.edu/wp-content/uploads/sites/2443/2016/09/Marathon-Bombing-Leadership-Response-Report.pdf

McGuire, D., Cunningham, J. E., Reynolds, K., & Matthews-Smith, G. (2020). Beating the virus: An examination of the crisis communication approach taken by New Zealand Prime Minister Jacinda Ardern during the Covid-19 pandemic. *Human Resource Development International, 23*(4), 361–379.

McKee, M., Moran, C., & Zazove, P. (2020). Overcoming additional barriers to care for deaf and hard of hearing patients during COVID-19. *JAMA Otolaryngology–Head & Neck Surgery, 146*(9), 781–782.

Memmott, M. (2014, January 15). 5 years ago Sully landed on the Hudson and Twitter took off. *National Public Radio*. https://www.npr.org/sections/thetwo-way/2014/01/15/262767982/5-years-ago-sully-landed-on-the-hudson-and-twitter-took-off

Mian, A., & Khan, S. (2020). Coronavirus: The spread of misinformation. *BMC Medicine, 18*(1), 89.

Miller, A. N., Collins, C., Neuberger, L., Todd, A., Sellnow, T. L., & Boutemen, L. (2021). Being first, being right, and being credible since 2002: A systematic review of crisis and emergency risk communication (CERC) research. *Journal of International Crisis and Risk Communication Research, 4*(1), 1–27.

Murphy, P. (1996). Chaos theory as a model for managing issues and crises. *Public Relations Review, 22*(2), 95–113.

Prasad, A. (2021). Anti-science misinformation and conspiracies: COVID–19, post-truth, and science & technology studies (STS). *Science, Technology and Society, 27*(1), 88–112.

Reynolds, B., Hunter-Galdo, J., & Sokler, L. (2002). *Crisis and emergency risk communication*. Centers for Disease Control and Prevention.

Reynolds, B., & Seeger, M. W. (2005). Crisis and emergency risk communication as an integrative model. *Journal of Health Communication, 10*, 43–55.

Reynolds, B. J. (2010). Building trust through social media. CDC's experience during the H1N1 influenza response. *Marketing Health Services, 30*(2), 18–21.

Schismenos, S., Smith, A. A., Stevens, G. J., & Emmanouloudis, D. (2020). Failure to lead on COVID-19: What went wrong with the United States? *International Journal of Public Leadership, 17*(1), 39–53.

Seeger, M. W. (2006). Best practices in crisis communication: An expert panel process. *Journal of Applied Communication Research, 34*(3), 232–244.

Seeger, M. W., Heyart, B., Barton, E. A., & Bultnyck, S. (2001). Crisis planning and crisis communication in the public schools: Assessing post Columbine responses. *Communication Research Reports, 18*(4), 375–383.

Seeger, M. W., Sellnow, T. L., & Ulmer, R. R. (1998). Communication, organization and crisis. In M. E. Roloff (Eds.), *Communication yearbook* (Vol. 21, pp. 231–275). Sage.

Seeger, M. W., Sellnow, T. L., & Ulmer, R. R. (2003). *Communication and organizational crisis.* Praeger.

Seeger, M., & Ulmer, R. (2002). A post-crisis discourse of renewal: The cases of Malden Mills and Cole Hardwoods. *Journal of Applied Communication Research, 30*(2), 126–142.

Sellnow, T. L., & Vidoloff, K. G. (2009). Getting crisis communication right: Eleven best practices for effective risk communication can help an organization navigate the slippery path through a crisis situation. *Food Technology, 63*(9), 40.

Sutton, J. (2018). Health communication trolls and bots versus public health agencies' trusted voices. *American Journal of Public Health, 108*(10), 1281–1282.

Ulmer, R. R., Sellnow, T. L., & Seeger, M. W. (2007). *Effective crisis communication: Moving from crisis to opportunity.* Sage.

U.S. Department of Health and Humans Services. (2018). *CERC: Crisis + Emergency Risk Communication.* https://emergency.cdc.gov/cerc/ppt/CERC_Introduction.pdf

Veil, S. R. (2011). Mindful learning in crisis management. *International Journal of Business Communication, 48*(2), 116–147.

Veil, S. R., Buehner, T., & Palenchar, M. J. (2011). A work-in-process literature review: Incorporating social media in risk and crisis communication. *Journal of Contingencies and Crisis Management, 19*(2), 110–122.

Vossekuil, B., Fein, R.A., Reddy, M., Borum, R., & Modzeleski, W. (2002). The final report and findings of the "Safe School Initiative": Implications for the prevention of school attacks in the United States. *Department of Education, Washington, DC; United States Secret Service, Washington, DC (ERIC Document Reproduction Service No. ED466024).* https://www2.ed.gov/admins/lead/safety/preventingattacksreport.pdf

Wheatley, M. J. (2007). *Leadership for an uncertain time.* Barrett-Koehler.

Wu, Y. L., Shao, B., Newman, A., & Schwarz, G. (2021). Crisis leadership: A review and future research agenda. *The Leadership Quarterly, 32*(6), 1–22.

In-class Activities

1. Identify a crisis in the news that is likely to pose health risks. Compare three news stories from three different sources and analyze the stories for message content, identifying the credibility of the sources, timeliness of the information, and feasibility of the public ask.

2. Put students in small groups and assign them one of the following health crisis scenarios. Have them write a two-minute press conference statement following the six communication principles of the CERC model (see Table 14.2) and present it to the class:

   a. Deli meat has been recalled due to a listeria contamination. The CDC says more than 500 people are confirmed ill and four are in the hospital, including a three-year-old girl who is now in a coma. You're the communications specialist for the CDC.

   b. A train carrying anhydrous ammonia has derailed just outside the city. The immediate area has been evacuated, and hospitals are crowded with people complaining of burning eyes and throats. You're the public information officer for the fire department.

   c. A devastating tornado has hit your state. Power is out across town and likely will be out for the next several days. A large section of a manufacturing plant collapsed, trapping an unknown number of people. Temperatures are forecast to be below freezing tonight. You're the communications specialist for the city.

Discussion Questions

1. How do you think the metaphor of a zombie apocalypse can help crisis communicators prepare for a public health crisis?

2. How long do you think you could survive in your current home if a mandatory shelter-in-place order were issued and there were no running water? What supplies would you need to survive for 72 hours? A full week?
3. Do you currently follow any social media accounts that would post helpful information during a crisis, such as the CDC and the American Public Health Association? If so, why would you recommend that others should follow these accounts? If not, what are your hesitations about following such accounts?

Unit VI
Looking Forward

Dr. Cheryl Montgomery—A Force for Good

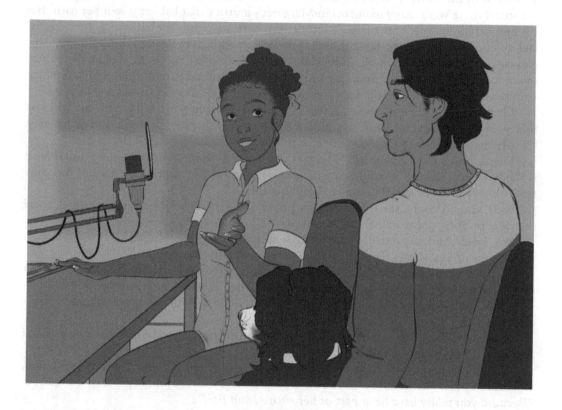

Somehow Cheryl had managed to tell her story in only an hour. Bryce's face hurt a little from smiling so much. And to Cheryl's delight, the butterflies were completely gone from her stomach.

"And now here we are," Cheryl said with a smile.

"Wow. What a journey," Bryce said. "And what interesting people you've had in your life," he noted.

"I really have," Cheryl replied. "And those are just the people I know. I've also been inspired by incredible individuals that I've never met. People whose success has centered communication in their work to promote public health."

"Who comes to mind?" asked Bryce.

"Oh, gosh, so many people. In recent years, Dr. Ala Stanford is at the top of the list. When her community of Philadelphia was devastated by the COVID-19 pandemic, she really stepped up to help. I first heard of her when *Philadelphia Magazine* reported that she rented a van, filled it with testing supplies, gathered a few volunteers, and began administering

DOI: 10.4324/9781003214458-35

COVID-19 tests to people in Black communities. She was motivated to do this," Cheryl elaborated, "when she realized that compared to people living in majority-white counties, people living in majority-Black counties were infected with COVID at three times the rate and dying at almost six times the rate. Her efforts eventually established the Black Doctors COVID-19 Consortium. Their mission is education and advocacy for the African American community. Dr. Stanford has been a model of equitable, community-based solutions during a public health crisis."

"That's a great example. What about from further in the past?" Bryce asked.

"Well, I would absolutely have to recognize the incredible Margaret Sanger, who, of course, was the women's right activist who coined the term 'birth control,' promoted awareness of the birth control pill, and founded the American Birth Control League. Like my story, there were many moments in Margaret's journey that led her down her path. But PBS reported that one of the larger motivational turning points for her was witnessing the lack of effective contraceptives that led many women who were facing unwanted pregnancies to resort to cheap, back-alley abortions that ended up killing them, especially women of color. Her group was the founding organization of Planned Parenthood, which now has community clinics all over the nation providing healthcare services to women in need."

"That's another great example. When you started sharing your story with us, you said that your grandmother, Helen, was probably the most influential person on your journey. Clearly that was true. Your accomplishments really pay tribute to her," Bryce stated.

"Thank you," Cheryl replied. "The fact that I get to share her story on a regular basis is the best gift. As hard as her death was, it may serve to help other women avoid the same fate. I know she'd be very honored to play that role."

"Well, and no doubt, she would be very proud of you. And your growing family. I heard that you recently got married?" Bryce asked.

"Yes, I did. And he's actually here today with our baby," Cheryl replied.

"Oh, great! Let's bring them in," Bryce said, waving to the door.

The door opened and in walked a man with hazel green eyes. In front of him trotted a happy puppy. The puppy got excited as Cheryl reached down to pick him up.

"Okay, welcome Dr. Juarez. We're excited you could join us today to talk about your amazing wife," Bryce said to Nathian.

"Great to be here. Thanks for letting me and Belarino join you today," Nathian responded as he scratched the puppy's ears.

"Well, I won't keep you long because we're almost out of time. But I'd love to ask you, what has it been like to have a front row seat to Cheryl's career journey?" Bryce inquired. "Because you really have been part of her entire adult life."

"Yes, I have. And it was special. From day one I knew Cheryl was a force—in a good way. When Helen was diagnosed with breast cancer, it was devastating to watch the whole family hurt," Nathian shared. "There was so much uncertainty. The healthcare system was difficult to navigate. Experiences with healthcare providers varied substantially with all the visits they had. There was just a lot. But the support that the Montgomery family provided each other was really something to witness. And Cheryl channeling her pain to help other women understand environmental health risks for breast cancer and receive treatment is, like I said, very, very special."

"That definitely seems to sum up the whole journey. And I see that we are out of time. Dr. Montgomery, thank you for being with us today. It's great to see how you used your graduate training in communication and medical degree together to serve your community. I'm sure I speak for all our listeners when I say that we wish you the best and can't wait to see what's next for you."

Nathian smiled and put his arm around Cheryl, who smiled back at him. The puppy, who was sitting in Cheryl's lap, jumped up and licked her face. Bryce, Nathian, and Cheryl all laughed for a minute before they stood up and left the podcast studio.

Notes

Learn more about the exemplary work Dr. Ala Stanford is doing with the Black Doctors COVID-19 Consortium: https://blackdoctorsconsortium.com/. Read more about her journey here: https://www.phillymag.com/healthcare-news/2020/08/08/ala-stanford-black-doctors-covid-19-consortium/

Learn more about the pioneering work of Margaret Sanger from PBS: https://www.pbs.org/wgbh/americanexperience/features/pill-margaret-sanger-1879-1966/

15 Your Next Steps in Health Communication

Congratulations! You've reached the last chapter! Like Cheryl Montgomery, you have persevered.

You've learned a lot about health communication throughout this book. You've learned about the discipline's foundations and the pernicious effects of discrimination that pervades the healthcare system. You've learned about the experiences and perspectives of patients, including patient-provider communication; uncertainty, decision making, coping, and health literacy; and health information seeking. You've learned about the experiences and perspectives of healthcare providers, the importance of social support and informal caregiving, and the complexities and challenges of end-of-life communication. You've also learned about some of the complexities and challenges of mental health and mental illness, intercultural health communication, and ethical issues in health communication. Finally, you've learned about health communication in the media, environmental health communication, and public health crises. That's a lot to digest, but you made it through. Gold star!

Now that you've reached this point in the book, we hope you have a more sophisticated understanding of health communication scholarship and its diversity. We also hope you've developed some appreciation for the array of theories that undergird health communication research, as well as the way that research can advance knowledge of health communication in all its forms. Whether researchers are designing and testing interventions to promote health, conducting in-depth interviews to develop a rich understanding of unique and personal healthcare experiences, or investigating and revealing issues of power inherent in the system and empowering marginalized people to promote social change—it's all important.

Important, too, is the application of research. The translational research that you've read about is having a real impact on the lives of others. It's helping patients to communicate more effectively with their physicians. It's helping healthcare providers to promote patient safety. It's helping people to improve their health literacy, to better navigate the healthcare system, to make healthier choices in life, and to avoid some of the unhealthier choices. As we said in the introductory chapter, health communication plays a *central role* in health promotion and disease prevention and treatment. It's a crucial role to play, and we hope you'll want to be a part of it.

To better prepare you for that role, we thought we'd take this last chapter to orient you to opportunities for graduate studies in health communication and non-academic career opportunities in health communication. We want to comment on our Montgomery family narrative, too. And we want to leave you with two personal calls to action. So, take a deep breath, and let's dive in one last time.

Health Communication Graduate Studies

Chances are very good that you're an undergraduate student, quite possibly one getting ready to graduate and never look back. If so, that's fantastic. Please accept our hearty

DOI: 10.4324/9781003214458-36

congratulations. We wish you well. But if you think that you might be interested in graduate education in health communication, you'll find these academic and professional resources of interest.

First, you'll need to find a place to study! You can find an extensive list of graduate programs in health communication and public health on the Society for Health Communication's website (see Society for Health Communication, 2016a). Many of the programs offer traditional master's and doctoral degrees, but several offer online or hybrid professional master's programs. If you're nervous about applying to graduate programs, we encourage you to visit your favorite professor during office hours to discuss the process. Faculty members are an invaluable resource for navigating graduate school applications. And we would be remiss if we didn't recommend considering the master's program at San Diego State University (where you could work with Dr. Record) before applying to the doctoral program at the University of Kentucky (where you could work with Dr. Harrington).

Let's say you've applied and been accepted into the graduate program of your choice. One of the things you'll want to do is to become involved in one or more of the professional organizations available to you. The discipline of communication has two major professional organizations: the **International Communication Association** and the **National Communication Association**. Both have health communication divisions. Three out of four regional communication associations have health communication interest groups: Eastern Communication Association, Southern States Communication Association, and Western States Communication Association. There also are health communication-focused organizations and initiatives peppering the scholarly landscape around the world. One we want to draw your attention to in particular is the **Society for Health Communication (Society)**.

Founded in 2016, the Society is an international organization whose mission is "to bring together health communication professionals and scholars to create meaningful connections, share knowledge across disciplines, promote health equity, and advance the science of health communication" (Society, 2016b, n.p.). At the time this book went to press, individual membership was free. The Society has a wealth of resources on its website, including information on graduate programs and job opportunities in health communication. They also offer a number of educational webinars. Examples include "The Golden Age of TV is Over: Developing Effective Youth Public Education Campaigns in the Digital Era," "Communicating About Disparities to Achieve Health Equity," and "Communicating on COVID-19 Vaccination – Past, Present, and Future."

As a graduate student, you'll definitely want to keep up with the literature and publish your own research. A good way to start is by reading *The Routledge Handbook of Health Communication* (Thompson & Harrington, 2022). Now in its third edition, the *Handbook* is an essential resource for any health communication graduate student. There also are several academic journals dedicated to publishing health communication scholarship, including *Health Communication* (the discipline's first and flagship journal), *Journal of Health Communication*, *Journal of Communication in Healthcare*, *Communication & Medicine*, and *Journal of Visual Communication in Medicine*. Scores of journals with broader scopes also publish health communication research (e.g., *American Journal of Public Health*, *Patient Education and Counseling*, *Qualitative Health Research*, *Social Science & Medicine*).

One more thing you'll want to do as a graduate student is attend professional conferences. Doing so allows you to network with other scholars and enhance your education through attending research panels and short courses. (It also can be a lot of fun. #NerdParties.) Table 15.1 provides a sample of conferences that feature health communication research. Of all these great conferences, you're most likely to find us (your favorite textbook authors) at the Kentucky Conference on Health Communication (KCHC) and the DC-area Health Communication Conference (DCHC). Should you ever attend, be sure to say hello!

Table 15.1 A Sample of Conferences with a Health Communication Focus

---

American Public Health Association annual meeting, Health Communication Working Group
  https://www.apha.org
DC-area Health Communication conference (DCHC)
  https://dchc.gmu.edu
Eastern Communication Association convention, Health Communication Interest Group
  https://www.ecasite.org
International Communication Association convention, Health Communication Division
  https://www.icahdq.org
International Conference on Communication in Healthcare
  https://each.international/eachevents/conferences/icch-2022
Kentucky Conference on Health Communication (KCHC)
  http://comm.uky.edu/kchc
National Communication Association convention, Health Communication Division
  http://www.natcom.org
National Conference on Health Communication, Marketing, and Media
  https://www.nchcmm.org
Society of Teachers of Family Medicine conference on medical student education
  http://www.stfm.org
Southern States Communication Association convention, Health Communication Division
  https://www.ssca.net
Western States Communication Association convention, Health Communication Interest Group
  https://www.westcomm.org

Considering Graduate School

There are many graduate programs with concentrations in health communication. If you're considering graduate school, consult the Society for Health Communication's website to see an extensive list of programs. Also meet with a faculty member to discuss which programs might be a good fit for you. Once in a graduate program, consider submitting to and attending professional conferences, such as the National Communication Association and International Communication Association conventions. Also strive to publish your research in health-focused academic journals.

Career Opportunities in Health Communication

Academic enlightenment is awesome, but you gotta pay the bills. So, what kind of careers are there in health communication? Plenty! Whether you have a bachelor's, master's, or doctoral degree, there is a job for you in health communication. To give you an idea of the breadth of opportunity, we're going to share some examples of jobs our former undergraduate students were interested in pursuing upon graduation with their bachelor's degrees. Table 15.2 lists the job title, the organization, and a very brief description of the organization. This is a *tiny sample* of the opportunities that are out there. If you're interested in a career in health communication, there is a place for you!

We'd like to take a moment to highlight one of the careers that we think is particularly important and promising in health communication: patient advocate. **Patient advocates**, or patient care advocates, serve as liaisons between patients and healthcare providers, and they help patients and families navigate the healthcare system. They become involved in

Table 15.2 Examples of Careers in Health Communication

Job Title	Organization	Organization Description
Communicable disease health educator	State Department of Public Health	Public health department
Communication specialist	Vanderbilt University Medical Center	Nonprofit academic hospital system
Community health worker or outreach coordinator	Center of Excellence in Rural Health	Nonprofit center to reduce health disparities in rural Kentucky
Corporate communications specialist	Teladoc Health Inc.	Multinational telemedicine and virtual healthcare company
Crisis manager	United Nations	International health organization
Health and wellness director	Living Care Lifestyles	Senior living community management company
Health communication specialist	Centers for Disease Control and Prevention	National public health agency
Healthcare facility administrator	Spero Health	Integrated healthcare services organization treating substance use disorders
Medical records clerk	Ciox Health	Healthcare information management company
Orthopedic medical devices sales representative	Zimmer Biomet	Medical device design, manufacturing, and sales company
Patient access representative	Conifer Health Solutions	Healthcare services company focusing on business outcomes
Patient care advocate	Employer Direct Healthcare	Medical care access facilitation company
Pharmaceutical sales representative	Access Pharmaceutical	Healthcare and pharmaceutical products/services company
Physical therapist technician	Baptist Health	Outpatient healthcare organization
Sales support associate	Prevail Infoworks	System integration and analytics software company
Social service worker	Department for Community Based Services	Government agency working to help families, children, and vulnerable adults
Wellness coach	Centerstone	Nonprofit health system treating mental health and substance use disorders

case management; billing and insurance navigation; home health and elder care; identification of mental health and substance use disorder services; and legal assistance such as workers' compensation, social security benefits, and malpractice litigation. Patient advocates can work through hospitals, insurance companies, and government agencies, and they also can set up a private practice.

Currently, there are a number of programs offering a range of patient advocacy training (Health and Patient Advocate Educational Programs, 2023). Certification in patient advocacy is offered through the Patient Advocate Certification Board (2022). There's also a professional organization, the **Alliance of Professional Health Advocates (Alliance)**. Founded in 2009, the Alliance describes itself as "the largest and most extensive professional and support organization for private, independent health and patient advocates and care managers" (Alliance of Professional Health Advocates, 2023, para. 1). Its goal is to serve as a resource for members to help them establish and navigate their patient advocacy efforts, including starting their own business. Average annual salary for a patient advocate ranges from $57,000 to $77,000 (Salary.com, 2022). If you're interested in helping patients and their families negotiate their way through this complicated healthcare system of ours, a career in patient advocacy might be right for you. Or like Nathian from our Montgomery family story, it could also be a first step in your career journey.

Patient Advocates

Patient advocate is one of many possible careers for a health communication major. Patient advocates serve as liaisons between patients and healthcare providers, and they help patients and families navigate the healthcare system. Depending on the position, they could be involved in case management; billing and insurance navigation; home health and elder care; identification of mental health and substance use disorder services; or legal assistance such as workers' compensation, social security benefits, and malpractice litigation.

The Montgomery Family

One of the unique aspects of this book is the Montgomery family narrative. As you now know, narrative plays a central role in health communication, with every patient having their own unique story. We hope that the trials and tribulations of the Montgomery family helped bring to life many of the topics we covered in our chapters. We also hope you realize that although our family narrative was fictional, there are kernels of truth in everything the members experienced.

For example, just as was true for Cheryl, women and people of color are often discouraged from pursuing certain career paths, such as going to medical school or earning a PhD. Yet, just like Cheryl, people are proving those naysayers wrong every day. And just as was true for Helen, the symptoms of women and people of color are often downplayed by healthcare professionals. But public health advocates are working tirelessly to raise awareness of these and other disparities. And just as was true for Monica, our most essential healthcare providers are burning out because healthcare systems don't optimally support providers (or patients). It will take all of us advocating for a healthcare system that protects patients and providers to make the changes we need. And just like Savannah, people are falling prey to the mis- and disinformation machines running rampant on the internet, and, sadly, the false beliefs resulting from exposure to mis- and disinformation have contributed to many people's deaths. Health communication efforts are being implemented across a variety of sectors, including public health, government, tech, and education, to monitor and correct mis- and disinformation, and some social media companies also appear to be upping their game. Until the mess is sorted out, though, it's up to every individual to remain vigilant and not fall for mis- and disinformation.

Calls to Action

As we wrap up this book, we have two calls to action for you, dear reader. First, we challenge you to move forward in your life with a clear eye to reducing discrimination and bias where you can. We realize that people can get extremely touchy about this, going on the defensive at the slightest suggestion that they might have any biases. Everyone has biases, though. Everyone is a product of their culture, and some biases are just a part of that. Therefore, having biases is not anyone's fault. However, when people learn about the nature of discrimination and how implicit bias affects everyone, working to overcome those biases then becomes a responsibility—assuming they want to be an ally (see Chapter 7). There are many tools to help in this respect.

For example, the National Institutes of Health (NIH; 2022a) offers resources to counter implicit bias. Although their goal is to reduce the negative impact of implicit bias in biomedical research, the principles taught in the course are broadly applicable. In addition, they present links to research studies on effective bias-reduction strategies that anyone can use. As noted in Chapter 2, these strategies include thinking of counter-examples of stereotypes in your social networks (Blair et al., 2001), imagining yourself in the position of someone being stereotyped (Galinsky & Moskowitz, 2000), being more mindful of situations that trigger implicit bias to then interrupt that thinking (Stewart & Payne, 2008), and taking implicit bias training courses, such as the one offered through NIH (2022b).

In addition, the Centers for Disease Control and Prevention (CDC; 2022) has developed a set of health equity guiding principles to promote inclusive communication. These principles are designed to help public health communication professionals address their audiences respectfully and inclusively and "ensure their communication products and strategies adapt to the specific cultural, linguistic, environmental, and historical situation of each population or audience of focus" (para. 3). They offer a two-page summary of the principles that you can download and reference to learn how to be more inclusive in your language use (see CDC, 2022). Even though the principles are meant for professional communicators, anyone can use them.

In addition to overcoming your own biases, it's important to help other people recognize and overcome theirs. As already mentioned, this can be a very delicate task because biases can be especially charged topics. But there are resources available to help you engage in these conversations, many of which center on the idea of **calling in instead of calling out.** The Harvard Office for Equity, Diversity, Inclusion & Belonging (EDIB; 2023) defines calling in as "an invitation to a one-on-one or small group conversation to bring attention to an individual or group's harmful words or behavior, including bias, prejudice, microaggressions, and discrimination" and calling out as "bringing public attention to an individual, group, or organization's harmful words or behavior" (p. 1). The authors of the Creative Equity Toolkit (n.d.), a diversity resource created in Australia, further explain the differences (para. 1):

> While call outs can be important ways to speak truth to power and call racist people to account, call-out (or cancel) culture is also criticised. Call outs can be performative and a way to 'signal virtue' that is more interested in self-aggrandisement than in achieving real change, especially on social media. The concept of 'calling in' seeks to refocus challenges to racism by talking to the person privately and aiming for change, rather than shame.

Call outs are not wrong, per se. For example, Loretta Ross, African American academic, feminist, and activist, says that call outs "are justified to challenge provocateurs who deliberately hurt others, or for powerful people beyond our reach. Effectively criticizing such people is an important tactic for achieving justice" (Ross, 2019, para. 16). But in everyday interaction, either in person or especially on social media, calling out people who use insensitive language or make other missteps, quite possibly unintentionally and without malice, can easily be perceived as confrontational and result in feelings of defensiveness and not being open to listening. Calling in is intended to be a less confrontational approach to engaging in conversations about charged topics. Both the Harvard EDIB and the Creative Equity Toolkit provide resources for how to call people in, including suggested phrases and ways to recognize the need to do so.

Beyond these resources, you can take steps yourself to raise your awareness and reduce implicit bias in several ways. One way is to learn about the history of all the "isms," either through taking classes at your school or learning on your own. This textbook's companion website lists several resources (e.g., books, movies, podcasts) that might interest you. Another way is to expand your social networks to be more inclusive of diversity in all its forms: race, sex, gender, disability, age, size, religion, political affiliation, and more. One strategy to accomplish this is to join a volunteer effort working to promote issues of social justice and civic good. You'll make new friends and contribute to society at the same time, a win–win! The ball is in your court now. The next step is yours.

Second, we urge you to become a strong advocate for your own healthcare. Part of this involves learning how to communicate effectively with providers. Don Cegala's PACE system, which we discussed in Chapter 3, is a start. We present it for you in Table 15.3. You might consider using it as a guide for future medical visits.

Table 15.3 PACE: Preparing for Your Next Medical Visit

To get more out of your medical visit, be prepared and use PACE:
P = Present detailed information about how you are feeling.
Be specific: Are you experiencing pain? If so, is it a sharp pain or a dull ache? Does it come and go or is it constant? Has anything helped alleviate the pain? What have you tried?
A = Ask questions.
Thinking about what you want to ask before your office visit and writing it down will make sure you ask what is important to you. You may want to ask, "How serious is my condition? What should I do if it gets worse? How long before I start feeling better?"
C = Check for understanding.
It's really important that you understand everything the doctor is telling you about your condition, the treatment, and any medications that are prescribed. It's your responsibility as a patient to speak up if you don't understand something. Ask the doctor to repeat or clarify any information that is unclear. Then repeat or paraphrase what they told you to make sure you understand.
E = Express concerns about the recommended treatment.
If you have concerns about the recommended treatment, speak up. For example, do you have concerns about being able to swallow pills? Are you concerned about the cost of a prescription? Are you worried about screening recommendations?
Be honest with your doctor by explaining how you are following the treatment. For example, are you taking all, some, or none of your medication, or are you doing all, some, or none of your at-home physical therapy? If you are having trouble with recommended treatment, be sure to explain why and offer to work with your doctor to find a modified or alternative treatment.
Before your next visit, answer the following:

What is the purpose of your visit?

_____

What are your symptoms? Be specific:

_____

What do you hope to get out of your doctor's visit?

_____

What questions/concerns do you have?

_____

List of medications:

_____   _____   _____

_____   _____   _____

In addition, remember that although healthcare providers are the ones with expertise in medicine, nursing, and other health professions, *you* are the one with expertise in your own body. You've lived in it your whole life, and you know when something's wrong. And when something *is* wrong, it's your responsibility to make yourself heard. If you think that a healthcare provider is not understanding you or perhaps not taking you seriously, keep trying or find another provider who will listen to you (they *are* out there!). Not getting the care you need could result in quite serious consequences. The story of Alice Tapper (2022) is a case in point. Alice is the daughter of CNN correspondent Jake Tapper. In November of 2021, when she was a high school student, she started experiencing stomach cramping, fever, chills, and vomiting bad enough to land her in the emergency room. The doctors there were at a loss, so she was transferred to another hospital. Upon the advice of her pediatrician, her parents told the doctors there to check for appendicitis. Because Alice's pain was throughout her abdomen and not localized to the right side, they rejected that diagnosis out of hand and instead said Alice had a viral infection. Alice kept getting sicker and sicker, and she was in incredible pain. However, the doctors wouldn't listen to her or her parents. Finally, in desperation, her father called the hospital administrator. With the administrator's intervention, the doctors performed tests that revealed no viral infection but instead, guess what, a perforated appendix. Alice was rushed to emergency surgery and fortunately survived. The same is not true of all children and teens with appendicitis, though, because, as Tapper notes in her article, the diagnosis is missed in up to 15% of that population, particularly those under the age of 5 years and girls. We urge you to read Alice's story and to either be your own advocate or call on someone who can advocate for you.

You also need to be your own advocate when it comes to navigating the health insurance "system" and avoiding (as best you can) catastrophic medical bills. We recommend that you become a regular listener to the podcast *An Arm and A Leg* (Weissmann, 2018–present) and sign up for their newsletter. Also watch the video that Brian David Gilbert (2022) produced explaining health insurance terms. Knowledge is power, and in this crazy healthcare system of ours, you need all the power you can get. And when push comes to shove, if you need help from an expert, you can look into finding a patient advocate through the AdvoConnection (2023) directory. Let's face it. As an unattributed quote we found in a meme on the internet advises, "By virtue of being a human, you have a body that needs attention. At some point, your check engine light is going to go on." When it does, it will be best to be prepared.

Calls to Action

Work to reduce discrimination and bias by engaging in self-reflection and advocating for social justice. As a patient, be an advocate for yourself or find someone to advocate for you.

Conclusion

At this point, we'll bring things to a close. We sincerely hope that you'll be able to take what you've learned from this book and apply it in your life. Whether you pursue further study in health communication, have a career in the field, or find yourself in the role of patient, caregiver, health media consumer, advocate, or ally, you should now be a more informed and enlightened participant. If you haven't already, be sure to check out our online resources where you'll find additional information, stories, and resources covering all the topics in this book—and more. And in the inimitable words of Garrison Keillor, "Be well, do good work, and keep in touch."

References

AdvoConnection. (2023). *The AdvoConnection directory.* https://advoconnection.com/

Alliance of Professional Health Advocates. (2023). https://aphadvocates.org/

Blair, I. V., Ma, J. E., & Lenton, A. P. (2001). Imagining stereotypes away: The moderation of implicit stereotypes through mental imagery. *Journal of Personality and Social Psychology, 81*(5), 828–841.

Centers for Disease Control and Prevention. (2022). *Health equity guiding principles for inclusive communication.* https://www.cdc.gov/healthcommunication/Health_Equity.html

Creative Equity Toolkit. (n.d.). *Call out & call in racism.* https://creativeequitytoolkit.org/topic/anti-racism/call-out-call-in-racism/

Galinsky, A. D., & Moskowitz, G. B. (2000). Perspective-taking: Decreasing stereotype expression, stereotype accessibility, and in-group favoritism. *Journal of Personality and Social Psychology, 78*(4), 708–724.

Gilbert, B. D. (2022, September 26). *A terrible guide to the terrible terminology of U.S. health insurance.* https://armandalegshow.com/episode/brian-david-gilbert/

Harvard Office for Equity, Diversity, Inclusion & Belong. (2023). *Calling in and calling out guide.* https://edib.harvard.edu/calling-and-calling-out-guide

Health and Patient Advocate Educational Programs. (2023). *Master list of health and patient advocacy educational courses, programs, and organizations.* https://healthadvocateprograms.com/master-list/

National Institutes of Health. (2022a). *Implicit bias.* https://diversity.nih.gov/sociocultural-factors/implicit-bias

National Institutes of Health. (2022b). *Implicit bias training course.* https://diversity.nih.gov/sociocultural-factors/implicit-bias-training-course

Patient Advocate Certification Board. (2022). *Are you ready? Become a board certified patient advocate today.* https://www.pacboard.org/

Ross, L. (2019, August 17). I'm a Black feminist. I think call-out culture is toxic. *The New York Times.* https://www.nytimes.com/2019/08/17/opinion/sunday/cancel-culture-call-out.html

Salary.com. (2022). *Patient advocate salary in the United States.* https://www.salary.com/research/salary/posting/patient-advocate-salary

Society for Health Communication. (2016a). *Degrees and certificates in health communication.* https://www.societyforhealthcommunication.org/degrees-and-certificates

Society for Health Communication. (2016b). *About the Society.* https://www.societyforhealthcommunication.org/about-the-society

Stewart, B. D., & Payne, B. K. (2008). Bringing automatic stereotyping under control: Implementation intentions as efficient means of thought control. *Personality and Social Psychology Bulletin, 34*(10), 1332–1345.

Tapper, A. (2022, December 15). I almost died last year from a medical problem that was entirely preventable. *CNN Opinion.* https://www.cnn.com/2022/12/15/opinions/appendicitis-misdiagnosis-girls-tapper/index.html

Thompson, T. L., & Harrington, N. G. (Eds.). (2022). *The Routledge handbook of health communication* (3rd ed.). Routledge.

Weissmann, D. (2018–present). *An Arm and A Leg.* Podcast. https://armandalegshow.com/

In-class Activities

1. The chapter describes how the healthcare experiences of the Montgomery family happen in real life. Put students in small groups and have them come up with examples from their own lives of character experiences from the story.

2. Have students pair up, designating one person as the doctor and one person as the patient. Present the class with the following scenario:

   The "patient" should think about a medical condition and pretend that they have that condition. Using the PACE criteria presented in Table 15.3, the patient should explain their symptoms to the "doctor." After five minutes, have the pairs switch roles. To conclude, facilitate a conversation about the experience.

Discussion Questions

1. What are your career plans after you finish your degree? How has this class helped shape this direction? How do you think this class will help you achieve your career goals?

2. How has what you learned in this class helped you think about what it means to be a patient? The next time you find yourself communicating with a provider, friend, or family member about your health, what will you do differently because of what you learned in this class?

3. How are health communication students, scholars, instructors, and practitioners uniquely situated to address discrimination and bias in the healthcare system? What about in communities? What about around the world?

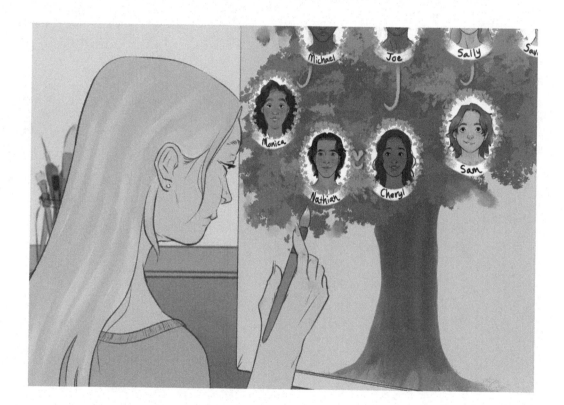

Author Index

Note: **Bold** page numbers refer to tables.

Subject Index

Note: **Bold** page numbers refer to tables; *italic* page numbers refer to figures.

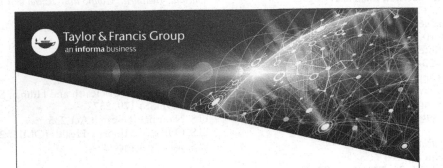

Printed in the United States
by Baker & Taylor Publisher Services